afoot & afield

Las Vegas
& Southern Nevada

A comprehensive hiking guide

SECOND EDITION

Brian Beffort

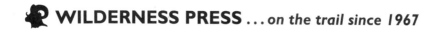
WILDERNESS PRESS ...*on the trail since 1967*

To Logan,
wishing you a lifetime of
exploration and wonder

Afoot & Afield Las Vegas & Southern Nevada: A Comprehensive Hiking Guide

1st Edition 2005
2nd Edition 2010
  5th printing 2018

Copyright © 2010 by Brian Beffort

Front cover photos copyright © 2010 by Kurt Kuznicki
Interior photos by author, except pp. 33, 73, 85, 87, and 92, which are copyright © 2010 by
  Kurt Kuznicki
Maps: Ben Pease, Pease Press
Cover design: Larry B. Van Dyke
Interior design and layout: Andreas Schueller and Lisa Pletka
Layout: Annie Long
Editor: Laura Shauger

ISBN 978-0-89997-651-8

Manufactured in the United States of America

Published by: **Wilderness Press**
  An imprint of AdventureKEEN
  2204 1st Ave. S., Suite 102
  Birmingham, AL 35233
  (800) 443-7227
  info@wildernesspress.com
  www.wildernesspress.com

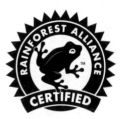

Visit our website for a complete listing of our books and for ordering information.

Distributed by Publishers Group West

Cover photos: Muddy's Hidden Valley (top); Trail Canyon, Mt. Charleston Wilderness
  (lower right); Telescope Peak (lower left)

Acknowledgments

My heartfelt appreciation goes to the many people who have helped me research and write this book. First and foremost, to Laura for her patience and fortitude while caring for our baby during my many days of research and writing; to the board members and staff of Friends of Nevada Wilderness, for their support, knowledge, and advice; to the people at Wilderness Press, for their excellent editing and guidance through the publishing process; to Dad and Wally, for their hospitality; to land management agency staff and volunteers, for their information and guidance; to all the volunteers and staff of the Nevada Wilderness Coalition and Nevada archaeological organizations, for their inspiration, dedication, and passion in protecting Nevada's natural and cultural legacies; and to everyone who has found beauty and adventure in Nevada's achingly beautiful deserts. You are part of what makes this place wonderful.

Las Vegas & Southern Nevada

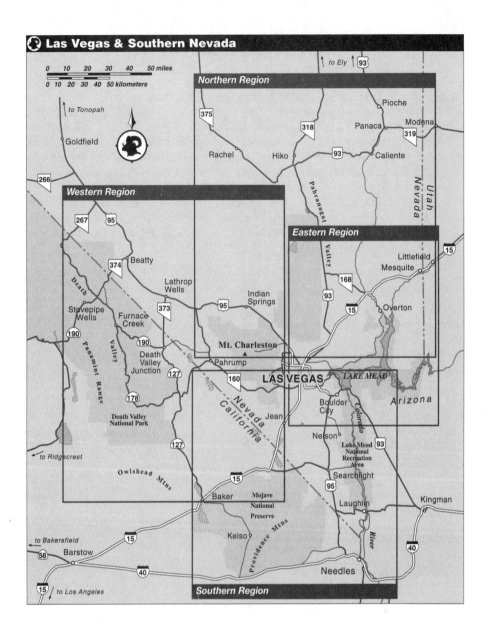

Contents

Preface

Saving Las Vegas

Southern Nevada is home to some of the country's most beautiful and fragile landscapes. Until recently, the region's scant water and ferocious summertime heat have kept all but a few from exploring the area's mountains, canyons, and valleys, leaving the landscape largely undisturbed.

Things are different now. Since 1987, the Las Vegas Valley has been one of the fastest-growing metropolitan areas in the country. In 1990, the population here was about 750,000 people. In 2010, it is fast approaching 2.2 million people. A natural consequence of this population growth is increasing numbers of people exploring the desert. Sadly, some of these people are destroying our beautiful desert with litter, vandalism, and irresponsible off-road vehicle driving.

This increased visitation could spell ruin for Southern Nevada's beautiful landscapes and for some of the vulnerable wildlife species that live here. Without water to help the land heal from impacts, the scars we inflict can last a long time. Roads left by miners a century ago look as though they were carved just recently, and the tracks of an all-terrain vehicle tearing up a ridge or across a valley can last a decade. For many plants and animals that live in the desert, the difference between life and death can be measured by a single rainstorm or a single square foot of undisturbed soil.

It might seem strange, then, for me to encourage more people to explore Southern Nevada. This desert does not need more people driving and hiking through it without regard to the scars they leave behind. But it does need more people who appreciate its fragile beauty and biological diversity, who will work to keep it beautiful into the future. I encourage you to join that latter group and hope this book will help you appreciate the stark beauty Southern Nevada has to offer and inspire you to treat it with care and respect.

This is Nevada, and I'm a gambling man. I'm betting that you will appreciate the Mojave Desert's unique beauty, if you don't already. I'm betting that you will learn to travel lightly on the land, that you will clean up after yourself and others, that you will share your love for the land with friends, and that you will help them appreciate it and learn to travel lightly as well. I'm betting that we can enjoy and explore the desert and still keep it beautiful for generations to come, and that we as a species can learn to keep our planet healthy and beautiful, so it can do the same for us.

Our challenge as humans in the early 21st century is to take responsibility for the impacts we inflict on the planet that sustains us. We Americans, who have become strong, independent, and resourceful in part thanks to the riches and beauty of our landscape, need to step up and become good stewards of the land, to care for the legacy we have inherited in order to pass it on to future generations.

Plus it's a lot more fun and rewarding to explore a beautiful landscape than a trashed one. And that's what this book is all about—getting outside and having fun amid Southern Nevada's natural wonders.

Please help me win my bet, because if I win, we all win.

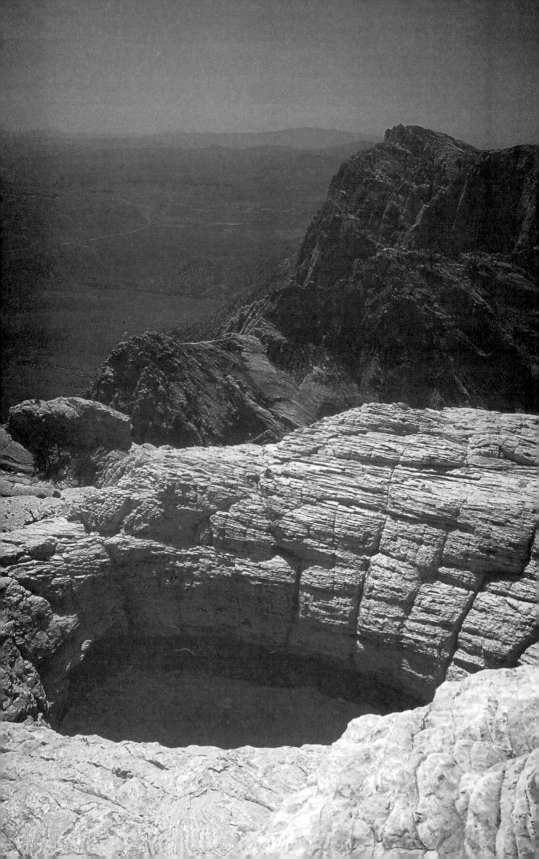

Introducing
Las Vegas & Southern Nevada

Congratulations! You're about to hit the jackpot.

Sure, the Strip's bright lights and casinos have a lot to offer, but if you enjoy natural wonders, you'll soon discover that Southern Nevada has more than just casinos. Within a couple hours' drive in any direction from the Strip, you'll find mind-bending geology, fascinating and colorful plants and animals, expansive views, and magical landscapes with myriad opportunities to hike, explore, and surround yourself with beauty and solitude.

Unfortunately, Nevada hasn't always gotten a lot of respect. Ever since pioneers opted for California's green valleys instead of Nevada's desert, the Silver State has had a reputation as desolate and inhospitable (and it can be, especially if you fail to plan and prepare accordingly—see Preparation & Equipment, page 14). The disrespect continues today, as our nation moves to store high-level radioactive waste at Yucca Mountain, only 90 miles north of Las Vegas. But it takes just one visit to appreciate what Nevada has to offer for this great region to get the respect it deserves.

Although Nevada can rarely be called lush, you'll find it can be stunningly beautiful when you see the landscape on its own terms. Consider a few facts you might not know about Nevada:

It is the **most mountainous state** in the country, with more than 300 ranges.

It is also the **driest state**. On average, some places in Nevada receive fewer than 4 inches of rain each year, which has created a unique desert ecosystem with a variety of interesting flora and fauna, as well as beautiful geologic formations.

Nevada is the **fourth most biodiverse state,** in part because of its incredible range of elevations, precipitation levels, and temperatures, which create life zones for a dizzying variety of plants and animals. More than 3,800 species of plants and animals are known to live in Nevada, and of these, hundreds are endemic species found nowhere else on Earth. The bulk of these endemic species live in Southern Nevada, thanks to its warm climate.

Nevada has **more public land than any state except Alaska.** Eighty-seven percent of Nevada's 71 million total acres is public and managed by the following agencies: Bureau of Land Management (48 million acres), National Park Service (775,000 acres), U.S. military (4.4 million acres, all off-limits to the public), U.S. Fish and Wildlife Service (2 million acres), U.S. Forest Service (5.8 million acres), and State Parks (133,000 acres).

Nevada is also **an extremely urban state,** with more than 90 percent of Nevada's nearly 3 million people living in metropolitan areas such as the Las Vegas Valley, leaving a whole lot of beautiful, empty country to explore.

The Desert Climate

Southern Nevada, the region covered by this book, is part of the Mojave Desert, which extends from the Sierra Nevada to the Colorado Plateau. Some scientists claim the Mojave isn't a true desert, that it's simply a transition zone between the lower, hotter Sonoran Desert to the south and the higher, cooler Great Basin Desert to the north. Others argue that because more than 200 plant and animal species live in the Mojave and nowhere else on Earth, it is a unique desert ecosystem in its own right.

Part of what makes the Mojave so special is its many mountain ranges. Elevations range from 282 feet below sea level in Death

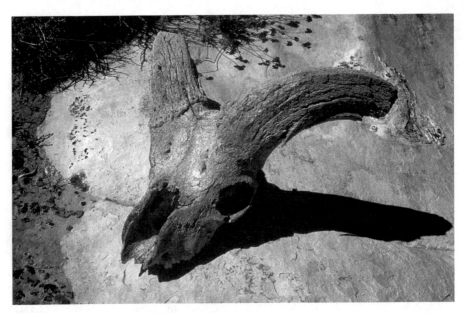

Please leave what you find, no matter how enticing.

Valley National Park to nearly 12,000 feet at the summit of Mt. Charleston, an hour's drive northwest of Las Vegas.

Weather also adds to the diversity. While valleys can remain parched—Las Vegas Valley receives an average of 4 inches of rain per year—precipitation levels change with altitude and aspect (exposure to sun). Winter and spring storms can deposit many feet of snow in the mountains, feeding creeks, canyons, and valleys below during runoff. Quick-tempered summer thunderstorms can drench one valley and leave the next one dry. Temperatures also vary, depending on the time of year, location, and elevation. The average low in January is 33°F, and the high in July is 104°F. As a rule, however, air cools between 3°F and 5°F for every 1000 feet of elevation gain.

Geology

The many rock formations in Nevada make geologists' eyes light up like a child's on Christmas morning, and they can make the rest of us wish we were geologists, just so we could understand more about the shapes and colors we see in the landscape.

What makes Nevada such a geologic wonderland? The scant rainfall keeps plants from blocking our view of the underlying geology, which tells stories about Earth's distant past. If we can understand these stories, we can learn what this region was like long ago and what happened to make it look as it does today.

To appreciate the major types of rock you'll encounter while exploring Southern Nevada, imagine what this area was like during several key periods of the ancient past. Between 540 million and about 250 million years ago, North America's West Coast was near the Nevada-Arizona border. There, sand and silt accumulated and eventually became sandstone and shale. Farther offshore, the shells of dying sea creatures formed layers that slowly transformed into limestone and dolomite after millions of years of pressure. You can see these ancient seabed sediments tower high above you at places like La Madre and Turtlehead peaks in Red Rock Canyon and in the Mormon Mountains.

During the age of the dinosaurs, between 250 million and 65 million years ago, the colliding Pacific and North American continental plates lifted Southern Nevada from the seas and began forming the Sierra Nevada to the west. Great shifting sand dunes covered much of the land from Nevada to Colorado. These dunes have since cemented into stone, creating brilliant sandstone formations at places like the Calico Hills in Red Rock Canyon, the Valley of Fire State Park, and along Northshore Road at Lake Mead National Recreation Area.

Over the last 65 million years, continental movements shifted. Southern Nevada and the Great Basin to the north began to pull apart, creating Nevada's signature basin-and-range character.

Between 17 million and 5 million years ago, volcanoes were active in the region, covering the landscape with black and dark brown basalts and lighter rhyolites that you'll see in the Eldorado Mountains along the Colorado River, and in the North and South McCullough mountains.

Over time, these rocks have thrust up, folded over, shuffled about, and eroded away to create the jigsaw puzzle of geology we see around Southern Nevada today. This is a simple and crude introduction to the area's geology. I go into more depth in specific trips, but much of the detail that makes Nevada's geology fascinating is beyond the scope of this book. If you want to learn more, check out the geology books and websites on page 265.

Plants

Two overwhelming factors affect living things in Southern Nevada: water and sun. Every living thing in the Mojave Desert has developed fascinating and beautiful strategies to deal with these two challenges.

Some plants, such as cacti, Joshua trees, and yucca, with relatively shallow roots take advantage of infrequent rains by soaking up as much water as they can when it comes, then storing it through long periods

Look carefully at rocks for fossils of ancient sea life.

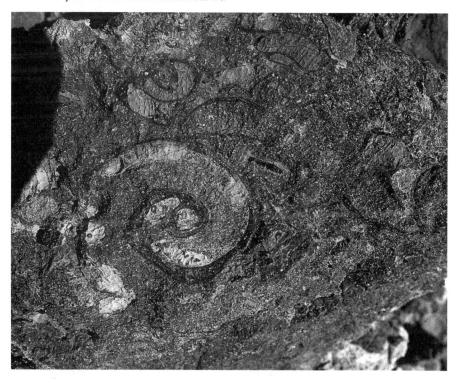

of drought. They in turn protect this treasure with painful spines.

Other plants, such as the mesquite bush, have deep root systems that reach for water underground. Some plants produce small leaves, with curved or thick, waxy skins to prevent water loss. Others cover their leaves with fine white hairs to reflect the harsh sun and prevent air movement, both of which steal precious moisture.

Perennial plants, such as grasses and some flowers, simply go dormant during periods of drought. Annuals, on the other hand, die each season. Their seeds, however, can wait through years of drought, until enough rain falls for them to grow again. They complete their entire life cycles quickly, producing seeds that can wait until the next life-giving rain. Annuals and perennials make up many of the wildflowers that paint the desert with color in the spring. Please help fragile plants survive by driving only on designated routes and not walking on or picking them.

As you travel throughout the Mojave Desert, you will pass through distinct vegetation zones, divided by soil type and elevation. Although each zone is typically dominated by one or two major species, a close inspection will often yield a wide diversity of plants and shrubs living in complex harmony. Here are a few of the vegetation zones in the Mojave, and the rough elevations at which they occur:

LOWER MOJAVE ZONE

Often dominated by white bursage, saltbush, creosote bush, and yucca, this zone ranges from saline valley bottoms to the lower slopes of alluvial fans, between sea level and 2500 feet in elevation. Cacti, such as barrel, fishhook, and prickly pear, are common, especially on rocky outcrops. Riparian areas in the Lower Mojave are often home to willow, mesquite, catclaw,

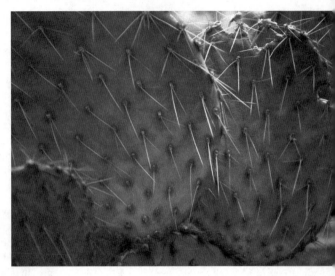

The Mojave is home to several species of beavertail cactus.

and ash. The noxious invader salt cedar (also called tamarisk) is taking over many riparian areas in this zone.

CREOSOTE-BLACKBRUSH ZONE

Blanketing many bajadas (alluvial slopes) between 2000 and 5000 feet in elevation across the Mojave are vast multilayered communities of well-spaced creosote bush and its common sidekick, blackbrush. Mojave yucca and desert almond may be present, as well as many cacti, such as cholla, barrel, red-flowered hedgehog, and beavertail.

JOSHUA TREE FORESTS

When conditions are right, Joshua trees will join the upper reaches of the creosote-blackbrush zone. These members of the lily family are found only in the Mojave and are therefore true indicators of the desert. Joshua tree forests stretch for miles on wide, gentle slopes between 3500 and 5500 feet in elevation, and where precipitation is between 8 and 10 inches per year. Very happy to have visitors, they regularly wave at passing cars. Make sure you wave back. Surround yourself with Joshua trees at the Wee Thump Joshua Tree Wilderness and at Mojave National Preserve's Teutonia Peak and Cima Dome.

PYGMY CONIFER FORESTS

Although you'll come across more as you move north, forests of single-leaf pinyon pine and juniper trees are common (depending on precipitation) between 5500 and 7000 feet in elevation, and they can occur as low as 3100 feet in the Virgin Mountains northeast of Las Vegas. Called pygmy forests because the trees are rarely taller than 20 feet, they are also home to ephedra, rabbitbrush, sagebrush, bitterbrush, and occasional cacti. Mountain mahogany joins these other residents in pygmy forests' upper elevations. You can see solid examples of these forests on the mid-elevation slopes of the Spring Mountains and on Grapevine Peak.

MONTANE FORESTS

Between 6000 and 9000 feet, precipitation is higher in this zone and some places support ponderosa pine, white fir, and aspen, with Douglas fir and spruce joining at higher elevations.

SUBALPINE ZONE

Above 8500 or 9000 feet in elevation, high-alpine forests dominate the landscape with bristlecone pines, limber pines, and whitebark pine.

ALPINE ZONE

Above timberline at 10,000 to 11,000 feet, trees disappear. Only the hardiest, ground-hugging bushes, forbs, sedges, and grasses grow beyond this point.

Scattered among these general vegetation zones are occasional niches—unique combinations of elevation, precipitation, sunlight, and soil—that are often home to unique, sometimes endangered species that live nowhere else on Earth. See more about enjoying these places without destroying them in the Leave No Trace section on page 18.

Animals

Every walking, flying, slithering, and scurrying creature in the desert plays an important role in this ecosystem and each employs impressive and sometimes dramatic strategies to survive this harsh climate. Animals, birds, and reptiles of the Mojave have developed physical and behavioral strategies to survive the desert's intense heat and lack of water. Most beat the heat by simply avoiding it—burrowing underground and coming out only at dawn, dusk, or night, when temperatures are cooler and the sun's radiation is less intense, making these the best times to see critters.

The Joshua tree forest at Cima Dome

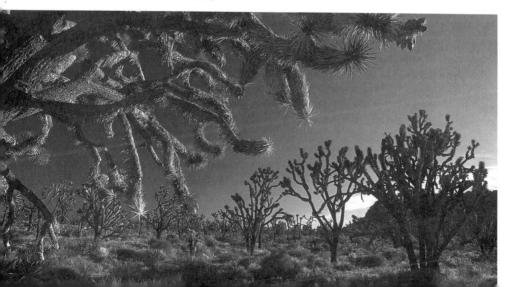

Animals in this region have developed many other survival strategies: Round-tailed ground squirrels and other rodents estivate (summer's version of hibernation) through the hottest summer months. Then, after waking for a few months, they head back underground to hibernate through winter. Jackrabbits and kit foxes have evolved large ears that pick up the slightest sounds of predator or prey and help dissipate heat.

Some animals, especially insects and rodents, get their moisture directly from the plants they eat. The desert tortoise escapes the heat by spending about 95 percent of its life in burrows underground, coming out only in spring and early summer to feed on grasses and flowers. It can live up to a year without drinking water.

There are hundreds of birds, animals, reptiles, amphibians, and insect species living in the Mojave. Here are a few of the most notable:

COUGARS

Also called mountains lions, these large cats historically have ranged throughout the Americas, from the Arctic Circle to the tip of South America, from sea level to above 10,000 feet in elevation. They also live in the mountains throughout Nevada. Their success stems from their stealth and razor-sharp teeth and claws.

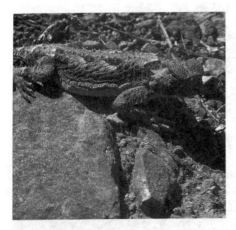

A horned lizard

With human population growth and encroachment on wild areas, human-cougar encounters have become more common. When they hear people approaching, most lions skedaddle without the people ever knowing they were around. They are also unpredictable, and attacks are possible. After generations of living in cities, we have forgotten that we, too, are part of the food chain and need to be cautious in lion country. Consider yourself lucky if you see a mountain lion under safe circumstances. I've been trying for years and have never seen more than tracks, but I've often wondered how many times they've watched me lumber by.

When traveling in cougar country, keep these tips in mind:

- Do not hike alone. Hike in groups and keep children and pets close.
- If you encounter a lion, do not run. You will trigger its instinct to chase, and they specialize in attacking from behind and severing the spine with surgical accuracy.
- Pick up children and pets, but do not turn your back on the cat or crouch down.
- Act large, wave your arms, make noise, be aggressive, and throw sticks and stones (but don't turn away to pick them up).
- If attacked, fight back as though your life depended on it (it does). Cougars have been repelled by aggressive defense.

CATTLE

Cattle graze on public land throughout Nevada, so do not be surprised if you come across cows when hiking. Please help keep cattle where they belong by closing any gates you pass through while driving to your trailhead or hiking.

WILD HORSES & BURROS

Descendants of horses and burros that escaped from Native Americans and European settlers over the years, wild horses and burros are now largely accepted as natural parts of the Western landscape. You might

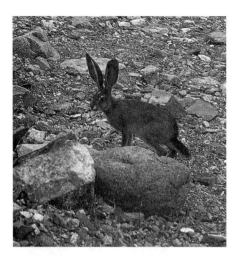

Jackrabbits' ears sense danger approaching *and* dissipate heat.

encounter them during your explorations, and they will likely scamper away.

COYOTES

The coyote is one of the few species that has thrived with the growing human population. Originally living only in the northwestern U.S., coyotes now range throughout North America. Coyotes vary greatly in size and color. They can be as small as 20 pounds or as big as 60. Their fur often has many colors, from gray to red, brown, and black. Coyotes usually keep their distance from people. Only coyotes that are sick or have been fed too often will approach people. If one approaches you, shout, throw sticks, and chase it away.

Although coyotes are often reviled as varmints, they deserve respect for their intelligence and ability to thrive despite our dominance of the landscape. Coyotes also play an important role in the ecosystem by helping keep the populations of rodents and sick wildlife in check. In some Native American oral traditions, the coyote plays an honored role as trickster and sometimes as the creator.

Today, the coyote's yips and howls add beauty and romance to the Wild West

landscape. There are no longer wolves in Nevada (although they might return soon), so if you thought you saw a wolf, it was probably a coyote or perhaps a kit fox, which is much smaller—more like a small dog with big ears.

RATTLESNAKES

Despite the fear they inspire in people, rattlesnakes are beautiful, fascinating, and misunderstood. They play an important role in Western ecosystems by controlling rodents, which carry diseases such as bubonic plague and hantavirus. In Southern Nevada, there are five species of rattlesnake: the Great Basin, the Mojave Green, the Sidewinder, the Panamint, and the Southwestern Speckled. There are also many species of nonvenomous snakes, such as bull snakes, racers, and king snakes.

As cold-blooded creatures, rattlesnakes avoid extreme heat or cold, so you are most likely to encounter them early mornings and late afternoons stretched across the trail and basking in the sun. In the heat of the day, they seek shade under rocks or bushes. They hibernate underground through the cold of winter and come out when the weather warms.

Rattlesnakes will likely feel the vibrations of your approach and move away before you arrive, but if you surprise them, they will curl up in a defensive coil, ready to strike, and ask you to buzz off with their rattling tails. Rest assured, they are much more afraid of you than you are of them. Rattlesnakes are not aggressive and will not bite unless you get too close. When you hear a rattle, stop immediately, spot the snake, and then move directly away.

Although national statistics are not gathered on the circumstances of snakebites, anecdotal reports from emergency room personnel reveal that most bites involve males under 30 years old, happen on the hand (the result of the victim messing with the snake), and involve alcohol. Luckily, snakes seem to sense human stupidity and can control the amount of venom they

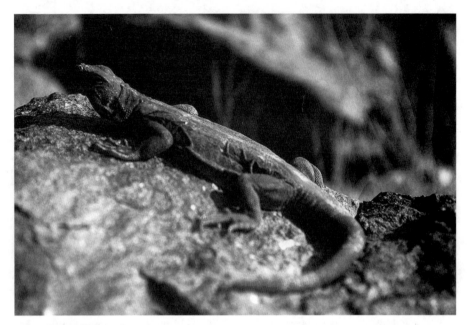

A female chuckwalla basking in the sun

release. Most bites are warnings that do not contain venom. Venomous snakes bit 1,927 people in the year 2000 (most were in the Southeast), and only two people died.

Rattlesnakes are exciting, beautiful parts of desert ecosystems and deserve your respect. If you encounter one in the wild, please don't kill it. Instead, make sure you're at a safe distance (they can only strike about half their own length, so triple that for good measure), give your pulse a minute to calm back down, say hello, and admire it. Both you and the snake will have a good story to tell friends when you get home. In the thousands of days I have spent exploring rattlesnake country, I have seen fewer than a dozen rattlesnakes.

SCORPIONS

Related to spiders, scorpions are venomous predators that prowl at night for other insects to eat. There are many species of scorpions in the U.S. and although they all inflict painful stings, only one species, *Centruroides exilicauda,* present in Southern

Nevada, is potentially dangerous (especially to small pets, children, and the elderly).

SPIDERS

There are many spiders in the desert, but only two are potentially dangerous: the black widow and the brown recluse. Tarantulas are large (as large as an adult human hand), but their bite is not usually dangerous.

Prehistoric People & Artifacts

Prevailing archaeological evidence shows that humans have lived in the Mojave Desert for at least 10,000 years and possibly much longer. This region, especially along the Colorado River, has always been a corridor of life, travel, and trade. Peoples from other regions also may have passed through, contributing influence from their own cultures.

The earliest people were hunter-gatherers, carrying their possessions on their backs, moving in small groups, and traveling from place to place with the rhythm of the seasons. They wore clothes made from animal skins and plant fibers, and they made tools from stone, animal bones, or horns. They either made temporary shelters or sought shelter in naturally occurring places such as caves.

In the distant past, when the climate was cooler and wetter, lakes filled low basins throughout the Mojave. Before the last ice age ended 10,000 years ago, animals such as mammoths, saber-toothed cats, camels, and ground sloths lived in the Mojave region, providing food and challenge for these early people.

Within the last few thousand years, other people came to the region, including the Hohokam, Ancestral Puebloans, Chemehuevi, Southern Paiute, Shoshone, Yuma (or Patayan), and Mojave peoples.

ANCIENT ROCK ART:
PETROGLYPHS & PICTOGRAPHS

As these people passed through and inhabited the Mojave, they left behind artifacts that help us understand what they ate, how they clothed and sheltered themselves, and what tools they used. Among the most mysterious and inspiring artifacts are the motifs and designs they carved (petroglyphs) or painted (pictographs) on rocks and canyon walls. Symbols found across the Southwest and into Mexico suggest a sharing of cultures over time. Others are unique to Nevada.

Archaeologists are able to classify the styles of rock art and to date them: Some

An agave roasting pit used by natives long ago

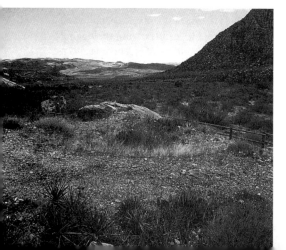

petroglyphs are fewer than 200 years old, while others date back thousands of years. Because different peoples may have contributed to the art at certain sites over time, and because several different cultural groups lived in the region at the same time, it's difficult to attribute these artifacts directly to one tribe or another. It's harder still to interpret their meaning. Every answer brings exceptions, questions, and alternative theories:

- Symbols near playas, springs, and streams seem associated with water.
- Those along trails may have been markers for travelers.
- Designs of bighorn sheep and other game may have been related to hunting.
- Some rock art panels may have recorded significant events or spiritual journeys taken by shamans (healers) or their initiates.
- Certain designs may have been symbols of clan or family affiliation or territory.
- Rock art in places with great echo qualities may be associated with indigenous groups that believed echoes were communication from the spirits.

Our contemporary ideas make it difficult to understand the original meanings of rock art. We see and interpret things differently than people who lived vastly different lives so many years ago. Although it's fun to try to understand what rock art means, who made it, how long ago, and why, it's also fun to enjoy the mystery and uncertainty of expressions we might never fully understand.

As tempting as it may be to take home a souvenir, please do not move or touch the artifacts. They are fragile and irreplaceable and even a respectful caress leaves oils from your skin on the rock, which can break down the varnish and hasten the art's destruction. Once rock art is destroyed or stolen, it is gone forever, and we all lose the opportunity to enjoy and learn from it.

Numerous federal and state laws protect archaeological resources. It is illegal to remove any artifact, or to disturb or excavate an archaeological site on federal or state land without a permit. Plus many of these sites are sacred to tribes here today. Please respect them as you would your own place of worship and report any vandalism you see to the appropriate land management agency.

Wilderness

When Congress passed the Wilderness Act in 1964, it gave Americans the power to preserve for future generations the same wild landscapes that we inherited from our ancestors. Wilderness designation is the highest protection land can receive, safeguarding it from development, extractive industry, roads, and motorized vehicles. Wilderness preserves habitat for wildlife and native plant communities, protects our water supplies and clean air by preserving functioning watersheds, and gives us all the opportunity to pursue traditional, nonmotorized activities amid an untrammeled natural landscape.

Since the Wilderness Act passed, Americans have designated more than 106 million acres of wilderness across the country. Although that figure seems large, it represents only 5 percent of the country (2.5 percent of the Lower 48). In Nevada, which has more public land than any state outside Alaska, less than 5 percent is protected as wilderness. In California, the percentage is a more visionary 15 percent. As our population grows and industrialization continues unchecked, these wilderness areas remind us of where we came from and let us compare our way of doing things with nature's way.

On November 6, 2002, the Clark County Conservation of Public Land and Natural Resources Act designated 17 wilderness areas in Clark County (the county Las Vegas is in) and expanded the Mt. Charleston Wilderness Area, which was originally designated in 1989. In 2004, the Lincoln County Conservation, Recreation, and Development Act designated 14 wilderness areas in Lincoln County (the county immediately north of Clark). The majority of Death Valley

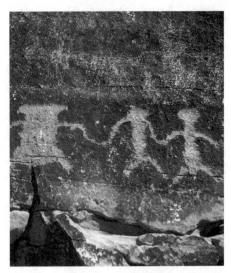

Please respect fragile petroglyphs from a distance.

National Park and Mojave National Preserve is also designated wilderness. Many of the hikes in this book are in wilderness and are listed in the chart below.

Confession: I'm biased. In my day job, I work for wilderness. I believe strongly that some of our landscape needs to be preserved free of permanent human impacts. Wilderness areas offer many benefits and are a legacy for future generations, who have as much right to enjoy nature as we do. Protecting the landscape that helped shape us as a people is also patriotic. We wouldn't be Americans without it, and America the Beautiful won't stay that way unless we work together.

There is a time and a place for highways, houses, shopping centers, mines, logging operations, and automobiles. There is also a time to get out of, or off of, our vehicles and walk, or to appreciate the view without driving in. And there is a time to give the plants, birds, animals, soils, and dynamic natural processes the space, solitude, and freedom they require to thrive according to their kind. If they flourish, we flourish, for ultimately we depend on them for our survival.

The benefits of wilderness and our responsibility to be good stewards of the land were summed up nicely by President Lyndon B. Johnson. When he signed the Wilderness Act on September 3, 1964, he said, "If future generations are to remember us with gratitude rather than contempt, we must leave them more than the miracles of technology. We must leave them a glimpse of the world as it was in the beginning, not just after we got through with it."

TRIPS BY WILDERNESS AREA	
WILDERNESS AREA	**TRIP(S)**
La Madre Mountain Wilderness	West 2, 3, 4, 6, 14, 16
Rainbow Mountain Wilderness	West 5, 7–11, 13
Mt. Charleston Wilderness	West 17, 20, 21, 25, 26, 27
Muddy Mountains Wilderness	East 7, 8, 17
Pinto Valley Wilderness	East 9, 11, 13
Jimbilnan Wilderness	East 14, 15
Lime Canyon Wilderness	East 24
Jumbo Springs Wilderness	East 25
Arrow Canyon Wilderness	North 8
Mormon Mountains Wilderness	North 9, 10, 11
Big Rocks Wilderness	North 15
Mt. Irish Wilderness	North 16
Black Canyon Wilderness	South 1, 2
Eldorado Wilderness	South 4
Ireteba Peaks Wilderness	South 6
Wee Thump Joshua Tree Wilderness	South 8
Spirit Mountain Wilderness	South 9
Bridge Canyon Wilderness	South 10
North McCullough Wilderness	South 12
South McCullough Wilderness	South 13

Note: Most of Death Valley National Park and Mojave National Preserve are designated as wilderness; however, because there are so many and most are unnamed, those areas are not included in this chart. If you're hiking away from a road or development in Death Valley or Mojave Preserve, you're probably in wilderness. If you're curious about wilderness in these parks, the Trails Illustrated maps for each of these parks (#221 and #256, respectively) indicate wilderness areas with green borders.

Comfort, Safey, & Etiquette

Exploring Southern Nevada's desert land-scapes can be enjoyable, inspiring, and healthy. If you're unprepared, unwise, or just plain unlucky, it can also be deadly. Luckily, preparation and commonsense can help maximize your enjoyment and minimize your risk, and that takes learning about the weather in the region, how to navigate the land, what to take on a trip, and proper trail etiquette.

Seasons & Weather

The Mojave Desert's brutal summer heat can make exploring uncomfortable, even dangerous. For this reason, fall, winter, and spring are the best times to hike in Southern Nevada. (Spring is particularly enjoyable because of all the wildflowers.) However, the region's generally dry, sunny weather makes exploring possible any time of the year. Although winter can be bitterly cold, warm days are frequent; cool trends are possible in summer.

Know how to avoid Southern Nevada's most unpleasant (or dangerous) weather with proper preparation, good timing, and a little help from the local weather service, and you should have an enjoyable time. For a forecast of today's weather in the Southern Nevada region, call the National Weather Service at (702) 263-9744.

PRECIPITATION

The Las Vegas Valley receives an average of four inches of rain per year; precipitation is greater in the mountains. The heaviest precipitation is split evenly between winter storms and summer thunderstorms. Snowfall is possible high in the mountains and down to the valley floor in winter months, and high-elevation snowfall can happen any day of the year.

Thunderstorms can also happen any time of year, but they prowl mainly June through October. They usually happen in the afternoon and evening and pose significant risk to hikers and explorers. Storms can build out of nowhere and unleash a fury of rain (I like the term "gulley washers"), dropping up to three inches or more of rain and hail in an hour. Lightning is a risk to anyone on open or high, exposed ground. Flash floods can sweep through canyons with deadly force (see the trips to Mary Jane Falls, page 78, and Bridge Spring Arch, page 221, for examples). Rain can also wash out roads or render them muddy and impassable.

If you watch the sky carefully, you can see thunderstorms coming before they hit. Growing cumulonimbus (towering puffy white clouds) indicate possible thunderstorm activity. Also watch for storms and lighting nearby or on the horizon. Be aware that distant mountains may drain to where you're standing, so even if no thunderstorms are nearby, a flash flood may be headed your way. Consider also that a dangerous storm may be sneaking up on you behind a nearby ridge or mountain. If puffy white clouds are growing anywhere in the sky, it's not a day to bag a peak or hike exposed ridges. Check with the local weather service to see what general trends are in store when you plan to explore. Avoid areas where storms are predicted.

If lightning is imminent:

- Seek lower ground.

- Avoid solitary trees, cave entrances, and metal objects. Stay at least 15 feet from other people.

- Crouch down and cover your ears.

- Avoid traveling along the bottoms of washes and canyons, and park and camp at least 40 feet above the bottom of a canyon or wash. If a flood comes, climb to higher ground immediately.

- Do not drive through flooded areas. The road may be washed out, and powerful currents may sweep you and your car away. If the water begins to rise over

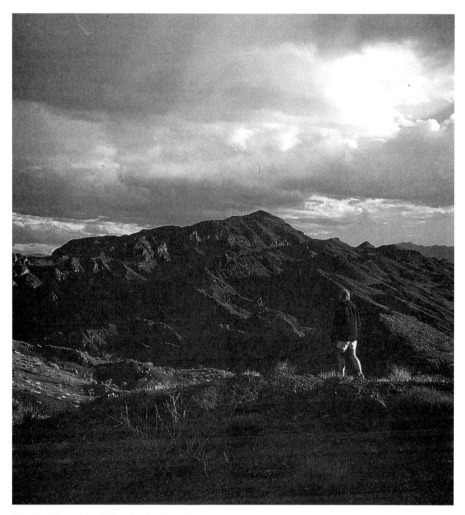

Enjoying the golden light of a clearing thunderstorm

the road, abandon your car and climb to high ground.

HEAT

On hot days in Southern Nevada, the temperature on the Strip can climb well above 100°F. It's not impossible to hike on these days; you just need to know where to go—into the mountains, where temperatures are cooler thanks to a condition known as the adiabatic lapse rate: Depending on the humidity, air cools between 3°F and 5°F for every 1000-foot climb in elevation. So that sweaty 100°F day on the

Strip (2200 feet) might translate to a cool 70°F at the top of Mt. Charleston (11,918 feet). Just make sure you're prepared for higher winds on exposed ridges and slopes, and avoid high places when thunderstorms are active.

Another option is to hike at night. The air is cooler, and the moon paints the landscapes a cool blue. The full moon rises with sunset about two weeks after the new (no) moon. My favorite nights to hike are two or three nights before a full moon, when the waxing gibbous moon is already high in

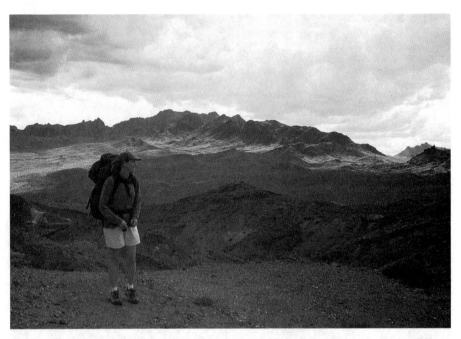

Backpacking at Lake Mead National Recreation Area

the sky at sunset and lights the way across the desert. Bring a headlamp in case clouds, canyons, or forest block the light.

If the day promises to be hot, begin your hike at first light. When you arrive at your destination, find a shady spot to wait out the heat of the day, then hike back when the sun sinks low and the temperature cools.

Preparation & Equipment

Although the area is beautiful, Southern Nevada's climate and terrain can be inhospitable, and even dangerous. Destinations like Red Rock Canyon and Valley of Fire have trails, restrooms, water, and rangers to help minimize your risk. Other destinations have no trails or services whatsoever. If you are new to exploring Southern Nevada, please stick to the more developed destinations, or go with someone who knows the area (several groups listed in Giving Back to the Land, page 20, offer guided hikes in this region) until you're more experienced and better prepared to explore Southern Nevada safely.

As you prepare for your trip, remember to pack the 10 essentials, plus a few other good things, that are useful to have when you're hiking and adventuring through Southern Nevada:

WATER & FOOD

Water is the one thing that can limit your exploration of the desert. It's essential for life, but it's extremely rare in this region and very heavy to carry. Follow these tips to ensure you return from your hike happy and hydrated:

If you are dayhiking, **plan to carry all the water you need,** at least two quarts per day per person. You'll need more on active and/ or hot days. At 8.3 pounds per gallon, water can add up quickly.

Don't count on springs, unless you know them well and have been to them recently. Many springs shown on maps have long since dried up.

Filter and/or treat all water you find at natural sources. Natural water sources across the West often contain microscopic bugs that can make you very sick.

In cold weather, **throw a few extra energy bars in your pack.** They're light and will help give you energy and sustenance when you need it. In hot weather, however, they turn to goop, in which case jerky or mixed nuts are best.

SUN PROTECTION

Long sleeves and pants, sunscreen (30 SPF or higher), a wide-brimmed sunhat (a baseball hat's not much better than a bare head), and quality sunglasses (rated to protect you against 100 percent of UVA and UVB rays) are all necessary.

SIGNAL MIRROR & WHISTLE

These are useful for attracting attention when you're injured or lost. Three short blasts on your whistle is the international signal for distress.

HEADLAMP

LED headlamps are more compact, lighter-weight, and last much longer than incandescent lights.

FIRST-AID KIT

In addition to the requisite bandages, antiseptics, and painkillers, make sure to include the following:

- **Comb.** Don't worry, your hair looks great, but it'll come in handy if you brush too close to a "jumping" cholla cactus. Deft comb work can remove cholla nodules without further injury.

- **Tweezers.** Use them to remove the individual cholla spines the comb left behind.

- **Duct tape.** This modern wonder can fix many things: ripped boots, backpacks, and clothing; delaminated soles; broken glasses, trekking poles, and tent poles; and it's a good item for securing splints, bandages, and other first aid items. Wrap a few feet around a trekking pole or water bottle, and you'll always have it ready when you need it.

EXTRA LAYERS

A warm hat, gloves, fleece jacket, and a wind/rain shell will keep you warm in case of the inevitable sudden storms, surprise sun-

sets, and unexpected winds. Hypothermia (when your heart, brain, and other core organs get too cold) can be life threatening. Don't underestimate the desert's ability to get brutally cold in winter and spring.

INSECT REPELLENT

Because of Nevada's low humidity, there are only 100 bugs in the whole state, but they are all waiting for you at the trailhead. If you find yourself in a buggy spot, your adversaries will likely be mosquitoes or "no-see-ums" (tiny biting flies). Insect repellent works well, especially if it contains DEET. If you are concerned about DEET's alleged toxicity (there is an ongoing debate about the danger of DEET, especially to children), spray your clothes instead of your skin, use a lower concentration of DEET, or choose an insect repellent with lemongrass, eucalyptus, or other natural repellent.

WATERPROOF MATCHES & FIRE STARTER

Fires can be used for emergency warmth at night or to signal rescuers when you're lost. Candle wax works well as a fire starter.

KNIFE

A Swiss Army–style knife with blades, can and bottle openers, screwdrivers, and other gadgets will come in handy many times over. Just make sure to place it in checked baggage at the airport, or you'll have to buy another after security takes it away from you.

CELL PHONE

A cell phone can be a lifesaver in an emergency situation. But like GPS units, they can also break, lose their power, or lose signal in deep canyons and remote locations. Think through your situation and try to avoid trouble before calling for help, which might incur steep charges for medical rescue transport. Unnecessary searches also risk the lives of rescuers and keep them from responding to more serious emergencies. Please avoid these unfortunate situations by planning and traveling carefully.

Cell phones also prevent you and others from fully experiencing the beauty and solitude around you. Please resist the urge to call your friends from a beautiful spot and reserve your cell phone for true emergencies.

GOOD BOOTS OR HIKING SHOES

Sturdy, comfortable shoes are your contact with the landscape, and thick soles protect against sharp rocks. In this region, footwear that breathes well is more important than waterproof boots, which don't provide ventilation. When buying boots, make comfort your highest priority. If your boots are uncomfortable, you won't have any fun, and the blisters that result can be excruciating and crippling.

TREKKING POLES

Four legs are better than two to help pull yourself up and ease yourself down, adding stability and speed along the way. Downsides include added cost, more stuff to deal with, and their tendency to interfere when you're climbing up or down cliffs and waterfalls.

LONG PANTS

It's tempting to wear shorts in warm weather, but on hikes without a trail, the sagebrush, bitterbrush, pinyon-juniper, and other plants can scratch your legs to heck. They'll also protect you from the sun's harsh UV rays.

DESERT GAITERS

These nylon covers help keep scree, debris, and annoying grass seeds from getting into your socks and shoes, saving you multiple stops to empty your shoes and hours of picking foxtails from your socks when you get home.

SURVIVAL: THE RULE OF THREES

You can survive for three minutes without air, three hours without shelter from extreme sun or cold, three days without water, and three weeks without food. This handy rule of thumb will help you establish your priorities when planning your desert travel.

Navigation

Staying found in the desert means planning ahead and being observant on your trip. Follow these tips to ensure safe travel:

Leave an itinerary of your trip and expected time of return with a responsible persom (include some leeway for delays). Ask this person to call for a search party if you're not in contact by a certain time. Make sure you contact that person upon your return.

Leave a similar itinerary on your dashboard, so folks at the trailhead will know whether to worry about you.

Beware of scale in the desert. The large rock formation next to you, or the canyon you're in, might disappear once you get farther away and see how many similar formations and canyons there are.

Park on a ridge or rise, rather than in a depression, so you can see your car from a distance when returning from your hike. Try to park near a prominent landmark, and be careful not to lose its place when that "prominent" landmark gets lost in such a vast landscape.

Pick a baseline—a prominent ridge, road, or power line—that you can use to find your way back. Watch the horizon. Draw a straight line from your destination, through your parking spot to the horizon behind, preferably to a prominent peak or feature on the horizon. Memorize this alignment. It might help you find your way back to your car.

Hike in a group for company and options if someone becomes injured. If the group plans to split up, make sure each group includes an experienced hiker. Choose a time and location to meet again, allow for delays, and then make every effort to make it there on time.

If you get lost, find shelter and stay near it. It's easier for search crews to find a stationary person than a moving target.

MAP & COMPASS

Desert landscapes can be deceiving and disorienting. These tools, used properly, will help you stay found, but remember that maps can be inaccurate or poorly labeled.

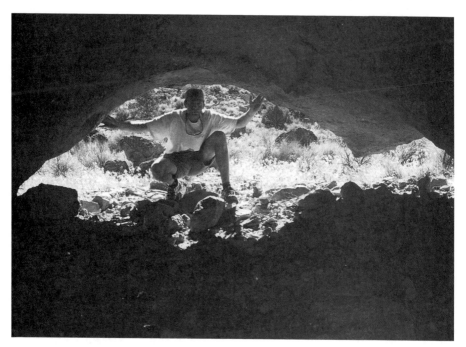

Some of the best discoveries aren't on any maps.

Roads on the map may have disappeared through nonuse, or new roads may have been established since the map was published. Similarly, the dot signifying a town won't tell you whether you can get gas and food, or whether you'll find a ghost town that hasn't had a living soul in 80 years.

I recommend the following:

Full-state atlases, such as Benchmark's road and recreation atlas, cover the entire state and offer enough details to help you navigate to your trailhead.

BLM 1:100,000-scale maps are good because they cover larger areas (most of a mountain range, for example), but they may not be detailed enough to help you navigate convoluted terrain.

USGS 7.5-minute maps provide good detail for specific areas, but several maps may be necessary to cover your chosen trip.

Maps on CD such as National Geographic's TOPO! series on Nevada allow you to explore the entire state seamlessly (no taping maps together on the floor), zoom back and forth among five different levels, add trails and landmarks, and get distance and elevation profiles for your route, and then print it out to take on your trip. All distance, hiking time, elevation, and GPS waypoint figures in this book are based on these maps.

Global Positioning System receivers can make navigation and communication easier, but they also pose definite risks. Batteries may run out, you might drop the unit, it could malfunction, or it may lose reception in deep canyons. GPS units also draw your attention to the LED readout rather than the landscape. While GPS is fun, bring a map and compass also.

Safety in Rattlesnake, Scorpion, or Spider Country

Watch where you walk. Avoid open-toed shoes and bare feet, especially at night.

Do not hike alone. It's nice to have people to rescue you quickly if you get bit or stung.

Avoid walking along the bottom of rocky ledges. Wear long pants and sleeves when traveling through brush.

Do not put your hands where you cannot see them. Gather firewood carefully.

When camping, **sleep in a tent or enclosure** and keep your shelter closed when you're not coming or going. Shake out your shoes and clothes in the morning to dislodge unwelcome visitors.

If you are bitten by a rattlesnake, stay calm. A majority of bites are "warning bites" and do not carry venom. Snakebites to your pet or children are more dangerous because the ratio of venom to body size is more likely to cause severe reactions. Do not cut and suck the wound, or use a suction device. The best first aid is simply to seek medical attention quickly and calmly.

If you're bitten by a spider, stung by a scorpion, or have an insect bite of unknown origin that keeps getting bigger, **seek medical attention immediately**.

Please help animals survive by **enjoying them from a distance.** Do not feed or approach any wild animal.

Trail Etiquette

There is a thin line between enjoying the landscape with respect and loving it to death. No matter how good our intentions are, simply being out in some of these areas can destroy them if we're not extremely careful.

Part of the reason I've written this book is to inspire people to love the desert and everything it offers, to share with others their love for this unique landscape, and to work to protect these areas from the impacts of what is the fastest growing population center in the country. If we cannot learn to protect our beautiful landscapes, these areas are doomed. If we work together, however, we can keep them beautiful and wild for us, our children, and our grandchildren's grandchildren to enjoy.

Leave No Trace

When driving, hiking, and exploring Southern Nevada, please follow these tips from the Leave No Trace Center for Outdoor Ethics:

Plan ahead and prepare. Know the regulations and concerns of the area you visit, including extreme weather, hazards, and emergencies. Visit in small groups and repackage food to minimize waste.

Travel and camp on durable surfaces, such as trails, rock, washes, gravel, and snow. Avoid trampling plants and living soils (see more about cryptobiotic soils on page 169). Protect riparian areas and help animals survive by camping, cleaning, and washing at least 200 feet from water. Do not cut switchbacks.

Dispose of waste properly. Pack out what you pack in and clean up after others. Deposit human waste in restrooms or in holes six to eight inches deep and at least 200 feet from water, camp, and trails. Use unscented, dye-free toilet paper (to keep animals from smelling it and digging it up), and bury it well.

Leave what you find. Examine and enjoy them, but leave cultural and historic artifacts, as well as neat rocks, plants, and other natural objects where you find them. Avoid introducing or transporting nonnative species (pick foxtails out of your socks once you get home, not at the next stop along the trail). Do not build structures or furniture or dig trenches around your tent when camping.

Minimize campfire impacts. Avoid building fires. Instead, use a lightweight stove for cooking and a candle lantern for light. Where fires are permitted, use established fire rings. Keep fires small and use only small, dead, downed wood that can be broken by hand. Put fires out completely. If camping high in desert ranges, please do not burn bristlecone. These trees can be thousands of years old, and the biomass they produce is scarce and precious to the soils at such high, harsh conditions.

Respect wildlife. Observe wildlife from a distance. Do not follow or approach wild animals, and never feed them. Feeding wildlife damages their health, alters natural behavior, and makes them bold and often dangerous to humans, which means they have to be killed. A fed bear is a dead bear.

Be considerate of others and respect the quality of their experience. Be courteous and yield to other groups on the trail. Step aside and downhill when encountering pack stock. Let nature's sounds prevail, and avoid loud noises and voices.

For more information about Leave No Trace principles, visit www.lnt.org or call (800) 332-4100.

Dogs

Hiking with Rover, Cassie, or Zack can be fun for both of you, but it can also be a bad idea: Brutal heat, scarce water, cacti, rattlesnakes, and paw-shredding limestone are just a few reasons to leave your dog at home.

Las Vegas, North Las Vegas, and Henderson all have leash laws requiring dogs to be on leash at all times. Dogs are allowed on BLM, U.S. Fish and Wildlife, and U.S. Forest Service lands, unless posted otherwise. Leashes are often required (or at least a common courtesy) in well-visited or developed areas. Even running free, your dog should be under voice control at all times. Dogs should not be allowed to harass or endanger wildlife, which have a hard enough time surviving in this harsh climate. Also be aware that the ride to and from your hike can be deadly, because car interiors can quickly reach 150°F on hot days, which can kill your dog in the few minutes it takes you to run into the store on the way home. It is both illegal and unwise to leave your dog unattended in the car for any time. If you bring your dog into the desert, please carry enough water and food for her. And at all times, it is courteous (and sometimes required) to clean up after your dog.

Here are dog regulations for some of the places mentioned in this book:

- **Red Rock Canyon National Conservation Area:** Dogs are allowed on trails and should be leashed to minimize conflicts with others. Leases are required at all times in campgrounds and at developed facilities like the visitors center, picnic areas, and overlooks.

- **Spring Mountains National Recreation Area:** Dogs must be under voice control in the backcountry and on leash in the more-visited Kyle and Lee canyons.

- **Mojave National Preserve:** Pets must be on a six-foot leash at all times.

- **Death Valley National Park:** Pets are not allowed in wilderness areas (most of the park) or on any trails. Pets must be on a short leash at all times on roads and in campgrounds.

- **Lake Mead National Recreation Area:** Pets are allowed on a six-foot leash at all times.

- **Valley of Fire State Park:** Pets are allowed on a six-foot leash at all times.

- **Wildlife refuges:** Pets must be under leash or voice control at all times, unless otherwise required.

Special Considerations in the Desert

Abandoned Mines

Mining has played a large part in shaping Nevada, and as a result, mining roads, buildings, tunnels, and shafts are scattered throughout the hills and mountains of the Mojave Desert. Exploring these remnants of our prospecting history can be a colorful and exciting part of exploring Southern Nevada. It can also be dangerous.

Most mining tunnels and shafts were unsafe when they were first built more than a century ago. Decades of rain, sun, wind, rust, and rot have made them even more so. Tunnels and shafts may be on the verge of collapse. Puddles on tunnel floors may contain poisonous chemicals or disguise vertical shafts. Tasteless, odorless, yet noxious gases may be present in tunnels. Miners may have left explosives or dangerous equipment behind unintentionally. For your own safety, please stay out of these areas.

Driving

Many of the hikes in this book require driving on dirt roads. Some are wide, smooth, well-maintained, and will make you want to drive 50 miles per hour. Others may be choked with rocks and ruts, allowing a top speed of 3 miles per hour. Rough routes can also tear up tires, oil pans, and other necessary car parts, leaving you stranded God-knows-where, a potentially dangerous and certainly expensive situation. And if you're driving a rental car, be aware that it probably has two-ply tires, which don't last long against sharp rocks. And double-check the fine print on your rental car's liability coverage; some companies do not cover your vehicle once it leaves the pavement.

When you're driving in the desert, follow these tips for a safe journey:

Fill your tank before leaving civilization for a long drive on remote roads. Confirm the location of your next/last gas station. A dot on the map doesn't necessarily mean there's a town (or gas or a phone).

Carry extra food and water. If venturing to a remote location, you should have several days of food and water in your car, just in case you break down and need it. Extra water is also good for quenching your thirst when you return from your hike, or for thirsty radiators.

Bring an extra spare tire, patch kit, and generator. A plug kit and air compressor that plugs into your car cigarette lighter helps repair small punctures but not large tears. One spare doesn't help if you get more than one flat.

Carry a jack, jumper cables, and spare tools.

Pack a shovel to dig yourself out of sand, mud, and snow.

Consider taking a tow cable, for generous souls to pull you out of that ditch, or for you to return the favor to others.

Bring a blanket or sleeping bag for cold nights when you get stuck.

Carry a tarp and cord to rig extra shade.

Stay on maintained and/or designated routes. Reckless, ignorant off-road vehicle use is one of the greatest threats to the desert landscape. It causes erosion; destroys fragile soils, critical plants, and wildlife habitat; and leaves ugly scars that can take centuries to heal (just look at some of the mining scars on desert hillsides).

Giving Back to the Land

All of the trips in this book are on public lands, and the ultimate responsibility for taking care of these lands belongs to the public, which means you and me. Please take to heart the Leave No Trace principles discussed on page 18. I also encourage you to give your time and/or money to conservation efforts in the region.

In Nevada, land management agencies and nonprofit organizations need volunteer help and financial donations to help protect natural and cultural resources. For a list of the government land management agencies, please refer to Appendix 3 (page 267).

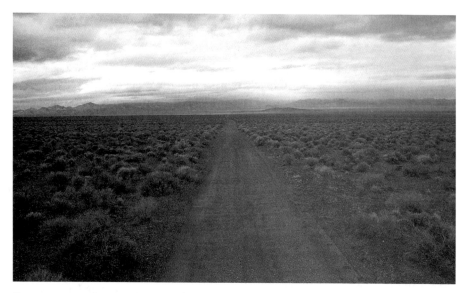

Commonsense and preparation can make lonely desert roads wonderful to explore.

If you are interested in volunteering your time or donating money to a nonprofit organization, consider some of these:

FRIENDS OF RED ROCK CANYON

This volunteer organization offers visitors interpretive presentations and organizes regular volunteer work parties at Red Rock Canyon. Contact them at (702) 255-8743 or www.friendsofredrockcanyon.org.

ARCHAEOLOGY SITE STEWARDS

These volunteers monitor petroglyphs and other archaeological sites to protect them from looters and vandals. Contact them at (702) 895-4863 or george.phillips@unlv.edu.

FRIENDS OF NEVADA WILDERNESS

This nonprofit organization is dedicated to protecting wild public lands across Nevada. In addition to public outreach, they also organize volunteer work parties to restore habitat in wilderness areas. Contact them at (775) 324-7667 or www.nevadawilderness.org.

RED ROCK AUDUBON SOCIETY

The Audubon Society is dedicated to protecting birds, other wildlife, and their habitats. The Red Rock Chapter organizes birding trips throughout the Mojave Desert. Contact them at (702) 390-9890 or www.redrockaudubon.org.

SIERRA CLUB TOIYABE CHAPTER

In addition to their conservation efforts across the state, the Sierra Club offers regular outings to beautiful spots around the region. Contact them at (702) 732-7750 or www.nevada.sierraclub.org/sngroup.

Using This Book

This book introduces you to the best of Southern Nevada's outdoor wonders, with trips for every ability and interest level. It includes the most popular destinations, such as Red Rock Canyon National Conservation Area, Valley of Fire State Park, Death Valley National Park, and Mt. Charleston. It will also help you discover places you might not have heard of, such as Anniversary Narrows, Arrow Canyon, Bowl of Fire, and the Wee Thump Joshua Tree Wilderness.

Although the book emphasizes hiking, there are also great scenic drives, historic ghost towns, horseback rides, mountain bike trails, and even a kayak float below Hoover Dam. Everything in this book is within a three-hour drive of Las Vegas, and all trips are possible in a single day, although some are better done overnight. All trips are in Nevada, except for those in Death Valley National Park and Mojave National Preserve, both of which are in California. Each trip includes a map (see legend below).

The trips in this book are divided into four general regions:

Western Region: West of Las Vegas Blvd., Interstate 15, and Highway 95. Includes Red Rock Canyon National Conservation Area, the Spring Mountains and Mt. Charleston, and Death Valley National Park.

Eastern Region: East of Las Vegas Blvd. and I-15, but north of Highway 93 through Boulder City. Includes Valley of Fire State Park and Lake Mead National Recreation Area.

Northern Region: East of Highway 95, west of I-15, and north of Las Vegas. Includes the Desert National Wildlife Refuge.

Southern Region: South of Las Vegas and Boulder City. Includes the McCullough Mountains, Sloan Canyon, the Eldorado Mountains, Spirit Mountain, and Mojave National Preserve.

This section outlines the information included with each trip entry. These quick reference guides help you gauge whether a particular trip is appropriate for you. Each trip includes a map, and the regional map at the beginning of each section in the book helps you see each trip's location relative to the others in that section. The general locator map on page iv gives you a perspective on the book's whole area.

Choosing a Trip

There are three ways to decide which trip is best for you:

- Choose a trip in the region you'd like to visit from the overview maps at the beginning of each section (Western Region, page 26; Eastern Region, page 122; Northern Region, page 176; Southern Region, page 214).

- Turn to Appendix 1 on page 263 and choose a recommended trip from the Best Trips by Theme suggestions.

- Choose a specific trip from the Table of Contents.

Explanation of Trip Summaries

Each trip entry includes a capsule summary, brief highlights, directions to the starting point, information about facilities and/or the trailhead, and the full description of the trip itself. The capsule summaries at the beginning of each trip entry include the following information:

DISTANCE & TRAIL TYPE

All distances given are round-trip, unless specified one-way. Trail types include loops, semiloops, and out-and-back hikes. If distances are longer or shorter than you'd prefer, don't let them keep you from enjoying the hike. Feel free to turn back early, or keep exploring beyond the listed destination. The point of this book is to get you out and exploring Southern Nevada. Only you can decide the distance that's best for you.

HIKING TIME

This figure is an estimate of the time an "average" person would take to complete the hike. But who is average? Your own hiking time will vary, depending on how fast you hike or how long you stop to rest and enjoy your surroundings.

ELEVATION

These figures show how much climbing and descending to expect for each trip (e.g., +150/-100 feet). For flat routes with very little change in elevation, one elevation figure is given (e.g., 100 feet).

DIFFICULTY

The hiking difficulty rating is based on the type of trail, the terrain, and the elevation gain/loss and is organized into four categories:

Easy: There may or may not be a trail, but the terrain is gentle and the route is easy to follow; *suitable for almost everybody.*

Moderate: Terrain is hilly, uneven, or challenging to navigate. There may or may not be a trail; *suitable only for physically fit people.*

Difficult: Terrain is steep, unstable, and otherwise challenging. Route-finding skills might be necessary. Occasional use of your hands might be required; *suitable only for fit and experienced desert hikers who want a challenge.*

Most Difficult: Climbing is necessary, requiring your hands, agility, strength, and balance. Exposure to painful or dangerous consequences if you fall might be involved; *suitable only for the most fit, agile, and experienced desert hikers.* This rating appears on hikes that require an occasional scramble up a boulder or waterfall, although the rest of the hike might be less difficult. See trip descriptions for specifics.

TRAIL USE

This section designates whether the trail is suitable for other uses, including backpacking and mountain biking, and whether it is good for kids and allows dogs. It will

also specify whether a map or compass is required for the journey.

BEST TIMES

Suggestions range from "cold" to "hot" and are intended to keep you out of the hottest valley bottoms on hot summer days, and off the highest, windiest peaks on cold winter days. Because everyone reacts differently to heat and cold, the best time for you to go is up to you. More specific times, such as early morning or during spring bird migrations, are mentioned if relevant. I use a different system for the Spring Mountains and Mt. Charleston, where winter snows make trails inaccessible (except to skis and snowshoes) between the first major snowstorm in the fall and early summer, when the snow melts. For these, I recommend the best months to visit—June through October, for example. Similarly, I recommend particular seasons to visit Mitchell Caverns/Providence Mountains State Recreation Area, Mary Beale Nature Trail, and Crystal Spring Trail in Mojave National Preserve to help you take advantage of both comfortable weather and hours of operation for the caverns.

AGENCY

Contact information for the responsible land management agency is listed here.

RECOMMENDED MAPS

This section lists the maps (beyond the simplified maps included with the hike description) necessary to navigate the route.

GPS WAYPOINTS

Global Positioning System waypoints are listed in UTM for the trailhead, destination, or notable features for each trip. (Most waypoints were determined using a computer mapping program.)

VEHICLE

Many trips in this book require a high-clearance or four-wheel-drive (4WD) vehicle to get to the trailhead, which will keep you from finding out the hard way, damaging your car, or getting stuck if you don't have such a vehicle. If passenger cars (low-clearance, two-wheel-drive) are OK, I'll say so.

A Final Word of Caution

Hiking anywhere outdoors entails risk, even on paved and patrolled trails. These risks are even greater in the unforgiving environment of Southern Nevada. If the desert heat doesn't get you, the sun, sharp rocks, twisting canyons, lightning, flash floods, prickly plants, rattlesnakes, scorpions, elevation, or mountain lions might. Commonsense, physical fitness, and proper preparation can reduce these risks significantly, but risks cannot be eliminated.

Every attempt was made to make descriptions and instructions in this book accurate. Changing road, weather, and landscape conditions, not to mention human error (yours or mine), and bad luck could lead to dangerous situations, so be aware and plan for these risks when you go on your trip. You are responsible for everything that happens to you out there. Good luck, be careful, and have fun!

Now that all this is out of the way, it's time to hike! When you're done, head back to Vegas, take a shower, hit the buffet, catch a show, win some money, and call it a great day!

Oak Creek (Western Region: Trip 11) in Red Rock Canyon National Conservation Area

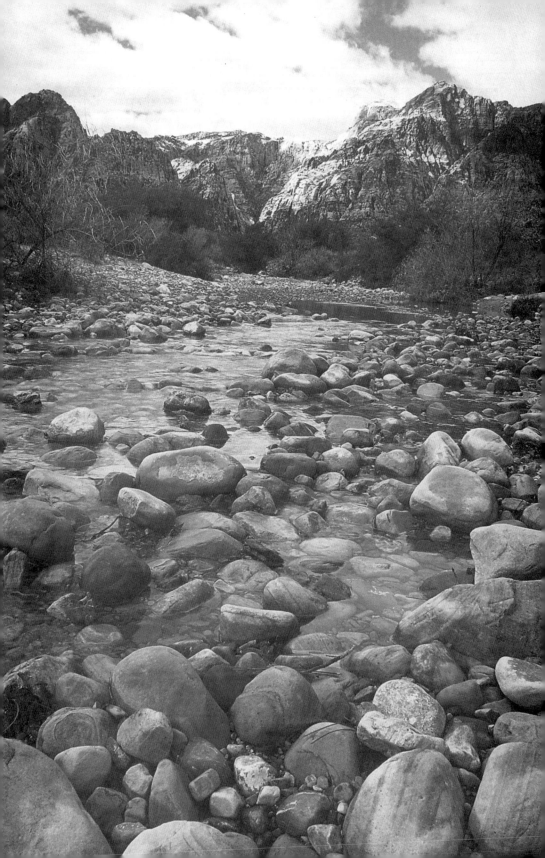

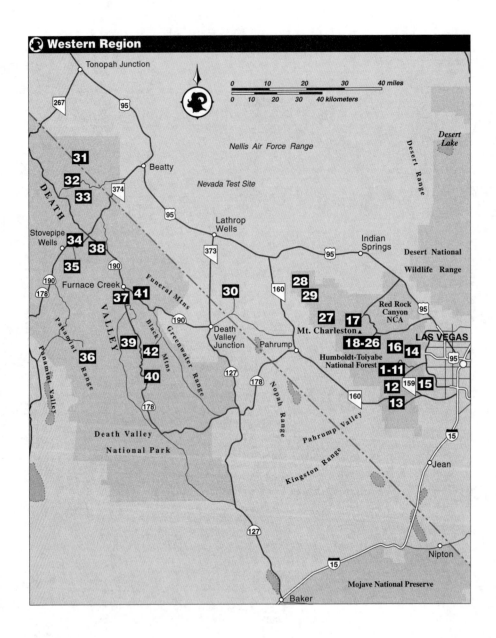

Tonopah Junction

267

95

Nellis Air Force Range

Desert Lake

31

Beatty

32

33

374

Nevada Test Site

Desert Range

95

Lathrop Wells

Stovepipe Wells

34 38

Indian Springs

Desert National

DEATH

35

190

Funeral Mtns

373

95

Wildlife Range

190

178

Furnace Creek

37 41

190

28

160

29

30

Red Rock Canyon NCA

95

VALLEY

Death Valley Junction

27

17

LAS VEGAS

Pahrump

Mt. Charleston

Black Mtns

Greenwater Range

39

18-26

95

Pahrump Range

42

36

40

127

Humboldt-Toiyabe National Forest

16

14

1-11

Panamint Valley

178

178

12

159

15

13

Nopah Range

160

Death Valley

National Park

Pahrump Valley

15

Kingston Range

Jean

127

Nipton

15

Mojave National Preserve

Baker

chapter 1

Western Region

INCLUDING RED ROCKS, SPRING MOUNTAINS, & DEATH VALLEY

Drive west from Las Vegas, and you'll discover places with breathtaking beauty and contrast, as well as pockets of life unlike any other on Earth. Here you'll discover the soaring, colorful cliffs, cool canyons, and hidden pockets of life in Red Rock Canyon; the cool forests of the Spring Mountains, capped by Southern Nevada's highest peak (11,918-foot Mt. Charleston); Death Valley, the largest national park in the Lower 48 and home to many geological wonders; and Badwater Basin, the lowest, driest, and hottest spot in the Western Hemisphere with surprising pockets of color and life.

Red Rock Canyon National Conservation Area

Red Rock's soaring and colorful sandstone cliffs, cut by deep canyons, rival the best any national park has to offer, and they're less than an hour from the Strip, making this the first obvious destination for everyone in Las Vegas. Whether you're planning a quick scenic drive or days of exploration, Red Rock Canyon will reward you with its beauty and mystery.

Not only is Red Rocks visually impressive, it offers opportunities for visitors to explore the geology, plants, animals, and history of the Mojave Desert. The white, banded cliffs of Turtlehead Peak and La Madre Mountain began nearly 600 million years ago as sediments settling to the bottom of the sea. Time and pressure compressed them into carbonate rocks, such as limestone and dolomite.

The bright red, orange, yellow, and tan rocks of the Red Rock escarpment and the Calico Hills are petrified sand dunes from the age of the dinosaurs, between 65 million and 250 million years ago. They're known locally as Aztec Sandstone and get their vibrant colors from oxidized iron and other minerals in the rock. Rock climbers come from around the world to climb on this wonderful stone. You'll probably see them high above as you explore.

Usually, older rocks are underneath younger rocks. But about 65 million years ago, the colliding Pacific and North American continental plates at Red Rocks pushed the older carbonate rocks up and over the younger sandstones. The line where these rocks meet is called the Keystone Thrust, which is visible on the Keystone Thrust Trail, the Top of the Rainbow Mountain Escarpment, and the Bridge Mountain Trail.

Over the centuries, springs and streams in the area have nourished more than 700 species of plants and animals, as well as prehistoric people and pioneer settlers. The historic Spanish Trail passes just south of the conservation area, where Highway 160 now climbs up and over Mountain Springs Summit.

In 1990, Congress designated the national conservation area to protect the natural, scenic, and historic aspects of the area. Congress added additional protection by designating the Rainbow Mountain and La Madre Mountain wilderness areas in 2002 (see page 10 for a discussion on wilderness).

If you're visiting the Las Vegas area for the first time, please read the sections in the introduction about weather, wildlife, preparation and equipment, and special considerations for the desert. If you're looking for a great scenic drive to fill a few free hours, take the 13-Mile Scenic Drive, then turn right (south) at its exit to follow Highway 159/Blue Diamond Road back to Highway 160. Turn left (east), and follow 160 back to Vegas.

Spring Mountains National Recreation Area

The Spring Mountains, which border the Las Vegas Valley on the west and include the Spring Mountains National Recreation Area and the Mt. Charleston Wilderness, are the highest, wettest mountains in Southern Nevada, making them ideal for escaping the summer's heat. Rising to 11,918 feet at the summit of Mt. Charleston, these mountains receive many feet of snow in the winter. Designated by Congress in 1993, the Spring Mountains National Recreation Area comprises more than 316,000 acres and offers soaring peaks and cliffs, stately forests, deep canyons, and a remarkable diversity of plants and animals. Hiking, skiing, birding, backpacking, climbing, and simply enjoying the diverse beauty of these high-elevation forests are a few of the activities possible in the area.

Geologically, the bulk of the Spring Mountains is composed of layered and tilted limestone that formed some 500 million years ago as sediments settled in ancient seas. Reminders of the range's oceanic past in the form of fossils are scattered throughout the area.

The Spring Mountains and Mt. Charleston (the names are practically interchangeable) are perfect examples of "sky island" habitats. Many species of plants and animals are nourished by the higher precipitation, yet the wide, arid valleys below prevent animals from migrating and plants from spreading seed to other mountains. Over time, the plants and animals in this isolated habitat have evolved into a unique community.

The Spring Mountains are also among the most biologically diverse of all Nevada's mountain ranges. They are home to about 1,000 plant species (a third of the total found in the state), 37 of which are trees (more than on any other Nevada mountain range). Twenty-eight species of plants and animals (15 plants, 9 butterflies, 2 spring snails, 1 ant, and 1 mammal) are endemic to the Spring Mountains, and because they live in small, isolated communities, they are very vulnerable. Several of the above species are endangered.

Simply driving from Las Vegas into the Spring Mountains takes you through several of the many vegetation zones on the range: The creosote shrub–dominated lands of the low valleys give way to the blackbrush-sagebrush-Joshua tree zone, then to the pinyon pine-juniper pygmy forest, and finally to the ponderosa pine and white fir–dominated montane forests. Hiking higher on trails takes you into alpine forests dominated by bristlecone and limber pines.

A note on best time to hike the Spring Mountains: For most hikes in the book, I use general temperatures (for example, cold to warm) to guide you to the best hikes depending on the season and weather. This system is intended to keep you out of the low valleys on the hottest days, and off the highest peaks and ridges on the coldest days. Because the Spring Mountains receive so much snow in the winter, I use a more specific recommendation of spring through fall for all hikes in the Mt. Charleston area.

Death Valley National Park

At nearly 3.4 million acres, Death Valley National Park is the largest national park in the Lower 48, offering geologic wonders and tenacious forms of life on a grand scale. It is home to Badwater Basin, the driest, hottest, and lowest place in North America. But you'll soon discover this grand and varied landscape tells many stories in its soaring peaks, twisting canyons, shifting sand dunes, parched dry lakebeds, well-adapted plants and animals, and evidence of early American pioneers' grit and determination.

Exposed formations in Death Valley represent most of Earth's geologic eras as far back as 1.8 billion years, although they have often been bent, thrust, tilted, metamorphosed, and eroded into an enigmatic and beautiful jigsaw puzzle of form and color. Death Valley's geologic forces are dynamic and continue today, with water, wind, and occasional earthquakes that continue to shape the landscape of Death Valley.

On a smaller scale, the different soil types combine with elevation, sunlight, and precipitation to create numerous habitats for plants and animals to survive. Between the valley floor, where rainfall averages less than 2 inches per year, and the higher peaks, which receive up to 15 inches of precipitation, there are a variety of habitats for plants and animals.

Although life is often hard to find here, more than 1,000 plant species live in Death Valley National Park, including 13 species of cactus and 23 endemic species that are unique to this area. If you're lucky enough to visit in a wetter-than-normal spring, you might see blooming wildflowers paint entire slopes with color. Living among these plants are 51 species of mammals, 307 species of birds, 36 reptiles, 3 species of amphibians, and 5 species of fish. At lower elevations, where summer temperatures average well above 100°F, life may be nonexistent, or simply hiding. In cool canyons, near water and high in the mountains, life is more abundant.

Scattered throughout the park are also remnants of early pioneer history, mostly in the form of abandoned mines and ghost towns. Every rusting piece of metal and sun-baked piece of wood is part of this history—leave everything you find so others may enjoy them too.

Herbert Hoover first designated Death Valley National Monument in 1933. In 1994, Congress expanded the acreage, designated it a national park, and protected 95 percent of it as wilderness. Please follow Leave No Trace principles when camping, hiking, and exploring Death Valley.

This book includes favorite Death Valley destinations on the eastern portion of the park, accessible in a day trip from Las Vegas. I hope you will return soon to explore more thoroughly. If you're new to exploring deserts, please turn to page 20 to learn about safe desert hiking.

If you want to see Death Valley in only one day (though I recommend spending more time there), you can do the park in a loop. Drive north from Las Vegas on Highway 95, turn left (west) and enter the park via Beatty or Scotty's Junction, drive south through Death Valley, then exit east via Furnace Wells and Death Valley Junction. From there, it's two hours back to Vegas, via Pahrump.

Looking to Las Vegas from Red Rock's Calico Hills

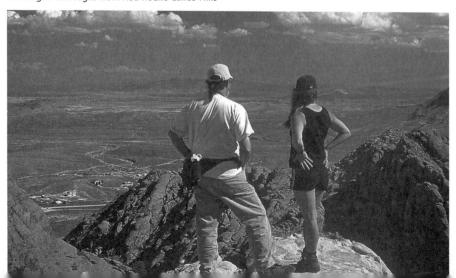

trip 1 Red Rocks: Sandstone Quarry to Calico Tanks

Distance	2.5 miles, out-and-back
Hiking Time	2 hours
Elevation	+/-580 feet
Difficulty	Moderate
Trail Use	Leashed dogs, good for kids
Best Times	Cool to warm
Agency	Bureau of Land Management, Red Rock Canyon National Conservation Area at (702) 515-5350; www.blm.gov/nv/st/en/fo/lvfo/blm_programs/blm_special_areas/red_rock_nca.html
Recommended Maps	*Las Vegas* 1:100,000; *La Madre Mtn.* 7.5-minute
GPS Waypoints	Calico Tanks: 36.161° N, 115.438° W
Vehicle	Passenger car OK

HIGHLIGHTS This scurry over jumbled sandstone leads to a hidden water pocket and a great view of Las Vegas. Calico Tanks is a great trip for families or those wanting a relatively short introduction to Red Rock Canyon, because it combines elements of the prehistory, history, geology, beauty, and fun that make Red Rocks famous.

DIRECTIONS There are two ways to approach Red Rock Canyon from Las Vegas:

1. From the north end of the Strip, take West Charleston Blvd./Highway 159 west for 17 miles to the entrance for the Red Rock Canyon Visitor Center and the 13-Mile Scenic Drive on the right (north) side of the road.
2. From I-15 on the south end of Las Vegas, take Highway 160 west for roughly 10 miles to Highway 159/Blue Diamond Road. Turn right onto 159 and follow it for about 10 miles as it circles clockwise through the Red Rock Canyon (with the Red Rock cliffs to your left) to the visitor center/scenic drive entrance on the left (north). This route takes about 30 minutes. From the entrance, drive 2.5 miles to the Sandstone Quarry Trailhead on the right (north) side of the road.

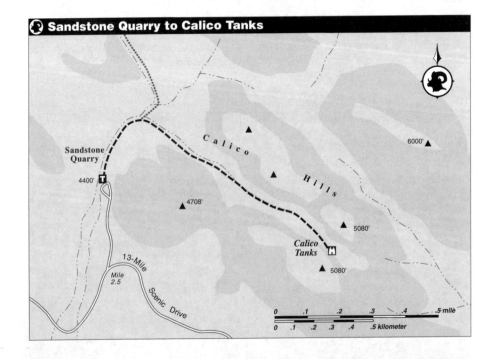

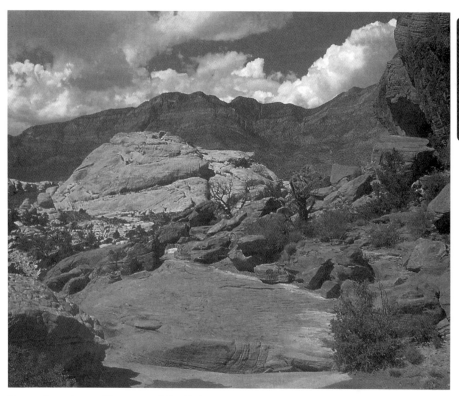

Contrasting colors and forms near Calico Tanks

FACILITIES/TRAILHEAD Restrooms are available at the trailhead and the visitor center at the entrance of the 13-Mile Scenic Drive. The only developed campground in the Red Rock Canyon is 2 miles east of the visitor center (1 mile south of West Charleston Blvd.) on Moenkopi Road. There are 71 individual sites and 5 group sites. Individual sites are first-come, first-served, but reservations are recommended for group sites. The campground has water, but no showers or shade. In the past, the campground has been closed during the summer because of low visitation and budget shortfalls. If you plan to visit in summer, call ahead to make sure it's open (702-515-5350). Backcountry camping in the Red Rock Canyon is allowed above 5000 feet, but permits are required (call 702-515-5050 for details). There are no developed campsites in the backcountry and fires are prohibited.

Hike north on the combination of Calico Tanks and Turtlehead Peak Trail from the parking lot, past Sandstone Quarry and an agave roasting pit farther up the trail on the left (north). Sandstone Quarry is the site where the Excelsior Stone Quarry mined sandstone blocks for construction between 1905 and 1912. The agave roasting pit is the remnant of an ancient native barbecue pit, where people roasted agave plants, as well as bighorn sheep, rabbit, and other game. The large circle of charred white rock around the pit shows that it was used for many years. Please preserve it by not walking on it.

Less than a mile after the quarry, when the trail forks, veer right (east) and follow the signs to Calico Tanks east over jumbled sandstone slabs to the largest of the tanks, a large pond in the rock. Calico Tanks are named for the water pockets in the sandstone. Throughout the desert Southwest, such pools are commonly referred to as *tinas* or *tinajas*, Spanish for "earthen jar" or "tank."

Animals love sandstone for its ability to hold water after storms, providing water sources in this otherwise parched landscape. Wildlife, such as bighorn sheep, depend on Calico Tanks' relatively constant water supply.

Even if you don't see bighorn on your visit here, take a close look at the water for another kind of wildlife. If the season and water are right, you should see myriad shrimp and other bugs swishing and flitting about. The shrimp are related to the famous sea monkeys (also known as brine shrimp), and they can survive long periods without water. Their eggs, like the seeds of plants, are able to survive for years of drought, waiting in the dust until life-giving rain falls. When water arrives, they sprout, mature, and breed in a matter of days, soon producing eggs that are once again ready to wait through dust and drought until water returns.

Although the going is, at times, unsteady on this trail, most hikers should be able to make it, especially with a helping hand or two. Once you have examined the pond, scramble to the far eastern side for a great view of Las Vegas Valley, and return the way you came.

trip 2 Red Rocks: Turtlehead Peak

Distance	4 miles, out-and-back
Hiking Time	2 to 4 hours
Elevation	+/-2000 feet
Difficulty	Difficult
Trail Use	Leashed dogs
Best Times	Cool to warm
Agency	Bureau of Land Management, Red Rock Canyon National Conservation Area at (702) 515-5350; www.blm.gov/nv/st/en/fo/lvfo/blm_programs/blm_special_areas/red_rock_nca.html
Recommended Maps	*Las Vegas* 1:100,000; *La Madre Mtn.* 7.5-minute
GPS Waypoints	Summit: 36.180° N, 115.446° W
Vehicle	Passenger car OK

HIGHLIGHTS This hike features sweeping views from a choice Red Rock Canyon peak. Although it's not an easy climb, Turtlehead Peak is one of the most accessible peaks listed in this book. If it's warm weather, you'll want to get an early start. If it's windy, bring a windbreaker to protect you at the summit.

DIRECTIONS There are two ways to approach Red Rock Canyon from Las Vegas:
1. From the north end of the Strip, take West Charleston Blvd./Highway 159 west for 17 miles to the entrance for the Red Rock Canyon Visitor Center and the 13-Mile Scenic Drive on the right (north) side of the road.
2. From I-15 on the south end of Las Vegas, take Highway 160 west for roughly 10 miles to Highway 159/Blue Diamond Road. Turn right onto 159 and follow it for about 10 miles as it circles clockwise through the Red Rock Canyon (with the Red Rock cliffs to your left) to the visitor center/scenic drive entrance on the left (north). This route takes about 30 minutes. From the entrance, drive 2.5 miles to the Sandstone Quarry Trailhead on the right (north) side of the road.

FACILITIES/TRAILHEAD Restrooms are available at the trailhead and the visitor center at the entrance of the 13-Mile Scenic Drive. The only developed campground in the Red Rock Canyon is 2 miles east of the visitor center (1 mile south of West Charleston Blvd.) on Moenkopi Road. There are 71 individual sites and 5 group sites. Individual sites are first-come, first-served, but reservations are recommended for group sites. The campground has water, but no showers or shade. In the past, the campground has been closed during the summer because of low visitation and budget short-

Turtlehead Peak

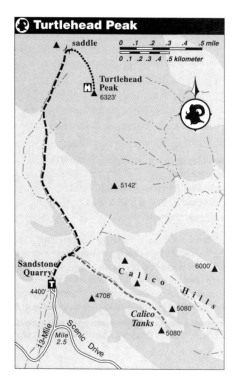

falls. If you plan to visit in summer, call ahead to make sure it's open (702-515-5350). Backcountry camping in the Red Rock Canyon is allowed above 5000 feet, but permits are required (call 702-515-5050 for details). There are no developed campsites in the backcountry and fires are prohibited. There is no water available on this hike, so bring all you'll need (1 gallon per person, per day; more in summer).

Hike north on the combination Calico Tanks and Turtlehead Peak Trail from the parking lot, past Sandstone Quarry, an agave roasting pit on the left (west) side of the trail, and the fork to Calico Tanks. Take the left fork, following the Turtlehead Peak Trail north up the drainage to the saddle to the left (west) of Turtlehead Peak.

There is not a developed main trail up the steep drainage west of the peak, but you can follow a series of use trails weaving back and forth. Follow the one heading toward the saddle and try not to trample plants or cause undue erosion. Once on the saddle, turn right (east) and climb the sloping sheets of limestone to the peak.

At the top, you'll be treated to one of the best views anyone could wish for—a sweeping clockwise panorama across the Red Rock escarpment to the banded white cliffs of La Madre Mountain and around to Las Vegas. On the back (north) side of Turtlehead Peak sits Brownstone Canyon with La Madre Mountain rising majestically farther north.

Return the way you came.

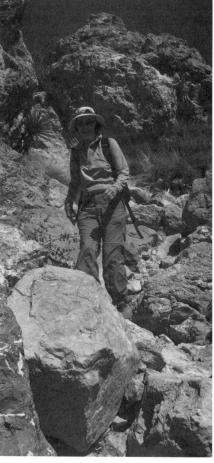

Hiking down Turtlehead Peak

trip 3 Red Rocks: Brownstone Canyon

Distance	5 miles, out-and-back
Hiking Time	4 to 8 hours
Elevation	+/-2400 feet
Difficulty	Most difficult
Trail Use	Leashed dogs, backpacking option
Best Times	Cool to warm
Agency	Bureau of Land Management, Red Rock Canyon National Conservation Area at (702) 515-5350; www.blm.gov/nv/st/en/fo/lvfo/blm_programs/blm_special_areas/red_rock_nca.html
Recommended Maps	*Las Vegas* 1:100,000; *La Madre Mtn.* 7.5-minute
GPS Waypoint	Top of the one of main formations: 36.112° N, 115.261° W
Vehicle	High-clearance or 4WD vehicle recommended

HIGHLIGHTS This hike takes you to a quiet corner of Red Rock Canyon National Conservation Area to a place of exquisite beauty, solitude, and mystery. It also takes you away from development and crowds—a perfect destination for a challenging dayhike or backpack. Brownstone Canyon is part of the 47,000-acre La Madre Wilderness Area and the Red Rock Canyon National Conservation Area.

Short, moderately easy hiking into Brownstone Canyon is, for the time being, impossible, because a subdivision has blocked the road leading to Brownstone's eastern trailhead (call Summerlin and urge them to provide public access to your public lands). What we have all lost in easy access, fit hikers have gained by the beauty of this alternate route—up and over the saddle west of Turtlehead Peak.

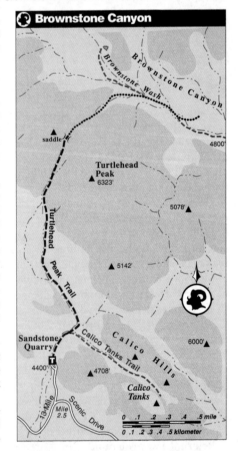

DIRECTIONS There are two ways to approach Red Rock Canyon from Las Vegas:

1. From the north end of the Strip, take West Charleston Blvd./Highway 159 west for 17 miles to the entrance for the Red Rock Canyon Visitor Center and the 13-Mile Scenic Drive on the right (north) side of the road.

2. From I-15 on the south end of Las Vegas, take Highway 160 west for roughly 10 miles to Highway 159/Blue Diamond Road. Turn right onto 159 and follow it for about 10 miles as it circles clockwise through the Red Rock Canyon (with the Red Rock cliffs to your left) to the visitor center/scenic drive entrance on the left (north). This route takes about 30 minutes. From the entrance, drive 2.5 miles to the Sandstone Quarry Trailhead on the right (north) side of the road.

FACILITIES/TRAILHEAD Restrooms are available at the trailhead and the visitor center at the entrance of the 13-Mile Scenic Drive. The only developed campground in the Red Rock Canyon is 2 miles east of the visitor center (1 mile south of West Charleston Blvd.) on Moenkopi Road. There are 71 individual sites and 5 group sites. Individual sites are first-come,

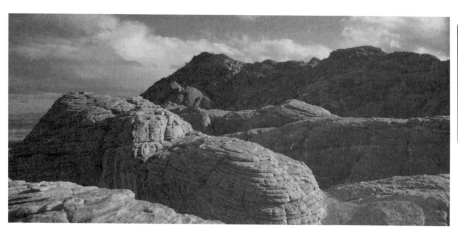

Some of the many sandstone formations in Brownstone Canyon

first-served, but reservations are recommended for group sites. The campground has water, but no showers or shade. In the past, the campground has been closed during the summer because of low visitation and budget shortfalls. If you plan to visit in summer, call ahead to make sure it's open (702-515-5350). Backcountry camping in the Red Rock Canyon is allowed above 5000 feet, but permits are required (call 702-515-5050 for details). There are no developed campsites in the backcountry and fires are prohibited. There is no water available on this hike, so bring all you'll need (1 gallon per person per day; more in summer).

Hike north on the combination Calico Tanks and Turtlehead Peak Trail from the parking lot, past Sandstone Quarry, an agave roasting pit on the left (west) side of the trail, and the fork to Calico Tanks. Take the left fork, following the Turtlehead Peak Trail north up the drainage to the saddle to the left (west) of Turtlehead Peak.

There is not a developed main trail up the steep drainage west of the peak, but you can follow a series of use trails weaving back and forth. Follow the one heading toward the saddle and try not to trample plants or cause undue erosion. For a side trip, turn right (east) and climb the sloping sheets of limestone to Turtlehead Peak—the view is worth it, if your legs are up for it.

To hike into Browstone Canyon, hike down the north side of the saddle, following the prominent drainage as it heads northeast down into Brownstone. Once in Brownstone, let your curiosity and inspiration guide you to the various rock formations. There are many perfect spots to picnic, and many shelters and overhangs under which you can escape the sun.

Turtlehead Peak hides Brownstone Canyon from the crowds and development of the Red Rock Canyon Visitor Center and scenic drive. The sheer limestone cliffs of La Madre Mountain to the northwest and north make a stunning backdrop, rising 3000 vertical feet above the valley.

Ancient people lived throughout what is now Red Rock Canyon National Conservation Area for thousands of years, leaving behind agave roasting pits and other artifacts, which help us understand these people. These artifacts are fragile, irreplaceable, and protected by state and federal laws. Please do not walk on agave roasting pits or touch any artifacts. Leave them as you find them so others may enjoy them too.

The soils, rocks, and plants of Brownstone Canyon are also fragile. Please travel in washes or over hard stone as much as possible.

Return the way you came.

trip 4 Red Rocks: Keystone Thrust Trail

Distance	2.2 miles, out-and-back
Hiking Time	1 hour
Elevation	+/-460 feet
Difficulty	Moderate
Trail Use	Leashed dogs, good for kids
Best Times	Cold to warm
Agency	Red Rock Canyon National Conservation Area at (702) 515-5350; www.blm.gov/nv/st/en/fo/lvfo/blm_programs/blm_special_areas/red_rock_nca.html
Recommended Maps	*La Madre Mtn.* 7.5-minute; free maps available at entrance station
GPS Waypoints	Trailhead: 36.173° N, 115.476° W
Vehicle	Passenger car OK

HIGHLIGHTS Hike along this trail to see the intersection of great and colorful geologic eras. The Keystone Thrust Trail is part of the La Madre Mountain Wilderness Area, designated by Congress in 2002.

DIRECTIONS There are two ways to approach Red Rock Canyon from Las Vegas:

1. From the north end of the Strip, take West Charleston Blvd./Highway 159 west for 17 miles to the entrance for the Red Rock Canyon Visitor Center and the 13-Mile Scenic Drive on the right (north) side of the road.

2. From I-15 on the south end of Las Vegas, take Highway 160 west for roughly 10 miles to Highway 159/Blue Diamond Road. Turn right onto 159 and follow it for about 10 miles as it circles clockwise through the Red Rock Canyon (with the Red Rock cliffs to your left) to the visitor center/scenic drive entrance on the left (north). This route takes about 30 minutes. At mile 6 in the 13-Mile Scenic Drive, turn right (north) and follow the signed, unpaved road less than a mile to the White Rock Trailhead, which leads to the Keystone Thrust Trail.

FACILITIES/TRAILHEAD Restrooms are available at the trailhead and the visitor center at the entrance of the 13-Mile Scenic Drive. The only developed campground in the Red Rock Canyon is 2 miles east of the visitor center (1 mile south of West Charleston Blvd.) on Moenkopi Road. There are 71 individual sites and 5 group sites. Individual sites are first-come, first-served, but reservations are recommended for group sites. The campground has water, but no showers or shade. In the past, the campground has been closed during the summer because of low visitation and budget shortfalls. If you plan to visit in summer, call ahead to make sure it's open (702-515-5350). Backcountry camping in the Red Rock Canyon is allowed above 5000 feet, but permits are required (call 702-515-5050 for details). There are no developed campsites in the backcountry and fires are prohibited.

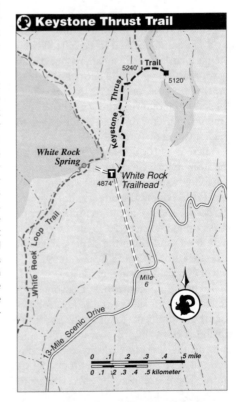

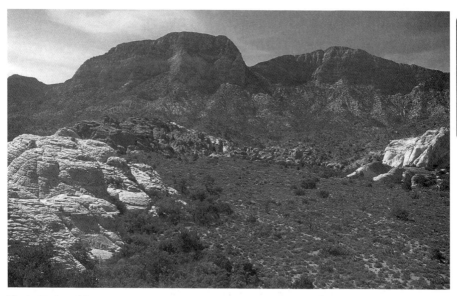

The La Madre Wilderness along the Keystone Thrust Trail

At the White Rock Trailhead, hike north from the parking lot to the end of the road, and then follow the Keystone Thrust Trail north up the wash. After a few minutes, follow the trail and a sign to Keystone Thrust, up a short flight of stairs, which climb right (east) out of the wash, then continue north to the crest of a small ridge and the high point of the trail.

A few yards after climbing out of the wash, look to the left and right of the trail for two agave roasting pits, which were basically barbecue pits used by Southern Paiute people as far back as 900 years ago. Please respect them from a distance.

At its high point, the trail veers to the east, drops into, and ends in a shallow canyon of pinkish sandstone, which is the Keystone Thrust. Here you will see that, even when it comes to rocks, what goes around, comes around. About 180 million years ago, during the age of the dinosaurs, a vast desert of sand dunes covered this region, stretching to what is now the Colorado Plateau. Deep underneath these sands are limestone layers created by sediments that settled in shallow seas about 500 million years ago.

Between 60 million and 65 million years ago, the Pacific and North American continental plates got into a shoving match. The conflict pushed up the Sierra Nevada to the west. The same forces pushed the deep limestone layers up and over the sand dunes in what is now Red Rock Canyon. Those limestone layers tower high above Red Rock Canyon to the north in La Madre Mountain.

Trapped by the limestone, minerals in the sand cemented the limestone together into sandstone. Since then, millions of years of ice, water, and wind have eroded the limestone away in some places, exposing the sandstone. The sandstone that was once on top is now back again. Erosion is still at work, sculpting the rocks and mountains of Red Rock Canyon into ever-changing forms.

Once you have admired these geologic formations, retrace your steps to return to the parking lot. From there, you can take a short side trip west and downhill a few hundred yards to White Rock Spring. A bench in the shade of a tree is a perfect place to enjoy the soothing sound of the trickling spring while looking out over the valley.

trip 5 Red Rocks: Children's Discovery & Lost Creek Trails

Distance	1.5 miles, loop
Hiking Time	30 minutes to 1 hour
Elevation	+/-300 feet
Difficulty	Easy to moderate
Trail Use	Leashed dogs, good for kids
Best Times	Cool to hot
Agency	Bureau of Land Management, Red Rock Canyon National Conservation Area at (702) 515-5350; www.blm.gov/nv/st/en/fo/lvfo/blm_programs/blm_special_areas/red_rock_nca.html
Recommended Maps	*Las Vegas* 1:100,000; *La Madre Mtn.* 7.5-minute
GPS Waypoints	Trailhead: 36.157° N; 115.493° W
Vehicle	Passenger car OK

HIGHLIGHTS This self-guided interpretive trail introduces kids of all ages to the many different features of the Mojave Desert at Red Rock Canyon, including petroglyphs, lessons of desert life, towering views, and a hidden waterfall in the canyon.

DIRECTIONS There are two ways to approach Red Rock Canyon from Las Vegas:

1. From the north end of the Strip, take West Charleston Blvd./Highway 159 west for 17 miles to the entrance for the Red Rock Canyon Visitor Center and the 13-Mile Scenic Drive on the right (north) side of the road.

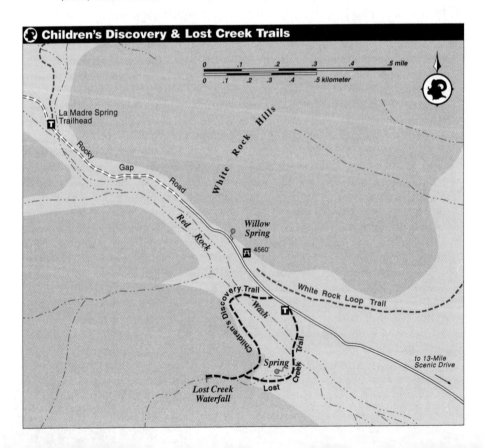

2. From I-15 on the south end of Las Vegas, take Highway 160 west for roughly 10 miles to Highway 159/Blue Diamond Road. Turn right onto 159 and follow it for about 10 miles as it circles clockwise through the Red Rock Canyon (with the Red Rock cliffs to your left) to the visitor center/scenic drive entrance on the left (north). This route takes about 30 minutes. At 7.5 miles on the scenic loop, turn right (west) into the Willow Spring Picnic Area.

FACILITIES/TRAILHEAD Restrooms are available at the trailhead and the visitor center at the entrance of the 13-Mile Scenic Drive. The only developed campground in the Red Rock Canyon is 2 miles east of the visitor center (1 mile south of West Charleston Blvd.) on Moenkopi Road. There are 71 individual sites and 5 group sites. Individual sites are first-come, first-served, but reservations are recommended for group sites. The campground has water, but no showers or shade. In the past, the campground has been closed during the summer because of low visitation and budget shortfalls. If you plan to visit in summer, call ahead to make sure it's open (702-515-5350). Backcountry camping in the Red Rock Canyon is allowed above 5000 feet, but permits are required (call 702-515-5050 for details). There are no developed campsites in the backcountry and fires are prohibited.

From the northwest corner of the parking area, follow the Children's Discovery Trail west, across the wash, as it circles south along the slope, past the mouth of Lost Creek Canyon (where a side trail leads to the Lost Creek Waterfall), then back to the car. The Lost Creek Trail also leaves from the parking lot and heads more directly toward the canyon mouth. Luckily, both trails lead

Cascade and shade at Lost Creek

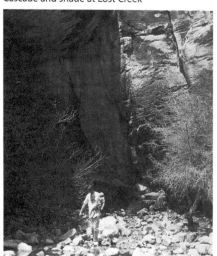

to the same place. Along the way, you'll have opportunities to learn about the different plants and animals of the desert, see rock shelters and rock art (petroglyphs), and enjoy views of the towering cliffs above.

After about a half mile, the Children's Discovery Trail meets the Lost Creek Trail, which leads into the Lost Creek box canyon. In early spring and after rain, a waterfall at the back of this box canyon fills the air with splashes to cool off the hottest days. Water is always a refreshing sight in the desert, and this is a great place to see it.

From the parking area, another optional trail leads a half mile west to an ancient agave roasting pit, once used by Paiute Indians to roast food such as agave and pine nuts and game such as rabbit and bighorn sheep.

The Children's Discovery Trail is a popular destination for school field trips, so plan to go early to avoid these crowds. Early in the day, you'll also enjoy cool temperatures and the wonderful song of canyon wrens singing from the cliffs. Kids, please remind your parents not to trample the sensitive plants in the area. The huge number of visitors to this trail makes it important for everyone to stay on the trail.

trip 6 Red Rocks: La Madre Spring & White Rock Loop

Distance	2.5 miles, out-and-back; 6.5 miles, loop
Hiking Time	2 to 4 hours
Elevation	+/-900 feet (out-and-back to spring); +/-1090 feet (loop)
Difficulty	Moderate
Trail Use	Leashed dogs, good for kids
Best Times	Cold to warm
Agency	Bureau of Land Management, Red Rock Canyon National Conservation Area at (702) 515-5350; www.blm.gov/nv/st/en/fo/lvfo/blm_programs/blm_special_areas/red_rock_nca.html
Recommended Maps	*Las Vegas* 1:100,000; *La Madre Mtn.* 7.5-minute
GPS Waypoints	La Madre Spring Pond: 36.180° N, 115.502° W
Vehicle	Passenger car OK (to Willow Spring Picnic Area); high-clearance or 4WD vehicle (to La Madre Spring Trailhead)

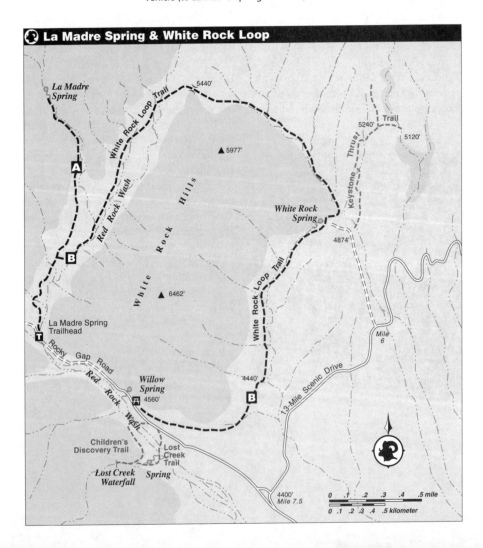

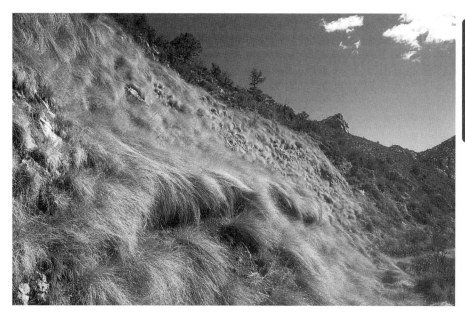

Life springs forth at La Madre Spring.

HIGHLIGHTS This loop takes you through a secluded pocket of life, around the rugged sandstone of Red Rock Canyon to La Madre Spring, where the water splashes life on this otherwise desert landscape. La Madre Spring is in the 47,000-acre La Madre Mountain Wilderness Area, designated by Congress in 2002.

DIRECTIONS There are two ways to approach Red Rock Canyon from Las Vegas:

1. From the north end of the Strip, take West Charleston Blvd./Highway 159 west for 17 miles to the entrance for the Red Rock Canyon Visitor Center and the 13-Mile Scenic Drive on the right (north) side of the road.
2. From I-15 on the south end of Las Vegas, take Highway 160 west for roughly 10 miles to Highway 159/Blue Diamond Road. Turn right onto 159 and follow it for about 10 miles as it circles clockwise through the Red Rock Canyon (with the Red Rock cliffs to your left) to the visitor center/scenic drive entrance on the left (north). This route takes about 30 minutes. Take the scenic loop and after 7.5 miles, turn right (west) into the Willow Spring Picnic Area. High-clearance vehicles can drive a half mile farther on the rough, unpaved Rocky Gap Road to the La Madre Spring Trailhead.

FACILITIES/TRAILHEAD Restrooms are available at the trailhead and the visitor center at the entrance of the 13-Mile Scenic Drive. The only developed campground in the Red Rock Canyon is 2 miles east of the visitor center (1 mile south of West Charleston Blvd.) on Moenkopi Road. There are 71 individual sites and five group sites. Individual sites are first-come, first-served, but reservations are recommended for group sites. The campground has water, but no showers or shade. In the past, the campground has been closed during the summer because of low visitation and budget shortfalls. If you plan to visit in summer, call ahead to make sure it's open (702-515-5350). Backcountry camping in the Red Rock Canyon is allowed above 5000 feet, but permits are required (call 702-515-5050 for details). There are no developed campsites in the backcountry and fires are prohibited.

From the paved parking area, hike west up Rocky Gap Road for a half mile to the La Madre Spring Trailhead, then follow the trail (an old access road) northeast as it climbs the gentle slope through blackbrush scrub, pinyon pine, and juniper trees. The sculpted sandstone of White Rock Hills rises to the south of the trail. The banded limestone cliffs of La Madre Mountain rise even higher to the north.

After a half mile, the trail forks, and you have two options:

A. For the shorter, out-and-back hike, take the left (north) fork for another mile, past old foundations to the right (south) side of the trail, and to the La Madre Spring drainage. The trail follows the drainage upstream to a small reservoir, then gets smaller and steeper as it climbs the drainage for another half mile to the spring.

La Madre Spring is a perfect example of what a little water can do to liven up a desert landscape. Even without the spring, plants at this higher altitude are healthy and abundant (relative to lower, drier valleys) thanks to the higher precipitation levels at this elevation. But when open water comes into the scene, life takes a quantum leap toward lush. Tall reeds, grasses, and other riparian plants choke the drainage, and water cascades happily into a series of pools, where birds and other wildlife come from miles to enjoy the water. When people are few, bighorn sheep will descend from the higher slopes to drink their fill.

Retrace your steps to the trailhead.

B. For the White Hills Loop, take the right fork, which heads east and runs clockwise around the rugged White Rock Hills, offering views of La Madre Mountain, Turtlehead Peak, the Calico Hills, and the Red Rock escarpment. The hike takes you past White Rock Spring and back to the Willow Spring Picnic Area.

trip 7 Red Rocks: North Peak

Distance	2.6 miles, out-and-back
Hiking Time	1 to 2 hours
Elevation	+/-770 feet
Difficulty	Moderate
Trail Use	Leashed dogs
Best Times	Cool to hot
Agency	Bureau of Land Management, Red Rock Canyon National Conservation Area at (702) 515-5350; www.blm.gov/nv/st/en/fo/lvfo/blm_programs/blm_special_areas/red_rock_nca.html
Recommended Maps	*Las Vegas* 1:100,000; *La Madre Mtn.* and *La Madre Spring* 7.5-minute
GPS Waypoints	North Peak: 36.134° N, 115.517° W
Vehicle	High-clearance or 4WD vehicle recommended

HIGHLIGHTS Rough drive aside, the summit of North Peak offers the best view in Red Rock Canyon for the least amount of effort. It also offers an interesting tour of the Keystone Thrust, one of the primary geologic features that makes Red Rock Canyon so impressive. North Peak is part of the Rainbow Mountain Wilderness Area, designated by Congress in 2002.

DIRECTIONS There are two ways to approach Red Rock Canyon from Las Vegas:

1. From the north end of the Strip, take West Charleston Blvd./Highway 159 west for 17 miles to the entrance for the Red Rock Canyon Visitor Center and the 13-Mile Scenic Drive on the right (north) side of the road.
2. From I-15 on the south end of Las Vegas, take Highway 160 west for roughly 10 miles to Highway 159/Blue Diamond Road. Turn right onto 159 and follow it for about 10 miles as it circles clockwise through the Red Rock Canyon (with the Red Rock cliffs to your left) to the visitor center/scenic drive entrance on the left (north). This route takes about 30 minutes. Take the scenic loop and after 7.5 miles, turn right (west) into the Willow Spring Picnic Area. The trailhead for this hike is at the summit of Rocky Gap Road (also known as Red Rock Summit), 5 miles from Willow Spring Picnic Area. Look for a trail sign on the left (south) side of the road, as well as a rough parking area for about 10 vehicles. Although the scenic drive is paved and accessible to all vehicles, Rocky Gap Road is rough and rocky. Attempting to drive it in a low-clearance vehicle will damage your car. Also, do not attempt to continue west on Rocky Gap Road, as it gets even rougher.

North Peak

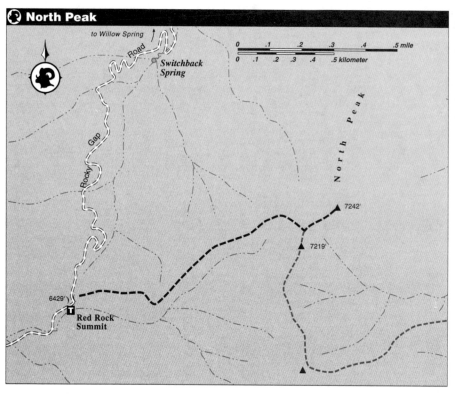

FACILITIES/TRAILHEAD The nearest restrooms are at the Willow Spring Picnic Area, which you pass on the way in, or at the visitor center at the entrance of the 13-Mile Scenic Drive. The only developed campground in the Red Rock Canyon is 2 miles east of the visitor center (1 mile south of West Charleston Blvd.) on Moenkopi Road. There are 71 individual sites and 5 group sites. Individual sites are first-come, first-served, but reservations are recommended for group sites. The campground has water, but no showers or shade. In the past, the campground has been closed during the summer because of low visitation and budget shortfalls. If you plan to visit in summer, call ahead to make sure it's open (702-515-5350). Backcountry camping in the Red Rock Canyon is allowed above 5000 feet, but permits are required (call 702-515-5050 for details). There are no developed campsites in the backcountry and fires are prohibited.

From the car, follow the Bridge Mountain Trail east about 1 mile to the top of the ridge. This first mile of the trail climbs through pinyon pine and juniper trees on the relatively gentle and rolling western slope of the Spring Mountains, and there's little indication of the sudden geologic change and world-class view waiting at the summit.

At the trail junction, turn left (northeast) and continue to the summit, following the sign to North Peak. The summit is 500-million-year-old limestone, which sits on top of Aztec sandstone that is hundreds of millions of years younger. Usually, older rocks are found beneath younger ones, which were deposited later. But collisions between the North American and Pacific continental plates about 65 million years ago shuffled the deck here and pushed the older rocks up and over the younger ones.

After admiring this geologic anomaly, retrace your steps to return.

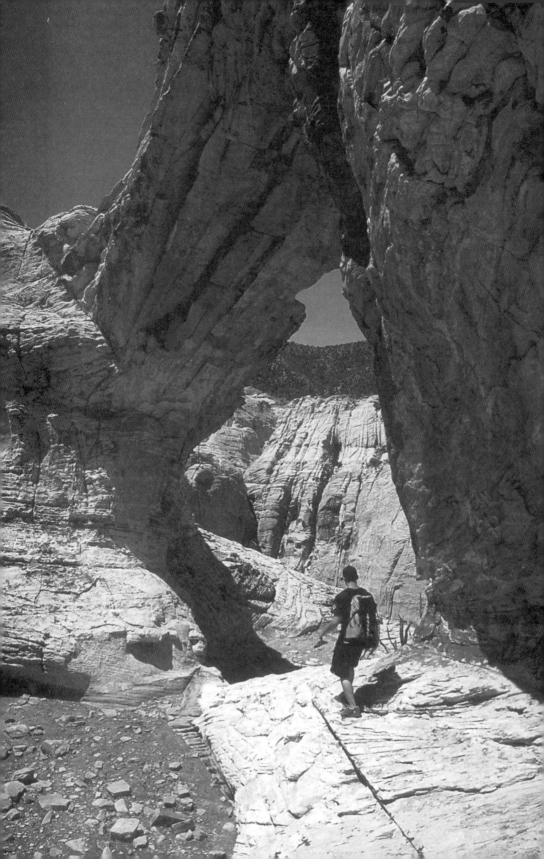

trip 8 # Red Rocks: Bridge Mountain

Distance	5 miles, out-and-back
Hiking Time	5 to 8 hours
Elevation	+/-3500 feet
Difficulty	Moderate (first 1.5 miles) to difficult (last mile)
Trail Use	Backpacking option
Best Times	Cool to hot
Agency	Bureau of Land Management, Red Rock Canyon National Conservation Area at (702) 515-5350; www.blm.gov/nv/st/en/fo/lvfo/blm_programs/blm_special_areas/red_rock_nca.html
Recommended Maps	*Las Vegas* 1:100,000; *Blue Diamond* and *Mountain Springs* 7.5-minute
GPS Waypoints	Bridge Summit: 36.131° N, 115.500° W
Vehicle	High-clearance or 4WD vehicle recommended

HIGHLIGHTS Bridge Mountain is one of the most difficult and memorable trips in this book. Reaching the peak requires climbing skills, agility, balance, and exposure to danger. But the adrenaline, sweeping views, and sense of accomplishment make the trouble worthwhile. Geological wonders and breathtaking views over Red Rock Canyon also abound on this difficult hike. Even if you don't bag the peak, the first 1.5 miles are well worth the hike for anyone who wants stunning views without the difficulty of the last mile to the summit. Bridge Mountain is part of the 25,000-acre Rainbow Mountain Wilderness Area, designated by Congress in 2002.

DIRECTIONS There are two ways to approach Red Rock Canyon from Las Vegas:

1. From the north end of the Strip, take West Charleston Blvd./Highway 159 west for 17 miles to the entrance for the Red Rock Canyon Visitor Center and the 13-Mile Scenic Drive on the right (north) side of the road.

2. From I-15 on the south end of Las Vegas, take Highway 160 west for roughly 10 miles to Highway 159/Blue Diamond Road. Turn right onto 159 and follow it for about 10 miles as it circles clockwise through the Red Rock Canyon (with the Red Rock cliffs to your left) to the visitor center/scenic drive entrance on the left (north). This route takes about 30 minutes. Take the scenic loop and after 7.5 miles, turn right (west) into the Willow Spring Picnic Area. The trailhead for this hike is at the summit of Rocky Gap Road (also known as Red Rock Summit), 5 miles from Willow Spring Picnic Area. Look for a trail sign on the left (south) side of the road, as well as a rough parking area for about 10 vehicles. Although the scenic drive is paved and accessible to all vehicles, Rocky Gap Road is rough and rocky. Attempting to drive it in a low-clearance vehicle will damage your car. Also, do not attempt to continue west on Rocky Gap Road, as it gets even rougher.

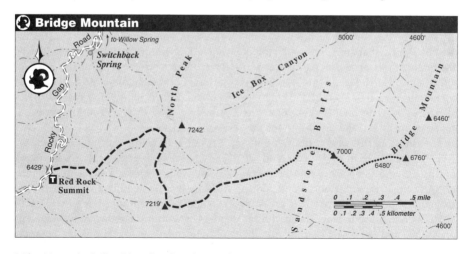

Bridge Mountain thrills with sculpted sandstone, dizzying heights, and world-class views.

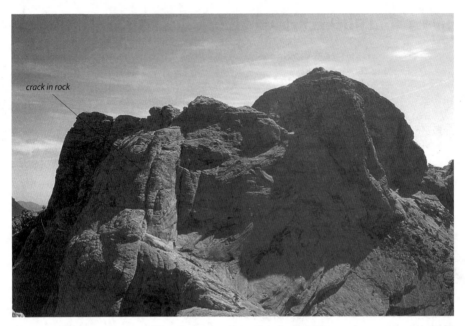
crack in rock

The route up Bridge Mountain follows the crack in the rock indicated above.

FACILITIES/TRAILHEAD The nearest restrooms are at the Willow Spring Picnic Area, which you pass on the way in, or at the visitor center at the entrance of the 13-Mile Scenic Drive. The only developed campground in the Red Rock Canyon is 2 miles east of the visitor center (1 mile south of West Charleston Blvd.) on Moenkopi Road. There are 71 individual sites and 5 group sites. Individual sites are first-come, first-served, but reservations are recommended for group sites. The campground has water, but no showers or shade. In the past, the campground has been closed during the summer because of low visitation and budget shortfalls. If you plan to visit in summer, call ahead to make sure it's open (702-515-5350). Backcountry camping in the Red Rock Canyon is allowed above 5000 feet, but permits are required (call 702-515-5050 for details). There are no developed campsites in the backcountry and fires are prohibited.

From the car, follow the Bridge Mountain Trail east about 1 mile to the top of the ridge. At the top, a trail sign points you either left to North Peak, or right to Bridge Mountain. Turn right (south) and continue along the ridge for another half mile. The trail then turns east and drops into the theater of sandstone just west of Bridge Mountain. Here, cliffs seem to drop away to the north, east, and south. The sandstone walls of North Peak rise to the north, and dome-shaped Bridge Mountain rises to the east.

Notice how the soil changes from whitish-gray to red and tan as you descend into the theater of sandstone (it's easy to miss while you're looking out at the dramatic views). This is the Keystone Thrust, the result of tectonic movement about 65 million years ago that pushed 500-million-year-old limestone up and over 150-million-year-old Aztec sandstone.

Until this point, the trail is moderate and accessible by most relatively fit hikers. If you're not interested or able to make the final push to the summit, the 3-mile round-trip hike to the sandstone theater west of the peak is rewarding in its own right and highly recommended. Beyond this point, the route becomes much more difficult, requiring both climbing and route-finding skills. Capable climbers might want to rope up with novice climbers to give them psychological support for the approaching climb.

From this point, your route takes you over open sandstone, where there is no trail. To stay on route, look for cairns and trail markers that look like two vertical parallel lines (like this: ||) spray-painted on the rock. On the northern slope of the sandstone theater (to your left as you're facing Bridge Mountain), look for a prominent water pool, or tinaja, in the sandstone, with ponderosa pine trees growing in it. Unlike limestone, sandstone holds water very well, which is why there are so many tinajas (some say tenayas) scattered throughout Red Rock Canyon. In the sometimes harsh climate of the Mojave Desert, these water pools mean survival to wildlife and plants. Although they might look inviting, please resist swimming in them. If only a few people jump in to cool off on a hot day, natural oils, insect repellent, and sunscreen can quickly accumulate in the water and render it poisonous to the animals that need it to survive.

From this tree-lined tinaja, head southeast and down 300 vertical feet to the saddle west of Bridge Mountain. Look for trail markers and for the easiest route down. Occasionally you will descend cracks in the rock and sometimes you will climb over open rock faces. When in doubt, scout around for the best route and for trail markers heading in the general direction of Bridge Mountain.

Once you reach the Bridge Mountain side (east side) of the sandstone saddle, look for a prominent crack heading straight up the rock for about 100 vertical feet. From the west side of the saddle, this route looks dangerous and difficult. Once you're there, however, it's not as difficult or dangerous as it appeared.

If climbing the crack becomes too difficult, you might climb the open rock to your right (south), where many foot- and handholds make climbing easier. The open rock, however, is more exposed and therefore more dangerous if you fall.

At the shelf on top of the crack, turn left (north) for a few steps, where a trail marker points out the best route to climb another 40 vertical feet to the next shelf. At that top, turn left (north) again, where you encounter a very beautiful bridge. Walk under the bridge, then climb the rock to the left (east). At the top, you have two choices:

1. Explore the Hidden Forest immediately to the south, walk east across the open stone a couple hundred yards, to where the rock slopes down and enters the forest in a large tinaja.

2. Continue to the summit of Bridge Mountain, veer right (southwest) and descend across the open stone to the low saddle, or lip, on the west side of the Hidden Forest. (The mountain rises to the south of the Hidden Forest.) From the lip, follow the rock layers and cairns diagonally (southeast) about a quarter mile up to the summit.

From either destination, carefully retrace your steps to return.

trip 9 Red Rocks: Ice Box Canyon

Distance	2.6 miles, out-and-back
Hiking Time	2 to 3 hours
Elevation	+/-600 feet
Difficulty	Moderate
Trail Use	Leashed dogs, good for kids
Best Times	Cold to hot
Agency	Bureau of Land Management, Red Rock Canyon National Conservation Area at (702) 515-5350; www.blm.gov/nv/st/en/fo/lvfo/blm_programs/blm_special_areas/red_rock_nca.html
Recommended Maps	*La Madre Mtn.* 7.5-minute; free map available at Red Rock National Conservation Area entrance station
GPS Waypoints	Waterfall: 36.143° N, 115.498° W
Vehicle	Passenger car OK

HIGHLIGHTS As the name implies, Ice Box Canyon is a good hike for a hot day. The trail takes you through a cool, shady box canyon with seasonal waterfalls in the heart of Red Rock National Conservation Area. The narrow canyon rarely sees sunlight, and the cool water and air pouring down from the mountains keep it significantly cooler than the open desert. But you will have to cross the open desert for a mile to get there, so it's a good idea to leave early to beat the heat. Ice Box Canyon is part of the Rainbow Mountain Wilderness Area, designated by Congress in 2002 to protect its natural beauty for generations to come.

DIRECTIONS There are two ways to approach Red Rock Canyon from Las Vegas:
1. From the north end of the Strip, take West Charleston Blvd./Highway 159 west for 17 miles to the entrance for the Red Rock Canyon Visitor Center and the 13-Mile Scenic Drive on the right (north) side of the road.

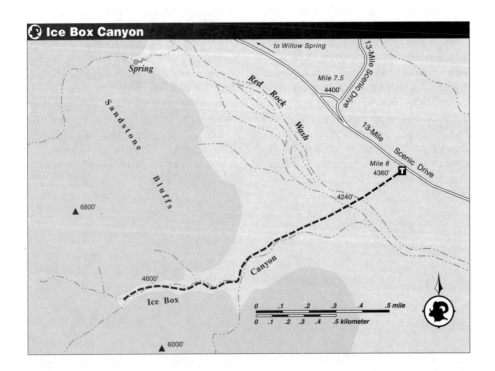

2. From I-15 on the south end of Las Vegas, take Highway 160 west for roughly 10 miles to Highway 159/Blue Diamond Road. Turn right onto 159 and follow it for about 10 miles as it circles clockwise through the Red Rock Canyon (with the Red Rock cliffs to your left) to the visitor center/scenic drive entrance on the left (north). This route takes about 30 minutes. Take the scenic loop and after 8 miles, turn right (west) into the parking area for the Ice Box Canyon Trailhead.

FACILITIES/TRAILHEAD The nearest restrooms are at the Willow Spring Picnic Area, which is a half mile before the turnoff to Ice Box Canyon, or at the visitor center at the entrance of the 13-Mile Scenic Drive. The only developed campground in the Red Rock Canyon is 2 miles east of the visitor center (1 mile south of West Charleston Blvd.) on Moenkopi Road. There are 71 individual sites and 5 group sites. Individual sites are first-come, first-served, but reservations are recommended for group sites. The campground has water, but no showers or shade. In the past, the campground has been closed during the summer because of low visitation and budget shortfalls. If you plan to visit in summer, call ahead to make sure it's open (702-515-5350). Backcountry camping in the Red Rock Canyon is allowed above 5000 feet, but permits are required (call 702-515-5050 for details). There are no developed campsites in the backcountry and fires are prohibited.

From the parking area, the trail heads west across the open desert and into the canyon. Once in the canyon, travel becomes more difficult, and scrambling is necessary to follow the wash to the pools and falls. Rocks may be slippery and dangerous when wet. Please be careful.

The trail ends in a box canyon, where waterfalls cascade down the steep rock in spring and after rain. The ponderosa pine forest at the canyon mouth survives here because of the cool air and water of Pine Creek. Bring your own water, or plan to treat or filter the water in the canyon, which might contain nasty bugs or disease.

After enjoying the cool shade and splashing water, retrace your steps to return.

trip 10 Red Rocks: Pine Creek Canyon

Distance	3 to 5 miles, out-and-back
Hiking Time	2 to 5 hours
Elevation	+/-600 feet
Difficulty	Moderate
Trail Use	Leashed dogs, good for kids
Best Times	Cold to warm (early morning or late afternoon in summer)
Agency	Bureau of Land Management, Red Rock Canyon National Conservation Area at (702) 515-5350; www.blm.gov/nv/st/en/fo/lvfo/blm_programs/blm_special_areas/red_rock_nca.html
Recommended Maps	*Blue Diamond* 7.5-minute; free maps available at Red Rock National Conservation Area entrance station
GPS Waypoints	Wilson Homestead: 36.123° N, 115.483° W
Vehicle	Passenger car OK

HIGHLIGHTS Pine Creek Canyon offers some of the best of the Red Rock Canyon National Conservation Area—beautiful and diverse plant communities nestled at the bottom of monolithic canyon walls. The ponderosa pine forest at the mouth of the canyon is a remnant from the last ice age, but it survives here thanks to the cool air and water flowing down Pine Creek Canyon. Pine Creek Canyon is part of the Rainbow Mountain Wilderness Area, designated by Congress in 2002 to protect its natural beauty for generations to come.

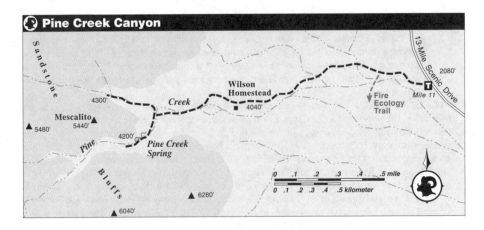

DIRECTIONS There are two ways to approach Red Rock Canyon from Las Vegas:

1. From the north end of the Strip, take West Charleston Blvd./Highway 159 west for 17 miles to the entrance for the Red Rock Canyon Visitor Center and the 13-Mile Scenic Drive on the right (north) side of the road.

2. From I-15 on the south end of Las Vegas, take Highway 160 west for roughly 10 miles to Highway 159/Blue Diamond Road. Turn right onto 159 and follow it for about 10 miles as it circles clockwise through the Red Rock Canyon (with the Red Rock cliffs to your left) to the visitor center/scenic drive entrance on the left (north). This route takes about 30 minutes. Take the scenic loop and after 11 miles, turn right (west) into the parking area for the Pine Creek Trailhead.

FACILITIES/TRAILHEAD Restrooms are available at the trailhead and the visitor center at the entrance of the 13-Mile Scenic Drive. The only developed campground in the Red Rock Canyon is 2 miles east of the visitor center (1 mile south of West Charleston Blvd.) on Moenkopi Road. There are 71 individual sites and 5 group sites. Individual sites are first-come, first-served, but reservations are recommended for group sites. The campground has water, but no showers or shade. In the past, the campground has been closed during the summer because of low visitation and budget shortfalls. If you plan to visit in summer, call ahead to make sure it's open (702-515-5350). Backcountry camping in the Red Rock Canyon is allowed above 5000 feet, but permits are required (call 702-515-5050 for details). There are no developed campsites in the backcountry and fires are prohibited.

From the parking area, the trail drops south into the wash, then veers west to follow Pine Creek toward the canyon.

After about a quarter mile, you pass the start of the Fire Ecology Trail on the left (south). This mile-long loop through an area burned by the BLM is a nice detour, especially if you enjoy level hiking through varied plant life. Plant species that thrive along the Pine Creek Trail include blackbrush, yucca, cholla, prickly pear cactus, bitterbrush, scrub oak, willow, sagebrush, manzanita, yerba buena, silk tassel, pinyon pine, and juniper, not to mention the myr-

iad wildflowers that bloom in spring—not bad for a desert.

Continuing west, the trail passes ponderosa pine trees and the remains of the house of Horace Wilson, who homesteaded the canyon in the 1920s. Wilson built a house among these pines, with glorious Pine Creek Canyon as his backyard. He abandoned the homestead in the 1930s and all that remain today are a few cement foundations.

After passing the homestead, the trail follows Pine Creek to the mouth of the canyon and the base of Mescalito, a large pyramid-shaped monolith separating the north and south forks of Pine Creek Canyon. Here, you'll see ponderosa pine trees towering over the mouth of the canyon. Ponderosas don't normally grow at this low elevation (about 4000 feet); they're more common above 5000 feet, where the air is cooler and precipitation is higher. But this forest is a remnant of the last ice age, 10,000 years ago, when Southern Nevada was cooler and wetter.

As you enter the canyon, the terrain gets more difficult, and numerous unofficial trails weave back and forth across the creek and up and down the slope. Sometimes, you might have to boulder-hop along the creek. Other times, large boulders or thick brush will force you to climb up the slopes above to continue. Luckily, it's difficult to get lost in these narrow canyons. When deciding which way to go, please choose to travel on durable surfaces and avoid trampling plants whenever possible.

As you hike, keep your eyes and ears open for rock climbers high on the cliffs above, which attract climbers from around the world. Please don't climb the cliffs without training, experience, and proper gear.

Less than a half mile later, the canyon forks. Veer left (southwest) to follow the main trail into the south fork of Pine Creek (to the left, south, of Mescalito). The farther you go, the more difficult travel gets, so go only as far as you're interested or able to travel.

It's possible to veer right at the canyon fork, to the north of Mescalito, but travel is very difficult and recommended only for agile rock-hoppers and scramblers. However, watery pools and shady grottos reward the adventurous.

Retrace your steps to return.

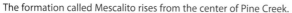

The formation called Mescalito rises from the center of Pine Creek.

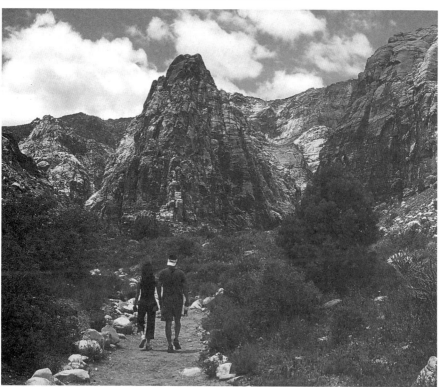

trip 11 Red Rocks: Oak Creek Canyon

Distance	2 to 3 miles, out-and-back
Hiking Time	2 to 3 hours
Elevation	+/-600 feet
Difficulty	Moderate
Trail Use	Leashed dogs, good for kids
Best Times	Cold to warm
Agency	Bureau of Land Management, Red Rock Canyon National Conservation Area at (702) 515-5350; www.blm.gov/nv/st/en/fo/lvfo/blm_programs/blm_special_areas/red_rock_nca.html
Recommended Maps	*Blue Diamond* 7.5-minute; free maps available at Red Rock National Conservation Area entrance station
GPS Waypoints	End of trail overlook: 36.103° N, 115.481° W
Vehicle	Passenger car OK

HIGHLIGHTS Oak Creek Canyon is one of several beautiful canyons cutting into the Red Rock escarpment. It receives fewer visitors than other canyons in the area, and the hike has two distinct personalities: The beginning approach across open desert offers sweeping views of the Red Rock escarpment and the freedom of open desert, and the canyon itself offers challenging hiking over jumbled boulders and steep slopes. Oak Creek Canyon is part of the 25,000-acre Rainbow Mountain Wilderness Area, designated by Congress in 2002 to protect its natural beauty for generations to come.

DIRECTIONS There are two ways to approach Red Rock Canyon from Las Vegas:

1. From the north end of the Strip, take West Charleston Blvd./Highway 159 west for 17 miles to the entrance for the Red Rock Canyon Visitor Center and the 13-Mile Scenic Drive on the right (north) side of the road.
2. From I-15 on the south end of Las Vegas, take Highway 160 west for roughly 10 miles to Highway 159/Blue Diamond Road. Turn right onto 159 and follow it about 10 miles as it circles clockwise through the Red Rock Canyon (with the Red Rock cliffs to your left) to the visitor center/scenic drive entrance on the left (north). This route takes about 30 minutes.

There are two trailheads accessing Oak Creek Canyon:

A. Take the scenic drive for 8 miles, then turn right (west), following the sign to Oak Creek Trailhead, which is less than a mile along the unpaved access road to the parking lot and trailhead. From the parking lot, follow the Oak Creek Canyon Trail (an old jeep trail) southwest for 1 mile to the canyon mouth.

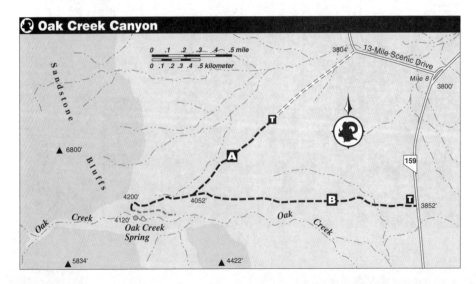

B. About 1 mile south of the exit of the Red Rock Canyon 13-Mile Scenic Drive, park on the west side of 159, by the locked gate and a jeep track heading west toward the cliffs. From the car, hike west on the jeep track about 1 mile to the canyon mouth. The track will cross other trails along the way, but keep your sights on the canyon.

FACILITIES/TRAILHEAD Restrooms are available at the first trailhead and at the visitor center at the entrance of the 13-Mile Scenic Drive. The only developed campground in the Red Rock Canyon is 2 miles east of the visitor center (1 mile south of West Charleston Blvd.) on Moenkopi Road. There are 71 individual sites and 5 group sites. Individual sites are first-come, first-served, but reservations are recommended for group sites. The campground has water, but no showers or shade. In the past, the campground has been closed during the summer because of low visitation and budget shortfalls. If you plan to visit in summer, call ahead to make sure it's open (702-515-5350). Backcountry camping in the Red Rock Canyon is allowed above 5000 feet, but permits are required (call 702-515-5050 for details). There are no developed campsites in the backcountry and fires are prohibited.

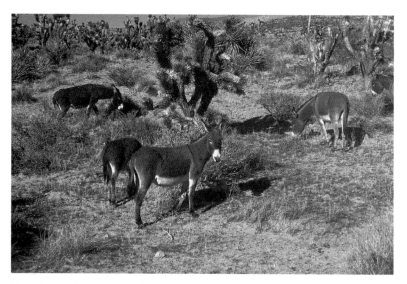

These feral burros are descendants of those that escaped from settlers and prospectors long ago.

Both trails in this description join as you near the mouth of Oak Creek Canyon. Blackbrush scrub, cholla, and a few Joshua trees accompany you as you hike toward the canyon. When you get to Oak Creek, the willow, scrub oak, and silk tassel growing along it will appear lush by comparison.

At the canyon mouth, the jeep trail does a hairpin turn back toward the east, and there's a nice viewpoint at the end, where the towering palette of color in Rainbow Mountain and Mt. Wilson dominate the horizon.

To travel west into the canyon, follow a use trail that drops into the wash. Continuing beyond this point requires scrambling and route-finding abilities. Oak Creek Canyon receives direct sun most of the day in late spring and summer, so don't expect ample shade to escape the heat. However, if you do go this way, you may be rewarded: The Oak Creek wild burro herd travels regularly into the canyon, and you might see a few of them ambling by.

Bighorn sheep are also common in the area, but chances are, they'll scamper to safety high above before you get anywhere near. Keep an eye open for them high on the slopes.

Once you have hiked as far as you're able or interested, retrace your steps to return.

trip 12 Spring Mountain Ranch State Park

Distance	Up to 3 miles, out-and-back or loop
Hiking Time	1 to 4 hours
Elevation	Up to +/-300 feet
Difficulty	Easy (with one difficult option)
Trail Use	Good for kids
Best Times	Cool to warm
Agency	Spring Mountain Ranch State Park, (702) 875-4141, http:// parks.nv.gov/smr.htm
Recommended Maps	*BLM Las Vegas* 1:100,000; free brochure map at entrance station
GPS Waypoint	Lawn between parking lot and ranch house: 36.414° N, 115.275° W
Vehicle	Passenger car OK

HIGHLIGHTS Celebrity history and natural beauty make for a scenic and relaxing visit at Spring Mountain Ranch State Park. There are more than 500 acres and several miles of paths and trails to explore. The higher elevation means 10°F to 15°F of relief from the heat in downtown Las Vegas, and guided hikes and tours make a visit to this state park an easy alternative to a strenuous hike on a hot day.

DIRECTIONS Spring Mountain Ranch State Park is near the southern end of Red Rock Canyon National Conservation Area. From southern Las Vegas, follow Highway 160 west for 10 miles to the Blue Diamond/Highway 159. Turn right (west) onto 159 and follow it west for about 5.5 miles to the park entrance on the left (west) side of the road.

FACILITIES/TRAILHEAD There are restrooms and water at the picnic area, which is open from 8 A.M. to dusk. The ranch house is open from 10 A.M. to 4 P.M.

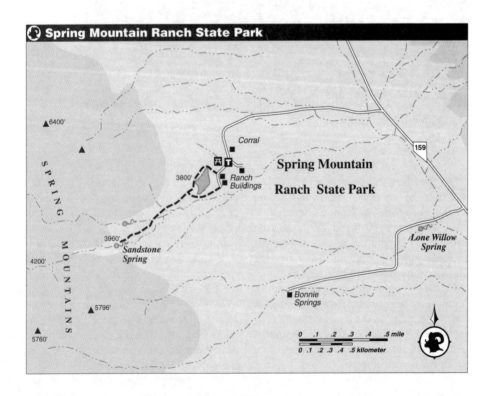

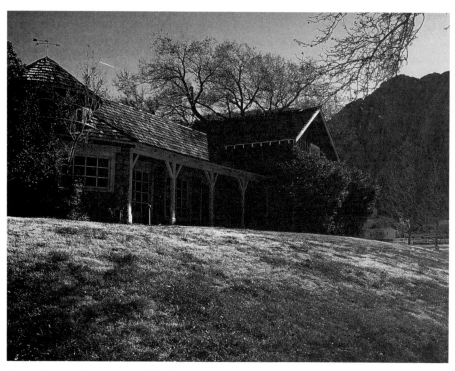

Spring Mountain Ranch is one of the finest pieces of real estate anywhere. Luckily, it's public.

Over the years, Spring Mountain Ranch State Park has served many roles. In the 1800s, the spring-fed creek and grassy meadows at the base of what are now called the Wilson Cliffs provided respite for travelers along the Spanish Trail. In 1876, former Fort Mohave Sergeant James B. Wilson and a partner filed on the property and named it the Sand Stone Ranch.

Later, as a working ranch and retreat for the wealthy, the ranch passed through the hands of notables such as Chet Lauck (who played Lum on the *Lum and Abner Radio Show*), Vera Krupp (the German movie star and one-time owner of the 33-carat Krupp Diamond, which is now worn by Elizabeth Taylor), and Howard Hughes.

In 1974, after overwhelming public objection to a proposed residential development, the Nevada Division of State Parks acquired the ranch. Today, the state park has shady picnic grounds, sprawling lawns, a visitor center housed in a historic ranch house, various historic buildings, and paths meandering around the grounds. The blacksmith shop and Sandstone Cabins on the property, built in the 1860s, are the second-oldest buildings in the Las Vegas area (the old Mormon Fort downtown is the oldest).

In addition to the meandering paths around the ranch, hikers will enjoy the Overlook and Ash Grove hikes. Fit, able hikers will enjoy the 2-mile (out-and-back) moderate hike, along a well-defined trail up to Sandstone Spring, at the mouth of Sandstone Canyon west of the ranch. The trailhead sits just above the lake on the west side of the ranch. The trail is well-defined, and the view up at the Red Rocks escarpment is breathtaking.

Guided tours of the property are also available, as are summer concerts and other performances. Call the state park for a hike schedule and other event details.

trip 13 Red Rocks: Top of the Rainbow Mountain Escarpment

Distance	2 miles, out-and-back (to ridge)
	6 miles, out-and-back or loop (to Sandstone Basin overlook)
Hiking Time	3 to 6 hours
Elevation	+/-1980 feet
Difficulty	Moderate
Trail Use	Leashed dogs, backpacking option
Best Times	Cool to hot
Agency	Bureau of Land Management, Red Rock Canyon National Conservation Area at (702) 515-5350; www.blm.gov/nv/st/en/fo/lvfo/blm_programs/blm_special_areas/red_rock_nca.html
Recommended Maps	*Blue Diamond* 7.5-minute
GPS Waypoints	Ridgeline northeast of parking area: 36.019° N, 115.487° W
	Sandstone basin: 36.051° N, 115.476° W
Vehicle	Passenger car OK

HIGHLIGHTS This hike makes the soaring views from the top of the Red Rock cliffs accessible to those who don't have a high-clearance, or 4WD, vehicle, and it's worth it, with peeks down through the steep canyons of the Red Rock escarpment and out east to Las Vegas. This hike explores the summit of the 25,000-acre Rainbow Mountain Wilderness Area, designated by Congress in 2002 to protect its natural beauty for generations to come.

There are also opportunities for side hikes out to the tops of the promontories along the way. However, this is an unofficial, cross-country route with neither trails nor signs. All hikers attempting this should be comfortable with desert route-finding. Bring extra layers to protect against the wind, which can whip enthusiastically over this ridgeline.

DIRECTIONS From I-15 at the southern end of Las Vegas, take Highway 160 west for 20 miles to the summit at the community of Mountain Springs. A quarter mile east of Mountain Springs, park at the unsigned pullout/parking area on the right (north) side of the road, across 160 from the gate to the Las Vegas Archers Spring Mountains Shooting Range.

FACILITIES/TRAILHEAD There are no facilities here. The closest restrooms and services are in Las Vegas.

Your goal is to hike to the top of the ridge about a mile to the east. Unfortunately, there are several jeep trails leaving the parking area, and all of them are unofficial and unsigned. Try to find the one that heads due north, then gradually turns to the east to a small communication tower on Peak 5827 on the map. It then climbs east to the ridgeline. The uncontrolled proliferation of off-road vehicle trails in this area makes it difficult to be precise about which trail to take; more trails appeared in the six-month period between my last two scouting trips to the trailhead.

After passing the small communications tower, the jeep trail peters out (although off-road vehicle riders seem determined to drive

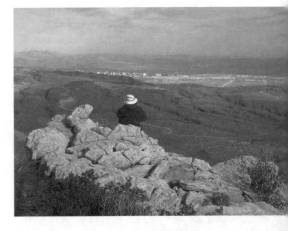

Views and solitude abound atop the escarpment.

⊙ Top of the Rainbow Mountain Escarpment

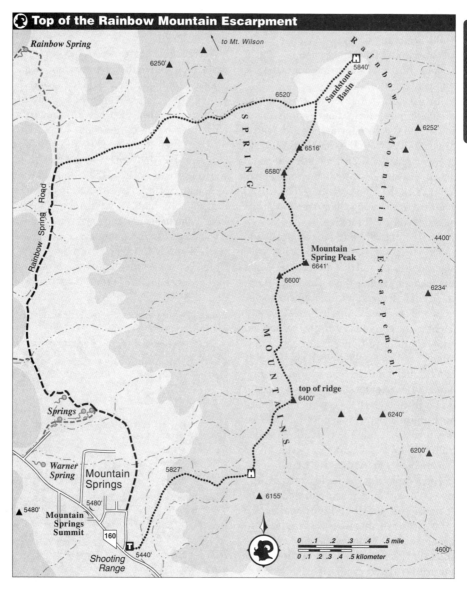

ever farther), but you should continue east. This route takes you through the pinyon, juniper, mountain mahogany, and cactus and, after about a mile, to the top of the ridge and into the Red Rock Canyon National Conservation Area and the Rainbow Mountain Wilderness, although there are no signs indicating the boundary. If your goal is a short hike with good views, turn around here and retrace your steps to return.

Once you are on the ridge facing north, it won't take long to notice the special geology here—the grayish blue of the limestone to your left, and the creamy reds, yellows, and browns of the Aztec sandstone to your right. The gray limestone is on top of the sandstone, despite the fact that the limestone is hundreds of millions of years older than the sandstone (usually older rocks are underneath the newer ones). This arrangement is possible thanks to the Keystone Thrust Fault. Beginning 65 million years ago, the pressure from continental plate movement began to thrust the older limestone over the younger sandstone.

To hike farther, turn left (north) and hike along the ridge. Again, there is no trail, but you shouldn't get lost if you stick to the ridge. About 2 miles from the car, keep your eyes open for a natural arch, or window, high on the eastern slope of Mountain Spring Peak (6641 feet), the highest peak you'll cross as you hike north along the ridge. You might miss it if you aren't looking.

After 3 miles, look to the northeast, and you'll see a sandstone basin below, this hike's destination. Hike down the slopes less than a mile into the basin. Once there, you'll find a population of ponderosa pine trees and manzanita shrubs—a wholly different plant community from the pinyon-juniper forest you hiked through a few minutes earlier. Depending on how recently rains came through, you might also find numerous water pockets, or *tinajas* (Spanish for "earthen jars"). Keep your eyes open for bighorn sheep throughout this hike, as they prefer these high slopes to the crowded trails below. Do not drink the water unless you are prepared to filter or treat it.

After exploring the basin, intrepid hikers could continue north along the ridge. A noble goal is Mt. Wilson, another 4.5 miles farther, with easy access to the summit and breathtaking views into First Creek and Oak Creek canyons. If you choose this alternative, retrace your steps back to the ridge before considering the two options below to return to the car.

Rocky Gap Road and the trailhead for North Peak and Bridge Mountain are 10 miles north of Highway 160 and would make a great destination for a two- or three-day backpack. However, you would need to arrange with someone to pick you up or use a car shuttle between Highway 160 and Rocky Gap.

To return to the car from the sandstone basin, you can either retrace your steps, enjoying continued views and less chance of getting lost, or you can hike west-southwest, up over the ridge, then down through the pinyon-juniper forest for about 1.5 miles to the unmarked Rainbow Spring Road. Turn left (south) on this jeep track, and it will lead you due south back to the community of Mountain Springs. This option is no more difficult, but finding the Rainbow Spring Road will challenge your orienteering skills. If you do get lost, head south, and you should reach Highway 160 after a few miles.

As you near the houses at Mountain Springs on Rainbow Spring Road, you will

Tinajas like this one provide life-giving water to wildlife during summer.

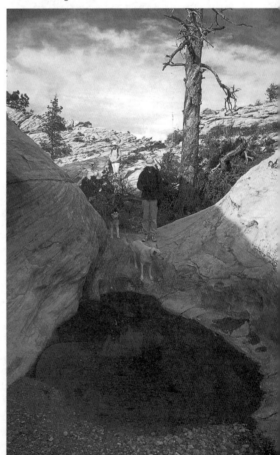

pass the tall grass of the springs. These higher-elevation (and therefore cooler) springs were used for centuries by natives, as evidenced by the many agave roasting pits in the area. Pioneer travelers along the Spanish Trail also stopped over at the springs as they moved between Las Vegas and Los Angeles.

Please respect the privacy of Mountain Springs property owners by steering clear to the north then east of the houses. Try not to let the maze of off-road vehicle tracks disorient you. Follow those that head east around the houses, then south to Highway 160 and your car.

trip 14 Red Rocks: Gateway Canyon

Distance	Up to 3 miles, loop or out-and-back
Hiking Time	2 to 3 hours
Elevation	+/-600 feet
Difficulty	Easy to most difficult
Trail Use	Leashed dogs, good for kids, backpacking option
Best Times	Cool to warm
Agency	Bureau of Land Management, Red Rock Canyon National Conservation Area at (702) 515-5350; www.blm.gov/nv/st/en/fo/lvfo/blm_programs/blm_special_areas/red_rock_nca.html
Recommended Maps	*Las Vegas* 1:100,000; *La Madre Mtn.* 7.5-minute
GPS Waypoint	Trailhead: 36.942° N, 115.252° W
Vehicle	Passenger car OK

HIGHLIGHTS Gateway Canyon hides behind the Calico Hills, off the beaten track of Red Rock Canyon National Conservation Area. Here you have a good chance of being surrounded by red rock majesty without the crowds. Gateway Canyon is part of the 47,000-acre La Madre Wilderness Area and the Red Rock Canyon National Conservation Area. The first mile is great for all ages; once in the canyon, travel becomes difficult—it's only for agile hikers and scramblers.

DIRECTIONS From Las Vegas, take West Charleston west toward Red Rock Canyon. One mile before (east of) the entrance to Red Rock Canyon, turn right (north), following the sign to Calico Basin, a small neighborhood tucked up against the east side of Red Rock's Calico Hills. Follow the road about a mile into Calico Basin. By the Red Springs Picnic Area, turn right (north) onto Calico Rd., then left (west) onto Assisi, then right (north) onto Sandstone, which ends after a half mile at a turnaround, and a gated section of gravel road that serves as a parking area.

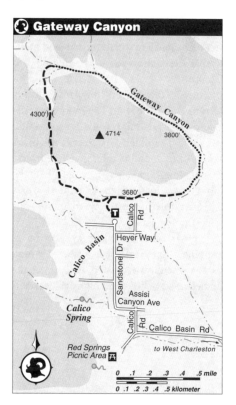

Gateway Canyon

At least that's what it looked like at press time. Don't be surprised to find a developed trailhead here, as Red Rock Canyon officials plan to build one.

FACILITIES/TRAILHEAD As of autumn 2010, there are no signs, restrooms, or other facilities here. The closest restrooms are at the Red Springs Picnic Area, or back down the road, across Highway 215 in Las Vegas.

Gateway Canyon sits on the other side of the jumbled sandstone ridge north of the parking area. These directions take you counterclockwise around this ridge.

From the parking area at the top of Sandstone Road, follow the unsigned, but distinct trail north to the boulders at the base of the ridge, then turn right (east), following the trail as it meanders through the boulders, then counterclockwise around the eastern toe of the ridge and into Gateway Canyon. There are many smaller trails heading off to various boulders, as this is a popular spot for climbers, so be attentive if you want to stay on track.

The first half mile of this hike is flat, easy, and suitable for all ages and abilities—a perfect morning or afternoon stroll. The boulders alone are worth the trip and make a great destination for kids to climb and explore.

Once in the canyon, the route quickly becomes more difficult. The route generally follows the wash, but specific routes around this or that boulder or waterfall might be harder to find, and climbing will be necessary at times. Luckily, you're in a canyon, and getting lost would take hard work. Consider this a great way to build your route-finding skills.

The sandstone in Gateway Canyon is stunning; stripes and polka dots were in high fashion when it was created. Also notice the tangled flood debris piled high against boulders and trees in the canyon, telling you *this is not the place to be during heavy rains.*

After a half mile or so of narrow canyon, the canyon opens up a bit. Look for Turtlehead Peak rising high above the canyon to the west. Once you see only 20 to 30 feet of sandstone lining the south (left) edge of the wash, break out those route-finding skills again, and look for routes out of the wash to the left (south). Although there are no signed trails, Gateway Canyon is popular with rock climbers, who have built cairns along the edge of the wash to mark their trails heading south up and over a prominent saddle and back to the parking area.

Once over the saddle, you will clearly see the parking area less than a mile to the southeast. Several trails crisscross the flats between the saddle and parking area, requiring attentive navigation to choose the straightest line back to your car.

Ancient people lived throughout what is now Red Rock Canyon National Conservation Area for thousands of years, leaving behind agave roasting pits, rock art, and other glimpses into their lives. These resources are fragile, irreplaceable, and protected by state and federal laws. Please do not walk on agave roasting pits or touch any artifacts. The soils, rocks, and plants throughout the area are also fragile. Please follow Leave No Trace principles whenever you travel and camp, by sticking to trails, washes, or stone whenever possible (read more about LNT and trail etiquette, page 18).

trip 15 Blue Diamond Hill

Distance	5 to 6 miles, out-and-back or loop
Hiking Time	3 to 5 hours
Elevation	+/-1500 feet
Difficulty	Moderate
Trail Use	Leashed dogs, map and compass
Best Times	Cold to warm
Agency	*BLM Las Vegas* at (702) 515-5000; www.nv.blm.gov/vegas
Recommended Maps	*Blue Diamond, NV* 7.5-minute
GPS Waypoints	Trailhead: 36.121° N, 115.433° W
	Las Vegas Overlook: 36.108° N, 115.398° W
Vehicle	Passenger car OK

HIGHLIGHTS Sitting literally across the street from Red Rock Canyon National Conservation Area, Blue Diamond Hill is the orphan twin of its more spectacular sibling to the west, but it should not be discounted. It offers not only secluded trails and interesting landscape, but also beautiful views of both Red Rocks and Las Vegas.

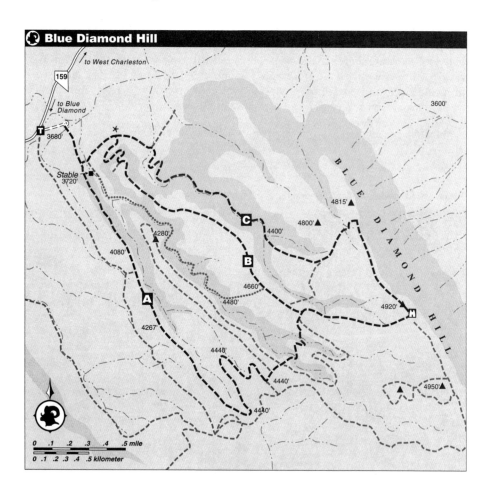

This would be a great option for a full moon (or a few days before full moon) hike. Leave late in the afternoon, enjoy sunset and a picnic dinner at the top, watch the lights wake up across the Las Vegas Valley, then let the moon's soft-blue light guide you back to the car. Bring extra layers in case it gets chilly, and a headlamp in case the moon's light somehow lets you down.

DIRECTIONS There are two ways to get to the trailhead from Las Vegas:

1. From northern Las Vegas, take West Charleston Blvd. west toward Red Rock Canyon National Conservation Area. After you cross Highway 215, drive another 6.3 miles and turn left (south) into the gravel parking area with a large sign: COWBOY TRAIL RIDES.

2. From southern Las Vegas, take Highway 160 west, then turn right (north) on Highway 159/Blue Diamond Road, which circles clockwise through the Red Rock Canyon for about 9.6 miles to the trailhead on the right (south) side of the road, which is marked by the same COWBOY TRAIL RIDES sign.

FACILITIES/TRAILHEAD There are no facilities here. The closest restrooms and services are in Las Vegas.

This region's popularity with mountain bikers and horse riders means that numerous trails crisscross Blue Diamond Hill, none of which are signed. All of these trails are unsigned, but they are obvious, wide, and easy to follow. Below are three of the many combinations possible. All other trails in the area are shown on the map, but faded back, to give you a sense of what's out there and keep you from getting confused when you come across them.

A. From the trailhead, hike southeast toward the main stable for the horse rides.

Pass to the right of the stables (keeping them on your left) to follow the wide horse trail that heads south up the ridge west of the canyon. The horse folks call this the Fossil Ridge Trail, although it is unsigned. About 1.5 miles south of the stables, the trail reaches the head of the canyon, then veers left (east), and meanders to the overlook, another 1.5 miles farther. From there, you can retrace your steps to return, or take B or C below.

B, C. From the trailhead, head southeast toward the main stable, as above, but half-

The unnamed canyons of Blue Diamond Hill offer beauty, solitude, and challenge.

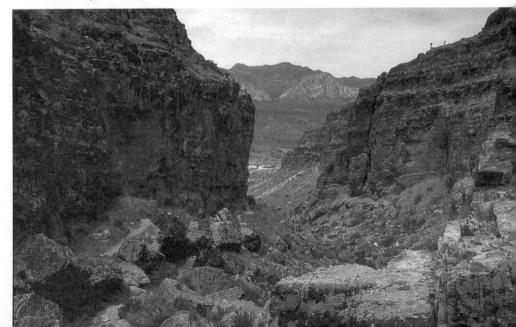

way between the car and the stable, turn left (east) onto a well-used horse trail, which takes you across a small drainage and then northeast across the flat country. Follow the trail as it circles clockwise around the point of the ridge. On the northeast side of the ridge, after you have been hiking about a half mile (indicated on the map by *), look south for a less well-used trail (B) that switchbacks south up the nose of the ridge (mountain bikers call this "Bone Shaker," but it applies more to their discomfort riding down, not to your breathlessness hiking up).

A few yards southeast of the junction with Option B (still on the flats), a faint trail (C) crosses a drainage, then heads southeast up into the canyon just east of B. Here and there, the trail disappears as the route crosses open rock. However, you will be in a narrow canyon. Continue upstream, look left and right for the trail to start again, and you should have no trouble finding your way. Both B and C head southeast to the viewpoint over Las Vegas. Option B is about 2 miles long, and C is about 1.5 miles long. Follow A, B, or C to return to your car.

Blue Diamond Hill is made of similar limestone layers as La Madre Mountain in Red Rock Canyon. As you hike, you will be able to see many layers in the canyon walls. Keep an eye out for fossils of ancient sea plants and shells, too, as these layers formed deep under the sea between 250 million and 500 million years ago.

When hiking out of the canyons and up on the gentler, open slopes, Blue Diamond Hill provides sweeping views of Red Rock Canyon. The overlook at the top offers a gorgeous view of Las Vegas. Despite the many trails and no signs to guide you, this open country makes it easy to get your bearings. Red Rock Canyon rises prominently to the west and north, and the trailhead is also visible from many high points. With a decent sense of direction or minimal compass skills, you should be able to navigate back to the trailhead if you get temporarily disoriented.

If you'd like a different type of adventure on Blue Diamond Hill, consider a horseback tour (call Cowboy Trail Rides at 702-307-2457) or a mountain bike ride (call Las Vegas Cyclery at 800-596-2953).

trip 16 Red Rocks: La Madre Mountain

Distance	Up to 10 miles, out-and-back
Hiking Time	6 to 8 hours
Elevation	+/-3500 feet
Difficulty	Difficult
Trail Use	Leashed dogs, backpacking option, map and compass
Best Times	Cool to warm
Agency	Bureau of Land Management, Red Rock Canyon National Conservation Area at (702) 515-5350; www.blm.gov/nv/st/en/fo/lvfo/blm_programs/blm_special_areas/red_rock_nca.html
Recommended Maps	*La Madre Mtn.* and *Blue Diamond NE* 7.5-minute
GPS Waypoints	Jeep track to parking: 36.259° N, 115.488° W Summit: 36.212° N, 115.459° W
Vehicle	Passenger OK

HIGHLIGHTS This unpretentious hike up a wash, through a pinyon-juniper forest becomes suddenly jaw-dropping when you reach the top; the world falls away, and you drink in amazing views from the crown peak of Red Rock Canyon National Conservation Area, thousands of feet above the valley

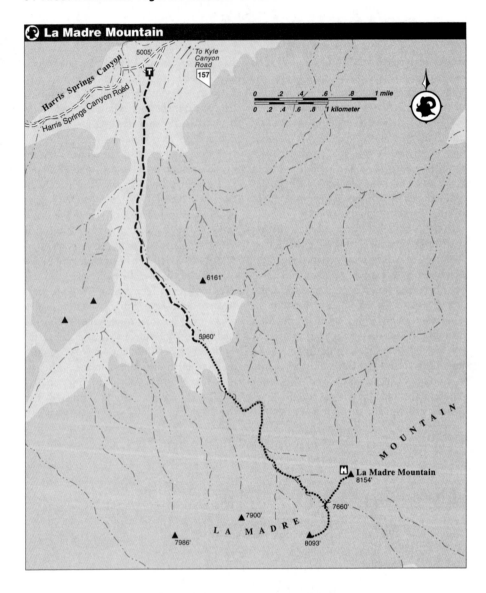

La Madre Mountain

below. You'll easily see why Congress designated La Madre part of the Red Rock Canyon National Conservation Area in 1990 and as the La Madre Mountain Wilderness in 2002. There is no water along this trip; bring all you'll need.

DIRECTIONS From U.S. 95 north of Las Vegas, turn left (west) onto Highway 157 toward Kyle Canyon. After 8.7 miles, turn left (south) onto a well-graded gravel road (Harris Springs Canyon). Follow this road as it leads south, then west for 2.7 miles to an unsigned, unmaintained jeep track heading left (south). Turn onto this track, and drive until you find a suitable parking spot (if you're in a passenger car, you might luck out with an additional mile or so of hiking). The wilderness boundary is 2 miles up this track, so please do not drive farther, even if someone else did (they drove into wilderness—a big no-no).

FACILITIES/TRAILHEAD There is no official trailhead (although there will be when the BLM gets around to it), and no other facilities here. The closest services are back down along Highway 95 toward Las Vegas.

From your car, continue following the jeep track as it heads south, then veers to the southeast at the western base of a prominent, rounded hill (point 6161 on the map—a good landmark for your return).

The hike up La Madre is difficult, but the views are sublime.

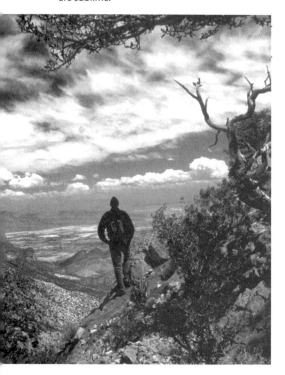

A. Climb northeast to the summit for 8154-foot La Madre Mountain, the tallest in the Red Rock Canyon. Though its view is sweeping and breathtaking, part of the view of Red Rock Canyon is blocked by Peak 8093 to the southwest.

B. Climb southwest to the summit of Peak 8093. Although not as high, this peak offers a more direct view of Red Rock Canyon proper.

If you're feeling strong, do both.

As you stand on top of the world, consider the many bands of limestone under your feet (which are, admittedly, easier to see from Red Rock Canyon to the south). These layers began as sediment settling in the sea between 250 million and 600 million years ago. About 65 million years ago, the colliding Pacific and North American continental plates pushed the older limestone of what is now La Madre up and over the much younger Aztec sandstone of Calico Hills and Red Rock escarpment to the south—known locally as the Keystone Thrust. Usually, older rocks are underneath younger rocks. Such is the power of Mother Earth. Science aside, it's beautiful.

Retrace your steps to return. And if you find my sunglasses sitting on a rock a mile or so back down the wash, let me know.

trip 17 Spring Mountains: Bristlecone Trail

Distance	Up to 6 miles, out-and-back or loop
Hiking Time	2½ to 3 hours
Elevation	+1091/-861 feet (from lower trailhead)
	+861/-1091 feet (from upper trailhead)
Difficulty	Easy to moderate
Trail Use	Leashed dogs, good for kids, mountain biking allowed, backpacking option
Best Times	Late spring to fall
Agency	U.S. Forest Service Spring Mountains National Recreation Area at (702) 515-5400; www.fs.fed.us/r4/htnf/districts/smnra
Recommended Maps	*Las Vegas* 1:100,000; *Charleston Peak* 7.5-minute
GPS Waypoints	Lower trailhead: 36.311° N, 115.676° W
	Upper trailhead: 36.306° N, 115.667° W
Vehicle	Passenger car OK

HIGHLIGHTS The Bristlecone Trail is a pleasant and beautiful hike through a diverse alpine forest in Lee Canyon in the Spring Mountains. It's suitable for the whole family, and perfect to escape the heat and stress of Las Vegas. As you hike, listen for the high trill of hummingbirds. Backpackers might enjoy a point-to-point backpack 15 miles north to Bonanza Peak Trailhead.

DIRECTIONS From Las Vegas, take Highway 95 north for about 45 minutes. About 14 miles past (north of) the Kyle Canyon/Highway 157 turnoff, turn left (west) onto Lee Canyon/Highway 156 and follow it west into Lee Canyon. There are two trailheads for this hike, one on each end of the trail:

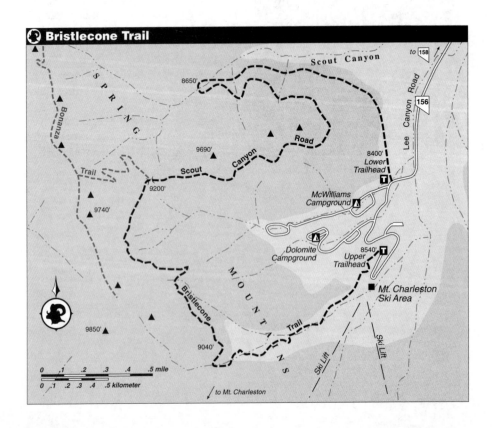

1. **Lower Bristlecone Trail:** To access the lower (east) trailhead, take Highway 156 for 14 miles west up Lee Canyon to the intersection with Highway 158 (Deer Creek Road). From there, continue west on 156 for 2.7 miles, then turn right (north) on an unsigned road for 200 yards to the trailhead (if you reach the roundabout and McWilliams Campground, you've gone too far).
2. **Upper Bristlecone Trail:** To access the upper (west) trailhead, follow Lee Canyon/Highway 156 to the end of the road, a half mile past the ski area, and 3.5 miles west of the intersection of 156 and 158. Park by the trailhead sign by the west end of the roundabout.

FACILITIES/TRAILHEAD The nearest water, toilets, and rangers are available at the Kyle Canyon Visitor Center on Highway 157. There are five campgrounds in the Spring Mountains, offering a total of 143 sites. Two are in Lee Canyon, two are in Kyle Canyon, and one is on Highway 158 between Kyle and Lee canyons. Both first-come, first-served and reservation sites are available. For more information, call (702) 515-5400. Unless otherwise posted, backcountry camping is allowed at least 100 feet from water (although I suggest camping at least 200 feet from water, as recommended by Leave No Trace and the State of Nevada). To protect the ancient bristlecone pine trees in the Spring Mountains, campfires are prohibited. Permits are required for camping in the Mt. Charleston Wilderness Area (register at trailheads).

From the lower (east) trailhead, hike north past the gate and follow the two-track trail (called Scout Canyon Road on maps) as it zigs and zags up Scout Canyon. After 3 miles, you'll pass the intersection for the Bonanza Trail, soon after which the trail becomes single-track and meanders south to the upper trailhead. The first 3 miles from the lower trailhead follow the remnant of Lee Canyon Road, which was built by the Works Progress Administration to access Clark Canyon and Pahrump on the east side of the Spring Mountains. Work stopped in 1942 during World War II, when road builders were assigned to other projects.

The "bottle brush" look of bristlecone pines makes these trees easy to identify.

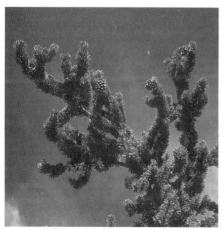

From the upper (west) trailhead, hike west along the northern edge of the ski area, where the trail wanders through aspen, ponderosa pine, and white fir. It then veers north to the high point, where it becomes a two-track trail that meanders northeast to the lower trailhead. For an enjoyable out-and-back option, start at the upper trailhead and hike for about 2 miles to the high point, passing a viewpoint and a stand of dead but very picturesque bristlecone snags along the way. Retrace your steps to return.

For hikers interested in a loop, the two trails are separated by a 0.8-mile walk along Lee Canyon Road.

Please stay on the trail and keep dogs on leashes, because the Bristlecone Trail passes through one of the only places on the planet where the rare Clokey's eggvetch grows. It has been a candidate species for protection under the Endangered Species Act.

Backpackers, consider this: Three miles from the upper trailhead, continue north on the Bonanza Trail north along the Spring Mountain Crest for a great one-night, point-to-point backpack to the community of Cold Springs, 15 miles north. This approach would require a car shuttle or a friend to pick you up. Campsites can be found among the bristlecones along the crest or at Wood Spring (roughly the half-way point), where you might also find water (the spring was flowing in October 2008).

To protect the ancient bristlecone pine trees in the Spring Mountains, all campfires are prohibited in the Mt. Charleston Wilderness; bring your camp stove. Please follow Leave No Trace principles whenever you travel and camp (see more about trail etiquette, page 18).

trip 18 Spring Mountains: Mummy Spring

Distance	6.4 miles, out-and-back
Hiking Time	3 to 4 hours
Elevation	+/-1800 feet
Difficulty	Moderate
Trail Use	Leashed dogs, but please consider leaving them at home to protect this enormously sensitive area.
Best Times	Late spring to fall
Agency	U.S. Forest Service Spring Mountains National Recreation Area at (702) 515-5400; www.fs.fed.us/r4/htnf/districts/smnra
Recommended Maps	*Angel Peak* and *Charleston Peak* 7.5-minute
GPS Waypoints	Raintree: 36.294° N, 115.623° N
Vehicle	Passenger car OK

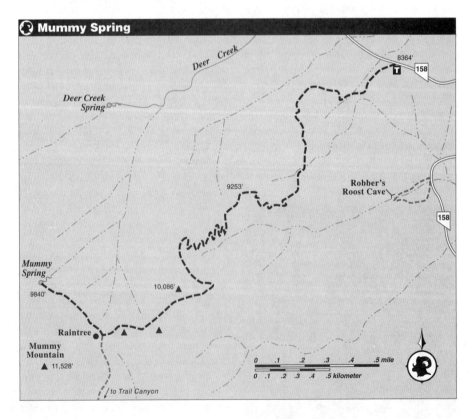

Along the way to Mummy Spring, the 3,000-year-old Raintree offers its wisdom.

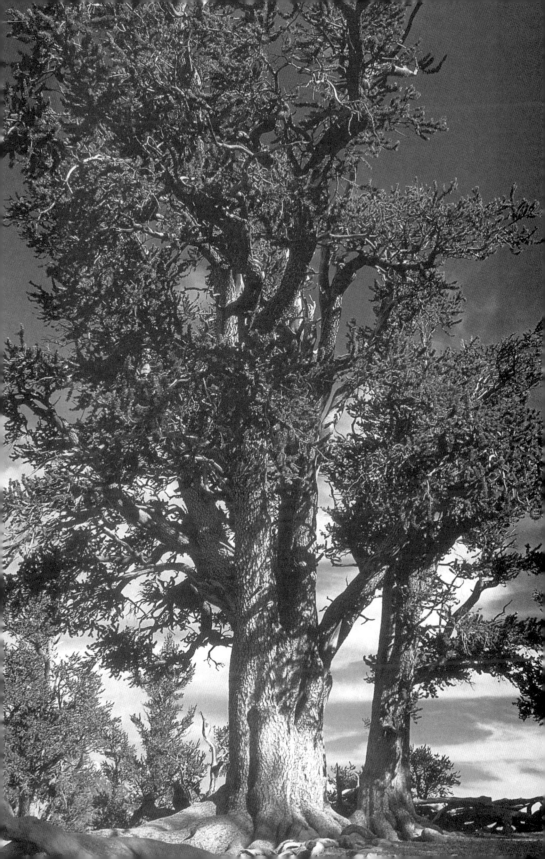

HIGHLIGHTS The hike to Mummy Spring is a tour through some of the Spring Mountains' most biologically diverse territory. The first section of the trail passes through a beautiful mixed forest of ponderosa, limber, and pinyon pines; mountain mahogany; white fir; and juniper. Above 9000 feet, bristlecones enter the mix.

DIRECTIONS From Las Vegas, take Highway 95 north about 30 minutes to Kyle Canyon Road/Highway 157. Travel west on 157 for about 17 miles to the intersection with Deer Creek Road/Highway 158. Turn right (north) onto 158 and follow it a little less than 5 miles to the signed NORTH LOOP TRAILHEAD on the left (west) side of the road.

FACILITIES/TRAILHEAD The nearest water, toilets, and rangers are available at the Kyle Canyon Visitor Center. There are five campgrounds in the Spring Mountains, offering a total of 143 sites. Two are in Lee Canyon, two are in Kyle Canyon, and one is on Highway 158 between Kyle and Lee canyons. Both first-come, first-served and reservation sites are available. For more information, call (702) 515-5400. Unless otherwise posted, backcountry camping is allowed at least 100 feet from water (although I suggest camping at least 200 feet from water, as recommended by Leave No Trace and the State of Nevada). To protect the ancient bristlecone pine trees in the Spring Mountains, campfires are prohibited. Permits are required for camping in the Mt. Charleston Wilderness Area (register at trailheads).

From the North Loop Trailhead, hike west for about 1.5 miles to a viewpoint from the ridge east of Mummy Mountain. The trail then switchbacks steeply through bristlecone pines to the top of the ridge.

At 2.7 miles, you reach an intersection under the tall cliffs of Mummy's Toe, where one of the Spring Mountains' celebrities—a 3,000-year-old bristlecone called Raintree—holds council. After paying your respects, veer right (northwest) at the intersection for another half mile to the springs. (A left turn at Raintree leads 2 miles to the intersection with the Trail Canyon Trail, then continues another 7 miles to the summit of Mt. Charleston.)

Mummy Spring, nestled in a cool, northeast-facing chute below Mummy Mountain, is a unique pocket of life in these mountains. Among the grasses, shrubs, and ferns grow several endemic sensitive and endangered species. To protect these species, the Forest Service would prefer that you didn't visit the springs. They've worked to prevent people from stomping across endangered species to reach the water, so please stay on the trail and bring your own water to drink.

To protect the ancient bristlecone pine trees in the Spring Mountains, campfires are prohibited in the Mt. Charleston Wilderness; bring your camp stove. Please follow Leave No Trace principles whenever you travel and camp (see more about trail etiquette, page 18).

Once you have admired the spring from a respectful distance, retrace your steps to return.

trip 19 Spring Mountains: Robber's Roost

Distance	0.3 mile, loop
Hiking Time	30 minutes to 1 hour
Elevation	+/-280 feet
Difficulty	Moderate
Trail Use	Leashed dogs, good for kids
Best Times	Late spring to fall
Agency	U.S. Forest Service Spring Mountains National Recreation Area at (702) 515-5400; www.fs.fed.us/r4/htnf/districts/smnra
Recommended Maps	*Angel Peak* 7.5-minute
GPS Waypoints	Roost: 36.301° N, 115.611° W
Vehicle	Passenger car OK

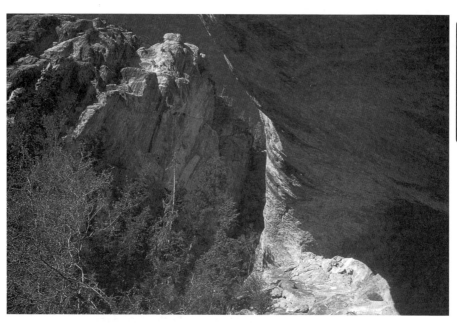

Erosion of the rock's weaker layers formed the shelter at Robber's Roost.

HIGHLIGHTS This hike to a lush canyon and a shady rock shelter that once served as a hideout for thieves promises fun for everyone.

DIRECTIONS From Las Vegas, take Highway 95 north about 30 minutes to Kyle Canyon Road/Highway 157. Travel west on 157 for about 17 miles to the intersection with Deer Creek Road/Highway 158. Turn right (north) onto 158 and follow it about 3.9 miles to the signed trailhead on the left (west) side of the road. Parking is across the street on the right (west) side of the road.

FACILITIES/TRAILHEAD The nearest water, toilets, and rangers are available at the Kyle Canyon Visitor Center. There are five campgrounds in the Spring Mountains, offering a total of 143 sites. Two are in Lee Canyon, two are in Kyle Canyon, and one is on Highway 158 between the two canyons. Both first-come, first-served and reservation sites are available. For more information, call (702) 515-5400. Unless otherwise posted, backcountry camping is allowed at least 100 feet from water (although I suggest camping at least 200 feet from water, as recommended by Leave No Trace and the State of Nevada). To protect the ancient bristlecone pine trees in the Spring Mountains, campfires are prohibited. Permits are required for camping in the Mt. Charleston Wilderness Area (register at trailheads).

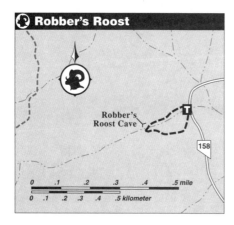

From the parking area, cross Deer Creek Road and follow the trail west as it climbs a quarter mile to a beautiful overhang/shelter in the limestone cliffs. At the shelter, cross the creek to follow the trail southeast as it loops back to the road.

Legend has it that thieves along the Mormon Trail in the 1800s used the shelter to hide out, stash their stolen goods, corral their horses, and keep an eye out for attackers. Formed because one layer of limestone was weaker than others and eroded away over the millennia, the dramatic cliff certainly looks like a good place to be a fugitive. It's also a great place for the kids to explore to see if there's any treasure still hidden about.

Adding to the historic romance is the beautiful diversity of the plants and trees in this canyon. Numerous shrub species and at least seven kinds of trees surround you on the hike, including pinyon pine, juniper, white fir, mountain mahogany, and ponderosa pine. In summer, look for columbine and other wildflowers. Early in the morning, listen to the many birds this diverse mountain forest attracts.

trip 20 Spring Mountains: Fletcher Canyon

Distance	3.5 miles, out-and-back
Hiking Time	2 to 3 hours
Elevation	+/-1030 feet
Difficulty	Easy to moderate
Trail Use	Leashed dogs (but please keep them from harassing the endangered Palmer's chipmunk), good for kids
Best Times	Late spring to fall
Agency	U.S. Forest Service Spring Mountains National Recreation Area at (702) 515-5400; www.fs.fed.us/r4/htnf/districts/smnra
Recommended Maps	*Angel Peak* and *Charleston Peak* 7.5-minute
GPS Waypoints	Roost: 36.301° N, 115.611° W
Vehicle	Passenger car OK

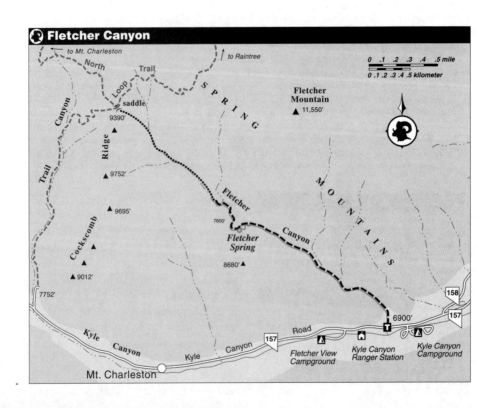

HIGHLIGHTS This hike explores a beautiful slot canyon high in the Spring Mountains. Slot canyons usually bring to mind lower-elevation deserts. Leave it to the miracles of nature to build one high in the mountains. Because limestone is soluble in water (most major cave systems in the world are in limestone), it's a wonder there aren't more such high-elevation slots in Nevada's many limestone mountains. This place is beautiful, but it is not the place to be during a flash flood. If thunderstorms are active, hike somewhere else.

DIRECTIONS From Las Vegas, take Highway 95 north about 30 minutes to Kyle Canyon Road/Highway 157. Take the exit for 157 west and drive 17 to the intersection with Deer Creek Road/Highway 158. The trailhead is on the north side of 157 approximately a half mile west of the intersection. The trailhead has little parking, but there are several parking areas across the street within 100 yards of the trailhead.

FACILITIES/TRAILHEAD The nearest water, toilets, and rangers are available at the Kyle Canyon Visitor Center on Highway 157. There are five campgrounds in the Spring Mountains, offering a total of 143 sites. Two are in Lee Canyon, two are in Kyle Canyon, and one is on Highway 158 between the two canyons. Both first-come, first-served and reservation sites are available. For more information, call (702) 515-5400. Unless otherwise posted, backcountry camping is allowed at least 100 feet from water (although I suggest camping at least 200 feet from water, as recommended by Leave No Trace and the State of Nevada). To protect the ancient bristlecone pine trees in the Spring Mountains, campfires are prohibited. Permits are required for camping in the Mt. Charleston Wilderness Area (register at trailheads).

From the car, follow the trail northwest through the forest. The canyon is not visible from the trailhead, but as you hike you'll notice the hills rising above and getting closer on either side. The first mile of this trail passes through a beautiful and diverse forest of pinyon pine, juniper, manzanita, mountain mahogany, and oak. As you climb higher, white fir, ponderosa pine, and even bristlecone pine make their appearance, making this a beautiful respite from the baking asphalt of Las Vegas.

After a mile or so, the trail wanders back and forth across the creek as it enters the canyon. Follow the canyon until it splits. Large boulders block travel to the left, and a dry waterfall blocks travel to the right.

Retrace your steps to the trailhead.

For a more difficult option, arrange to have someone pick you up at the Trail Canyon Trailhead, a 3-mile drive from the Fletcher Canyon Trailhead, via Kyle Canyon and Echo roads. This option is only for experienced, agile hikers who are skilled with map and compass. Climb past the boulders in the left (south) fork of the canyon junction, then follow the drainage up to the northwest, out of the slot canyon. Continue in the drainage more than a mile to the saddle of Cockscomb Ridge, where you'll reach the saddle and Trail Canyon

Trail. Turn left (southwest) and follow Trail Canyon Trail another 2 miles down to its trailhead, where your prearranged ride will pick you up. Give yourself another one to two hours for this more difficult option.

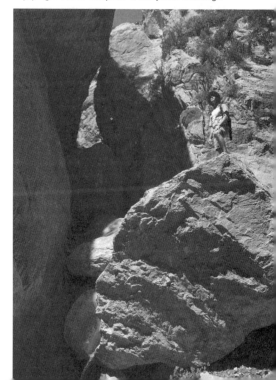

Enjoying Fletcher Canyon's beauty and challenge

trip 21 Spring Mountains: Trail Canyon

Distance	4 to 6 miles or more, out-and-back
Hiking Time	3 to 5 hours
Elevation	+/-2000 feet (to Cave Spring)
Difficulty	Moderate
Trail Use	Leashed dogs, backpacking option
Best Times	Late spring to fall
Agency	U.S. Forest Service Spring Mountains National Recreation Area at (702) 515-5400; www.fs.fed.us/r4/htnf/districts/smnra
Recommended Maps	*Charleston Peak* 7.5-minute
GPS Waypoints	Trailhead: 36.267° N, 115.656° W
	Cave Spring: 36.291° N, 115.652° W
Vehicle	Passenger car OK

HIGHLIGHTS Trail Canyon is a pleasurable hike onto the slopes below Mummy Mountain and to the east of Mt. Charleston. The intriguing geology, aspen, and pine forests, as well as views across the valley reward all who work their muscles and lungs to climb this slope. Trail Canyon is part of the 56,600-acre Mt. Charleston Wilderness Area.

DIRECTIONS From Las Vegas, take Highway 95 north about 30 minutes to Kyle Canyon Road/Highway 157. Take the exit for 157 west and drive 18.5 miles to the Kyle Canyon Visitor Center. From the visitor center, follow Highway 157 west for 1.8 miles. At the hairpin curve, continue straight (west) onto Echo Road for a half mile to the trailhead on the left (north) side of the road.

FACILITIES/TRAILHEAD The nearest water, toilets, and rangers are available at the Kyle Canyon Visitor Center. There are five campgrounds in the Spring Mountains, offering a total of 143 sites. Two are in Lee Canyon, two are in Kyle Canyon, and one is on Highway 158 between the two canyons. Both first-come, first-served and reservation sites are available. For more information, call (702) 515-5400. Unless otherwise posted, backcountry camping is allowed at least 100 feet from water (although I suggest camping at least 200 feet from water, as recommended by Leave No Trace and the State of Nevada). To protect the ancient bristlecone pine trees in the Spring Mountains, campfires are prohibited. Permits are required for camping in the Mt. Charleston Wilderness Area (register at trailheads).

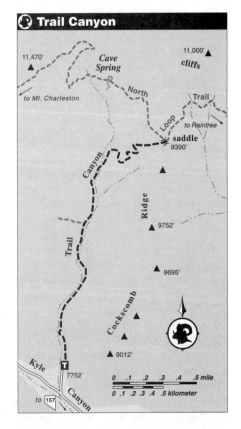

From the car, hike north up the Trail Canyon Trail for 2 miles to the intersection with the North Loop Trail, where you'll see towering ponderosa pine trees. There are many places to turn around on this hike, but the views get better the farther you go.

A right (east) turn will take you 2 miles to Raintree and Mummy Spring. A left (west) turn will lead another half mile to Cave Spring and onward to the summit of Mt.

Charleston (9 miles from trailhead). Cave Spring offers mysterious caves at the base of the cliffs. Another mile beyond that, the trail reaches the top of the ridgeline, where you'll find stunning views of Mt. Charleston and the twisted geology in its south ridge. After 6 miles, the trail traverses through the crags and cliffs of Devil's Thumb on its way to the final ascent of the peak.

If your goal is to summit Mt. Charleston, be prepared for a very long day, and bring plenty of water, food, extra layers, and the 7.5-minute map for the area (recommended above). Only fit, experienced hikers should attempt Mt. Charleston.

To protect the ancient bristlecone pine trees in the Spring Mountains, campfires are prohibited in the Mt. Charleston Wilderness; bring your camp stove. Please follow Leave No Trace principles whenever you travel and camp (see more about trail etiquette, page 18).

Whichever way you choose to go, retrace your steps to return.

Trail Canyon offers stunning views of Mt. Charleston's twisted geology.

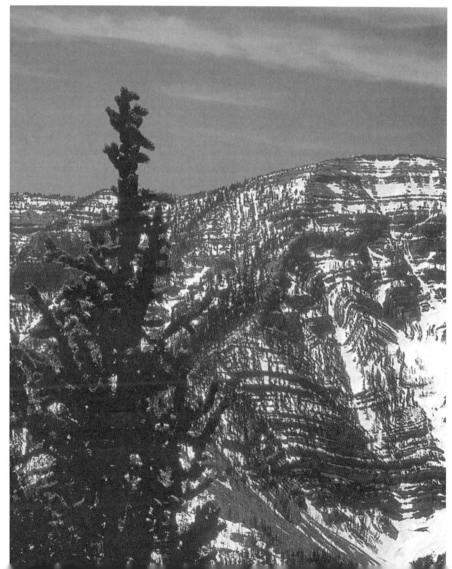

trip 22 Spring Mountains: Mummy Mountain

Distance	10 miles, out-and-back
Hiking Time	6 to 8 hours
Elevation	+/-3820 feet
Difficulty	Difficult
Trail Use	Backpacking option, map and compass
Best Times	Late spring to fall
Agency	U.S. Forest Service Spring Mountains National Recreation Area at (702) 515-5400; www.fs.fed.us/r4/htnf/districts/smnra
Recommended Maps	*Charleston Peak* 7.5-minute
GPS Waypoints	Mummy Peak: 36.299° N, 155.649° W
Vehicle	Passenger car OK

HIGHLIGHTS At 11,528 feet, Mummy Mountain is the second-highest peak in the Spring Mountains. With its shining limestone cliffs, it's also a prominent landmark that looks like a mummy lying on its back when viewed from Highway 95 to the northeast. Although the off-trail section of the climb is quite a huff, the view makes up for it—sweeping from the picturesque Sisters peaks to the north, to the Nevada Test Site and the Nellis Air Force Range to the northeast, to the Desert National Wildlife Refuge to the east, and to Las Vegas to the southeast. Griffith and Charleston peaks mark the high points of the Spring Mountains to the south and west. Mummy Mountain is within the 56,600-acre Mt. Charleston Wilderness Area.

DIRECTIONS From Las Vegas, take Highway 95 north about 30 minutes to Kyle Canyon Road/ Highway 157. Take the exit for 157 west and drive 18.5 miles to the Kyle Canyon Visitor Center. From the visitor center, follow Highway 157 west for 1.8 miles. At the hairpin curve, continue straight (west) onto Echo Road for a half mile to the trailhead on the left (north) side of the road.

FACILITIES/TRAILHEAD The nearest water, toilets, and rangers are available at the Kyle Canyon Visitor Center. There are five campgrounds in the Spring Mountains, offering a total of 143 sites. Two are in Lee Canyon, two are in Kyle Canyon, and one is on Highway 158 between the two canyons. Both first-come, first-served and reservation sites are available. For more information, call (702) 515-5400. Unless otherwise posted, backcountry camping is allowed at least 100 feet from water (although I suggest camping at least 200 feet from water, as

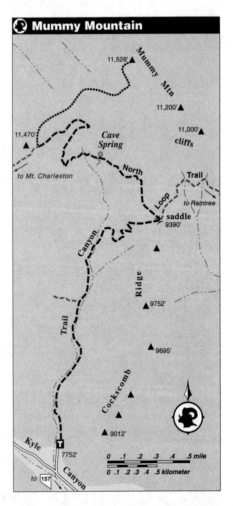

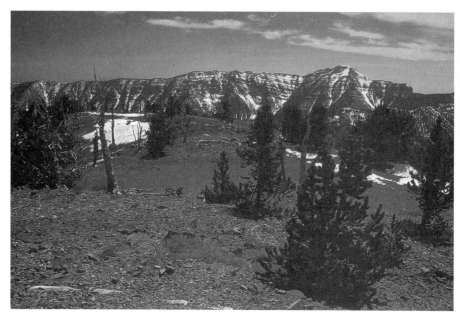

Mt. Charleston as seen from the top of the Mummy

recommended by Leave No Trace and the State of Nevada). To protect the ancient bristlecone pine trees in the Spring Mountains, campfires are prohibited. Permits are required for camping in the Mt. Charleston Wilderness Area (register at trailheads).

Hike north 2 miles up the Trail Canyon Trail, then turn left (west) onto North Loop Trail toward Mt. Charleston. About 1 mile past the intersection (a half mile past Cave Spring), as you near the top of the ridge in the middle of a stand of dead trees, the trail makes a switchback and skirts along the limestone cliff on the east side of the slope.

Continue another couple hundred yards on the trail, then turn right and scramble straight up the scree slope to the saddle at the top of the ridge. This section is difficult, and there is neither sign nor trail to guide you. Once on the ridgeline, turn right (east) and follow the ridgeline (there's a faint climbers' route) past bristlecones to the base of Mummy Mountain's summit cliff band.

Here, the route is more visible. It veers north for a quarter mile to a chute that climbs east to the summit. Follow it, and you're there. The summit plateau is wide and gentle, offering numerous campsites and picnic spots.

To protect the ancient bristlecone pine trees in the Spring Mountains, all campfires are prohibited in the Mt. Charleston Wilderness; bring your camp stove. Please follow Leave No Trace principles whenever you travel and camp (see more about trail etiquette, page 18).

Retrace your steps to return.

trip 23 Spring Mountains: Mary Jane Falls

Distance	3 miles, out-and-back
Hiking Time	2 to 3 hours
Elevation	+/-948 feet
Difficulty	Moderate
Trail Use	Leashed dogs, good for kids
Best Times	Late spring to fall
Agency	U.S. Forest Service Spring Mountains National Recreation Area at (702) 515-5400; www.fs.fed.us/r4/htnf/districts/smnra
Recommended Maps	*Charleston Peak* 7.5-minute
GPS Waypoints	Falls: 36.279° N, 115.671° W
Vehicle	Passenger car OK

HIGHLIGHTS This most popular hike in the Spring Mountains heads up challenging switchbacks to a refreshing waterfall. But avoid it during thunderstorms. In 1971, a sudden storm washed away the campground where the trailhead is now.

DIRECTIONS From Las Vegas, take Highway 95 north about 30 minutes to Kyle Canyon Road/Highway 157. Take the exit for 157 west and drive 18.5 miles to the Kyle Canyon Visitor Center. From the visitor center, follow Highway 157 west for 1.8 miles. At the hairpin curve, continue straight (west) onto Echo Road for one third of a mile. Then turn left (west) onto the unpaved access road, following the signs to the Mary Jane Falls Trailhead.

FACILITIES/TRAILHEAD Restrooms and information are at the trailhead. Information, water, toilets, and rangers are also available at the Kyle Canyon Visitor Center. There are five campgrounds in the Spring Mountains, offering a total of 143 sites. Two are in Lee Canyon, two are in Kyle Canyon, and one is on Highway 158 between the two canyons. Both first-come, first-served and reservation sites are available. For more information, call (702) 515-5400. Unless otherwise posted, backcountry camping is allowed at least 100 feet from water (although I suggest camping at least 200 feet from water, as recommended by Leave No Trace and the State of Nevada). To protect the ancient bristle-cone pine trees in the Spring Mountains, campfires are prohibited. Permits are required for camping in the Mt. Charleston Wilderness Area (register at trailheads).

From the car, follow the Mary Jane Falls Trail northwest, strolling leisurely through aspen, white fir, ponderosa pine, and mountain mahogany. Soon, you'll meet the split personality of the Mary Jane Falls Trail. After about 0.3 mile, the trail veers to the right (north) and becomes much more difficult, making a series of switchbacks up the steep slope to the falls.

While you're climbing, you'll see why cutting switchbacks is a bad idea. Many people do here, and the hillside has been ravaged, requiring many volunteer hours and taxpayer dollars to maintain. Please help the area remain beautiful by staying on the trail.

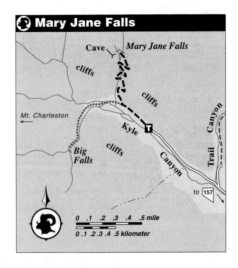

Mary Jane Falls

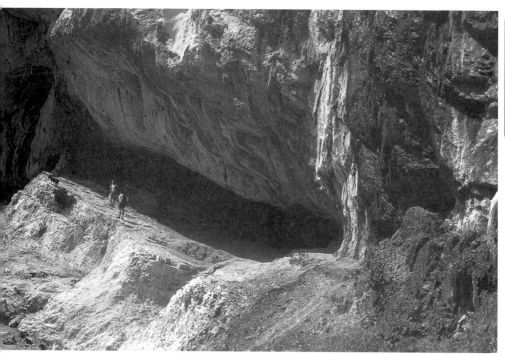

Hikers enjoy the splash and shade of Mary Jane Falls.

The reward for your toil is a refreshing shower under the falls, and beautiful views of Big Falls across the canyon and the twisted limestone layers rising above Big Falls on Mt. Charleston. A cave at the base of the cliff just southwest of Mary Jane Falls is worth the extra scramble to explore. Retrace your steps to return.

trip 24 Spring Mountains: Big Falls

Distance	2 miles, out-and-back
Hiking Time	2 to 3 hours
Elevation	+/-650 feet
Difficulty	Difficult
Trail Use	Leashed dogs
Best Times	Late spring to summer
Agency	U.S. Forest Service Spring Mountains National Recreation Area at (702) 515-5400; www.fs.fed.us/r4/htnf/districts/smnra
Recommended Maps	*Charleston Peak* 7.5-minute
GPS Waypoints	Falls: 36.279° N, 115.671° W
Vehicle	Passenger car OK

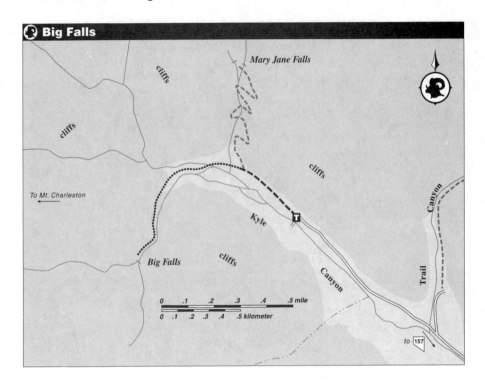

HIGHLIGHTS No signs point to this waterfall, but it is the most spectacular one in the Spring Mountains, and the route through jumbled boulders is fun for experienced hikers. While hundreds of thousands of people hike to nearby Mary Jane Falls, you won't get nearly the crowds here. Most of the Mary Jane hikers are beginners who don't belong boulder-hopping up to Big Falls. Interestingly, if you're fit and agile, getting to Big Falls might take less time than grinding up those switchbacks to Mary Jane. Under your experienced and watchful supervision, this would make a great hike for kids old enough to jump, climb, and scramble. However, please avoid it during thunderstorms, as this area is subject to flash floods.

DIRECTIONS From Las Vegas, take Highway 95 north about 30 minutes to Kyle Canyon Road/Highway 157. Take the exit for 157 west and drive 18.5 miles to the Kyle Canyon Visitor Center. From the visitor center, follow Highway 157 west for 1.8 miles. At the hairpin curve, continue straight (west) onto Echo Road for one third of a mile. Then turn left (west) onto the unpaved access road, following the signs to the Mary Jane Falls Trailhead.

FACILITIES/TRAILHEAD Restrooms and information are at the trailhead. Information, water, toilets, and rangers are also available at the Kyle Canyon Visitor Center. There are five campgrounds in the Spring Mountains, offering a total of 143 sites. Two are in Lee Canyon, two are in Kyle Canyon, and one is on Highway 158 between the two canyons. Both first-come, first-served and reservation sites are available. For more information, call (702) 515-5400. Unless otherwise posted, backcountry camping is allowed at least 100 feet from water (although I suggest camping at least 200 feet from water, as recommended by Leave No Trace and the State of Nevada). To protect the ancient bristlecone pine trees in the Spring Mountains, campfires are prohibited. Permits are required for camping in the Mt. Charleston Wilderness Area (register at trailheads).

This hike heads northwest along the Mary Jane Trail for the first half mile. When the Mary Jane Trail veers right (north) to begin its switchbacks, head left (west) instead and into the wash. There is no sign (to avoid encouraging unfit or unprepared hikers), but a well-used route should lead you diagonally and west across the wash. Your goal is to veer southwest up into Big Falls Canyon, which comes into the main wash about a quarter mile upstream.

Once in Big Falls Canyon, the route becomes harder to follow. The canyon sides are steep, and jumbled boulders in the wash prevent direct, easy hiking. Sometimes, you might be in the wash, and sometimes it's easier to go up the hill to either side, climbing around impassable boulders or steep drops in the wash. The canyon is well-defined, however. Stay in it, and it will lead you directly to the falls.

Once at the falls, you have an opportunity to cool off with a shower and enjoy the steep limestone walls around you before heading back.

In good snow years, this north-facing canyon has snow until late spring. If this is the case, snowshoes are recommended. Or plan to hike during a cool spell, when cold mountain temperatures keep the snowpack hard and easy to walk on. The snow cannot set during warm nights, and sinking up to your thighs with each step quickly stops being fun. If you end up hiking on snow, avoid walking directly above running water, which might have carved out invisible and dangerous holes in the snow underneath you. Retrace your steps to return.

The scramble to Big Falls is not for beginners.

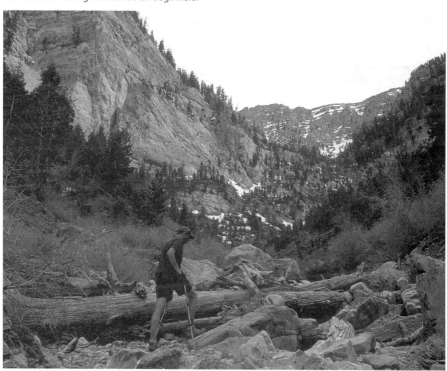

trip 25 Spring Mountains: Cathedral Rock

Distance	2.5 miles, out-and-back
Hiking Time	1 to 2 hours
Elevation	+/-920 feet
Difficulty	Moderate
Trail Use	Leashed dogs, good for kids
Best Times	Late spring to fall
Agency	U.S. Forest Service Spring Mountains National Recreation Area at (702) 515-5400; www.fs.fed.us/r4/htnf/districts/smnra
Recommended Maps	*Charleston Peak 7.5-minute*
GPS Waypoints	Cathedral Rock: 36.254° N, 115.648° W
Vehicle	Passenger car OK

HIGHLIGHTS Rising majestically 1000 vertical feet above the road below, Cathedral Rock offers a wonderful view (and possible vertigo) accessible by a relatively easy hike.

DIRECTIONS From Las Vegas, take Highway 95 north about 30 minutes to Kyle Canyon Road/Highway 157. Take the exit for 157 west and drive 18.5 miles to the Kyle Canyon Visitor Center. From the visitor center, follow Highway 157 west for 2.2 miles, following the hairpin curve to the signed ECHO PICNIC AREA on the right (south). Another trailhead is at Cathedral Rock Picnic Area (fee required) a few hundred yards farther up the road.

FACILITIES/TRAILHEAD Restrooms, picnic area, and information are at the trailhead. Information, water, toilets, and rangers are also available at the Kyle Canyon Visitor Center. There are five campgrounds in the Spring Mountains, offering a total of 143 sites. Two are in Lee Canyon, two are in Kyle Canyon, and one is on Highway 158 between the two canyons. Both first-come, first-served

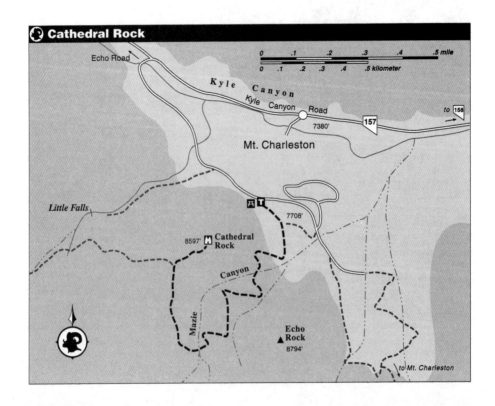

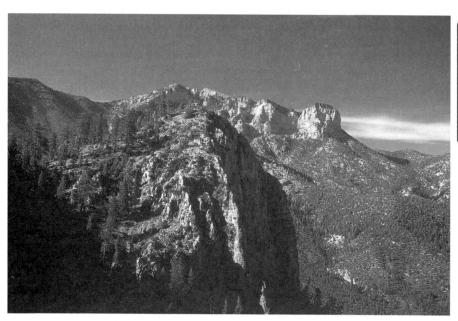

Cathedral Rock stands tall over the town of Mt. Charleston.

and reservation sites are available. For more information, call (702) 515-5400. Unless otherwise posted, backcountry camping is allowed at least 100 feet from water (although I suggest camping at least 200 feet from water, as recommended by Leave No Trace and the State of Nevada). To protect the ancient bristlecone pine trees in the Spring Mountains, campfires are prohibited. Permits are required for camping in the Mt. Charleston Wilderness Area (register at trailheads).

From your car, follow the Cathedral Rock Trail to the left as it climbs clockwise around to the back and top of Cathedral Rock, which rises directly above the parking area. Along the way, the trail passes through pine, fir, and aspen forest. Notice how the middle of Mazie Canyon, which rises to the south of Cathedral Rock, has only very small trees where it has any. Winter avalanches sweep the canyon clean and make sure nothing tall grows.

Near the top of Cathedral Rock, a small waterfall tumbles past the trail during spring snowmelt. The view is wonderful, but the edges are steep and deadly if you get too close. Keep children and dogs close to you.

Please resist feeding the chipmunks in the area. Although they look like any other chipmunk at first glance, they are the endangered Palmer's chipmunk, which live in the Spring Mountains and nowhere else in the world. If they get accustomed to human food, they will lose the motivation to forage for their natural diet during winter and might become extinct.

To protect the ancient bristlecone pine trees in the Spring Mountains, all campfires are prohibited in the Mt. Charleston Wilderness; bring your camp stove. Please follow Leave No Trace principles whenever you travel and camp (see more about trail etiquette, page 18).

Once you have enjoyed the view, retrace your steps to return.

trip 26 Spring Mountains: Mt. Charleston Peak Loop

Distance	18 to 22 miles (depending on specific routes), out-and-back or loop
Hiking Time	A long day or overnight
Elevation	See specific routes below for elevation
Difficulty	Most difficult
Trail Use	Leashed dogs, backpacking option, map and compass
Best Times	Late spring to fall
Agency	U.S. Forest Service Spring Mountains National Recreation Area at (702) 515-5400; www.fs.fed.us/r4/htnf/districts/smnra
Recommended Maps	*Las Vegas* 1:100,000-scale; *Charleston Peak* 7.5-minute
GPS Waypoints	Mt. Charleston peak: 36.271° N, 115.694 ° W
Vehicle	Passenger car OK

HIGHLIGHTS Named after Charleston, South Carolina, by the Dixie general of a mapping team in 1869, Southern Nevada's highest peak is more reminiscent of the Rocky Mountains than the Deep South. And what a great mountain! With its stately forests and soaring limestone cliffs, it's hard to believe Las Vegas is so close. Take a minute to give your respect to a bristlecone pine, many of which are more than 3,000 years old. Look for 500-million-year-old sea fossils along the way, and the wreckage of a crashed plane about a half mile south of the peak. In 1989, the Nevada Wilderness Protection

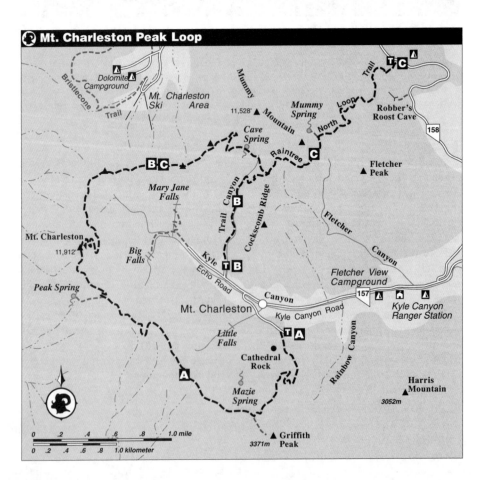

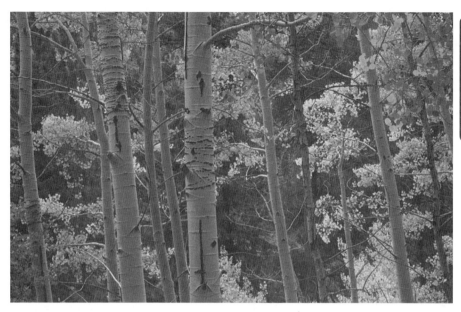

Aspens glow yellow and gold in fall.

Act designated about 43,000 acres of the mountain as the Mt. Charleston Wilderness Area. In 2002, Congress expanded the wilderness to its current 56,600 acres.

DIRECTIONS From Las Vegas, take Highway 95 north about 30 minutes to Kyle Canyon Road/Highway 157. Take the exit for 157 west and drive 18.5 miles to the Kyle Canyon Visitor Center. For directions to the three trailheads that provide access for the Mt. Charleston climb, see the specific routes below.

FACILITIES/TRAILHEAD Information only at the trailhead. Information, water, toilets, and rangers are also available at the Kyle Canyon Visitor Center on Kyle Canyon Road. There are five campgrounds in the Spring Mountains, offering a total of 143 sites. Two are in Lee Canyon, two are in Kyle Canyon, and one is on Highway 158 between the two canyons. Both first-come, first-served and reservation sites are available. For more information, call (702) 515-5400. Unless otherwise posted, backcountry camping is allowed at least 100 feet from water (although I suggest camping at least 200 feet from water, as recommended by Leave No Trace and the State of Nevada). To protect the ancient bristlecone pine trees in the Spring Mountains, campfires are prohibited. Permits are required for camping in the Mt. Charleston Wilderness Area (register at trailheads).

The three trailheads that provide access for a Mt. Charleston peak climb are described below. Whichever you chose, expect the Mt. Charleston high country to be significantly cooler than the Las Vegas Valley. The summit of Mt. Charleston is more than 8000 feet higher than the Strip, and air cools between 3°F and 5°F for every 1000-foot gain in elevation. When I camped there one May, Las Vegas was enjoying overnight lows around 60°F, but I was snuggled in my winter sleeping bag against wind and a low of 26°F on Charles-ton's south summit ridge. Don't forget your warm clothes and wind jacket, not to mention lots of water, food, and good sturdy boots. Cave Spring, 3 miles up from Trail Canyon, is the only water source available along the way, unless snow and runoff are present elsewhere.

As the highest peak in Southern Nevada, Mt. Charleston rewards visitors with incredible views in every direction, from Telescope Peak in Death Valley to the West; past the Nellis Air Force Range and the Desert National Wildlife Range to the Virgin

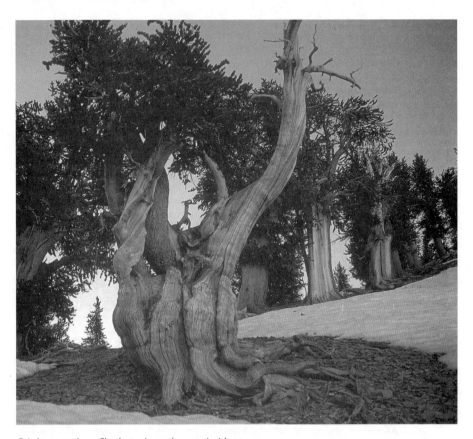

Bristlecones along Charleston's south summit ridge

Mountains to the east; and over the many peaks of the Spring Mountains stretching north and south.

A. South Loop Trail (18 miles, out-and-back; elevation gain/loss of +4640/-400 feet): The trailhead is at the Cathedral Rock Picnic Area (parking fee required). From the Kyle Canyon Visitor Center, follow Highway 157 west (follow the hairpin curve left at 1.8 miles) for 2.2 miles to the picnic area on the right (south). To avoid the fee, park at the Echo Picnic Area, a few hundred yards before the picnic area on the right (south) side of the road, then walk to the trailhead along the road.

The hike begins at the signed SOUTH LOOP TRAILHEAD in the Cathedral Rock Picnic Area. From the car, hike south on the well-maintained South Loop Trail through aspen, mixed conifers, and bristlecone pine trees as it climbs steeply for 3 miles to the summit ridge.

On the summit ridge, you'll find good undeveloped campsites among the bristlecones, if you plan to camp before summiting. Please camp only in established campsites, especially in the meadows. Plants have a hard enough time surviving here. Please avoid trampling them.

And to protect the ancient bristlecone pine trees in the Spring Mountains, all campfires are prohibited in the Mt. Charleston Wilderness; bring your camp stove. Please follow Leave No Trace principles whenever you travel and camp (see more about the trail etiquette, page 18).

Once on the summit ridge, follow the trail along the ridge northwest of the summit about 6 miles farther. Dedicated peak baggers will want to detour south once on the summit ridge to climb Mt. Griffith (11,057 feet), adding a mile to the trip. This detour rewards with soaring views over the southern Spring Mountains toward Mt. Potosi and the Las Vegas Valley.

To return, either retrace your steps or follow the trail as it zigzags down the northeast face and through the incredible scenery of Trail Canyon to either the Trail Canyon or North Loop trailheads (descriptions of these below). The easiest loop back to your car will be via Trail Canyon Trailhead and a 1.5-mile walk to South Loop Trailhead down Echo Road, then right up Kyle Canyon Road.

B. Trail Canyon Trail (18 miles, out-and-back; elevation gain/loss of +4900/-830 feet): This route begins at the Trail Canyon Trailhead. At the hairpin curve on Highway 157, 1.8 miles west of the Kyle Canyon Visitor Center, continue straight (west) onto Echo Road for a half mile to the trailhead on the left (north) side of the road.

From every angle Charleston rewards with beautiful mountain views.

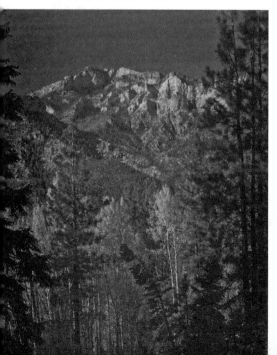

From the car, hike north on the Trail Canyon Trail, admiring the mixed forest of aspen and conifers around you and the sculpted cliffs rising above.

After 2 miles, the Trail Canyon Trail intersects with the North Loop Trail. Turn left (west), following the North Loop Trail through a stunning canyon to the summit of Mt. Charleston. Once on the summit, either retrace your steps to return, or descend via the South Loop Trail (described above), which heads south from the summit, then walk 1.5 miles northwest along the road back to the Trail Canyon Trailhead.

C. North Loop Trail: 24 miles, out-and-back; elevation gain/loss of +5130/-1650 feet): This route begins at the North Loop Trailhead on Deer Creek Road/Highway 158 (between Kyle and Lee canyons). From Las Vegas, take Highway 95 north about 30 minutes to Kyle Canyon Road/Highway 157. Travel west on 157 for about 17 miles to the intersection with Deer Creek Road/Highway 158. Turn right (north) onto 158 and follow it a little less than 5 miles to the signed NORTH LOOP TRAILHEAD on the left (west) side of the road. Deer Creek Road/Highway 158 is 1.5 miles downhill (east) of the visitor center.

To begin, hike west on the North Loop Trail. After 2.7 miles, at Raintree, veer left (southwest), following the North Loop Trail for another 2 miles to the intersection with the Trail Canyon Trail. Veer right (west) and follow the North Loop Trail another 9 miles to the summit of Mt. Charleston.

Despite its name, the North Loop Trail is not recommended as part of a loop hike to the summit of Mt. Charleston. At 12 miles one-way, the distance to the peak is farther than either the Trail Canyon or South Loop trails. It's also several miles from the other trailheads, making for an inconvenient shuttle between them. So once you get to the summit, retrace your steps to return.

Which Route Up Mt. Charleston Is Best?

With its shady aspen, ponderosa, and bristlecone forests, the north-facing South Loop Trail is better for hiking on a warm day, and campsites are numerous along the summit ridge south of the Mt. Charleston summit. The south-facing Trail Canyon Trail has more stunning views and better sun exposure on colder days. However, you'll encounter fewer campsites along the way if you plan to camp on your way up.

Whichever way you choose to hike up, Trail Canyon or South Loop, choose the other to descend, as each is unique and beautiful in its own right. The North Loop Trail route is the longest, and although it's beautiful, I do not recommend making it a loop hike unless you have a car shuttle to the South Loop Trailhead.

trip 27 Spring Mountains: Bonanza Peak

Distance	8 miles, out-and-back
Hiking Time	6 to 8 hours
Elevation	+/-2850 feet
Difficulty	Moderate
Trail Use	Leashed dogs, backpacking option
Best Times	Cool to warm (may have snow in the winter and spring)
Agency	U.S. Forest Service Spring Mountains National Recreation Area at (702) 515-5400; www.fs.fed.us/r4/htnf/districts/smnra
Recommended Maps	*Charleston Peak* 7.5-minute Official U.S. Forest Service and BLM map of the Spring Mountains National Recreation Area and Red Rock Canyon National Conservation Area
GPS Waypoints	Parking/trailhead: 36.382° N, 115.7507° W Bonanza Peak: 36.366° N, 115.7508° W
Vehicle	High-clearance or 4WD vehicle recommended; passenger car OK if you're careful

Storms high in the Spring Mountains can be dangerously cold and wet when it's dry and warm below. Always hike with extra layers.

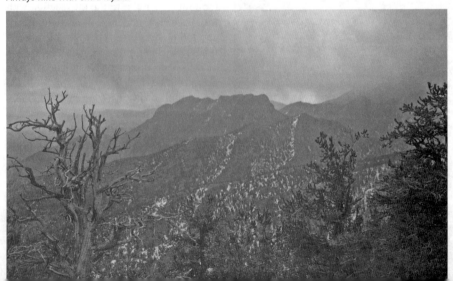

Bonanza Peak

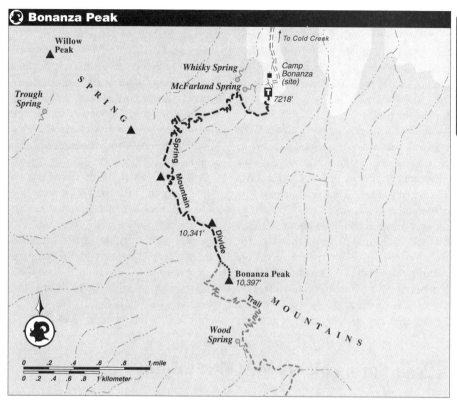

HIGHLIGHTS In a less-crowded corner of the Spring Mountains, the Bonanza Peak Trail offers a challenging hike along a well-defined trail through a mature, beautiful forest in the 57,000-acre Mt. Charleston Wilderness. The majestic views through the bristlecone pine trees along the crest of the range are worth the effort. Watch for elk, bighorn, and deer. Carry all your water, as there is no water along the way.

DIRECTIONS From Las Vegas, drive north on Highway 95, past the exits to Kyle and Lee canyons. About 5 miles north of Lee Canyon, turn left (west), following the sign to Cold Creek (a large correctional facility sits to the left as you make the turn). The trailhead is about 15 miles from U.S. 95. Pass through Cold Creek, following the signs and veering left (south) to the Bonanza Trailhead. At 14 miles, pavement becomes gravel, making your last mile slower and bumpier.

FACILITIES/TRAILHEAD The nearest facilities are at the Snow Mountain Indian Colony, a few miles south of the Lee Canyon exit on U.S. 95 back toward Vegas. There are no campgrounds in Cold Creek, but there are five campgrounds in the Spring Mountains, offering a total of 143 sites. Two are in Lee Canyon, two are in Kyle Canyon, and one is on Highway 158 between the two canyons. Both first-come, first-served and reservation sites are available. For more information, call (702) 515-5400. Unless otherwise posted, backcountry camping is allowed at least 100 feet from water. Permits are required for camping in the Mt. Charleston Wilderness Area (register at trailheads). To protect the ancient bristlecone pine trees in the Spring Mountains, campfires are prohibited in the Mt. Charleston Wilderness; bring your camp stove. Please follow Leave No Trace principles whenever you travel and camp (see more about trail etiquette, page 18).

From the trailhead, follow the trail (also called the Spring Mountain Divide Trail) south then north, back and forth, for 80 switchbacks as it climbs a side ridge to the main north-south crest of the Spring Mountains. Often the trail is on north-facing slopes, where the trail might hide under lingering spring snowdrifts. As you hike, watch the forest change from a mixture of white fir, Jeffrey pine, and mountain mahogany, to noble old-growth Jeffrey pines and finally to bristlecone along the crest. Once at the crest, turn left (south), following the trail another 1.5 miles or so toward the peak.

The last half mile or so is off-trail; the true trail passes just below and west of the peak on its way 10 miles farther south to the Bristlecone Trailhead in Lee Canyon (Trip 17). Bonanza Peak is not prominent, so it's easy to miss. A mile or so south of gaining the crest, watch carefully for unsigned routes (marked by cairns, perhaps) that veer left (southeasterly) from the trail to follow the summit ridge south to the summit. If the trail begins descending steeply as you're hiking south along the crest, you've gone too far. Retrace your steps to the highest point of the

trail, and find the best route up and east to the peak. Retrace your steps to return.

From the peak, enjoy views of the prominent Sheep Range in the Desert National Wildlife Range to the northeast; to the west, across Pahrump to the Funeral Mountains and Death Valley National Park; and to the southeast, look past McFarland Peak to Mummy Mountain with Mount Charleston capping it all.

A nice backpacking option: Continue south along the main trail for a great one-night, point-to-point backpack to Lee Canyon and the Bristlecone Trailhead. This approach would require a car shuttle or a friend to pick you up. Find campsites among the bristlecones along the crest or at Wood Spring (roughly the halfway point), where you might also find water (call the Forest Service first to make sure).

trip 28 Spring Mountains: Mt. Stirling

Distance	5 miles, out-and-back
Hiking Time	5 to 7 hours
Elevation	+/-2065 feet
Difficulty	Difficult
Trail Use	Leashed dogs, map and compass
Best Times	Cool to warm (may have snow in the winter)
Agency	U.S. Forest Service Spring Mountains National Recreation Area at (702) 515-5400; www.fs.fed.us/r4/htnf/districts/smnra
Recommended Maps	*Mt. Stirling* and *Niavi Wash* 7.5-minute Official U.S. Forest Service/BLM map of the Spring Mountains National Recreation Area and Red Rock Canyon National Conservation Area
GPS Waypoints	Parking area and trailhead: 36.478° N, 115.963° W Mt. Stirling summit: 36.453° N, 115.968° W
Vehicle	High-clearance or 4WD vehicle recommended

HIGHLIGHTS Mt. Stirling, the northernmost peak in the Spring Mountains, is a place of rugged beauty, solitude, and mystery. But you must pay for these joys with rough and confusing roads, no distinct trailhead, and the challenge of navigating challenging terrain with no trail. (Long pants and gaiters are recommended). This trip is for experienced desert travelers only. Stirling's summit is part of the 69,650-acre Mt. Stirling Wilderness Study Area (WSA). Once managed by the Bureau of Land Management, a majority of the WSA was transferred to the Forest Service in 1988 and is now part of the Spring Mountains National Recreation Area.

DIRECTIONS From Las Vegas, drive north on Highway 95, past the exits to Kyle and Lee canyons, to the community of Indian Springs. From the west end of Indian Springs, continue 11.2 miles farther on 95, then turn left (south) onto Forest Service Road 553. A small sign on 95 indicates FOREST SERVICE ACCESS. Drive 9 miles, trending south-southwest and following 553 at each intersection (there are

⊘ Mt. Stirling

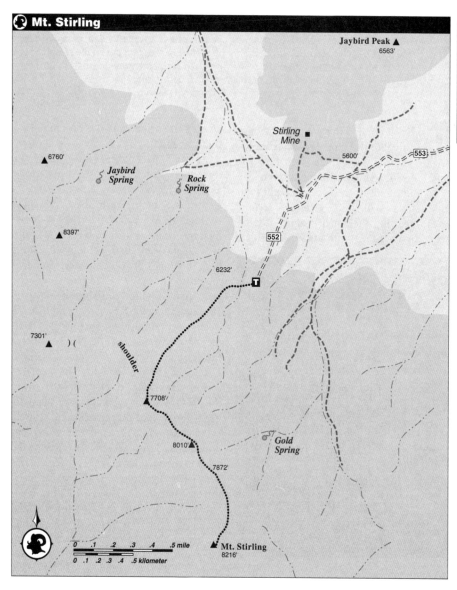

Jaybird Peak ▲
6563'

Stirling
Mine ■

5600'

553

▲6760'

Jaybird
Spring

Rock
Spring

552

▲8397'

6232'

T

7301'
▲) (

shoulder

7708'▲

8010'▲

Gold
Spring

7872'

0   .1   .2   .3   .4   .5 mile

0 .1 .2 .3 .4 .5 kilometer

▲ Mt. Stirling
8216'

many routes and forks in this country, but most are signed). Landmarks include a small power line at 0.9 mile and the signed national forest boundary at 5 miles. The route follows the drainage east then south of 6563-foot Jaybird Peak.

At 8.4 miles, Route 553 crests the ridge east then south of Jaybird and seems to end at an intersection where several signed routes come together. Continue southwest for another half mile on 552 to a parking area at the base of a small ridge, which climbs south toward the main ridge. You cannot see the summit from the parking area, because it's hiding a half mile beyond the high point on the ridge to your south.

FACILITIES/TRAILHEAD The nearest facilities are in Indian Springs on U.S. 95. There are five campgrounds in the Spring Mountains, offering a total of 143 sites. Two are in Lee Canyon, two are in Kyle Canyon, and one is on Highway 158 between the two canyons. Both first-come, first-served and reservation sites are available. For more information, call (702) 515-5400. Unless otherwise posted, backcountry camping is allowed at least 100 feet from water (I suggest camping at least 200 feet from water, as recommended by Leave No Trace and the State of Nevada, to leave room for wildlife to get to this life-giving resource). Campfires may be prohibited, depending on the season. Please do not touch rock art, because the oil from your skin can damage the stone's desert varnish. Please follow Leave No Trace principles whenever you travel and camp in the desert.

There is no trail to the summit of Mount Stirling, but the route is simple: southwest up to the main ridge, then turn left and follow it southeast to the summit. The ridge due south of the car is difficult with thick shrubs and rocky sections. I recommend crossing the small drainage to the west, then heading south up the next ridge, where a fire some years ago cleared out the thick shrubs.

As you hike, notice geology changing underfoot, with granite, shale, limestone, and quartzite all making an appearance (a good reason, perhaps, why there's mining in the region). Also notice the relic ponderosa pine trees once you climb higher. Attentive eyes might even find petroglyphs dating back thousands of years. Retrace your steps to return.

From the summit, you'll have a wonderful view south into the Spring Mountains, and a clear view northeast into the restricted territory of the Nevada Test Site, Nellis Air Force Range, and toward the infamous Groom Lake/Area 51/Dreamland. That not-so-secret, super-secret military base is where the UFO and alien bodies have allegedly been stored since they crashed in Roswell, New Mexico, in 1947, and where the government is allegedly reverse-engineering the UFO to enhance our military capacities. Less controversially, Area 51 is also where many military aircraft, such as the U2, the SR-71, and Stealth Bombers, have been tested and designed. That view has made Mt. Stirling a popular destination for camouflage-clad UFO and military-conspiracy theorists. Or perhaps it's the beautiful views and lonely terrain that draws them.

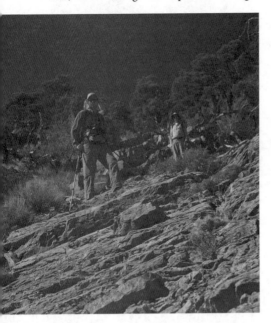

Hiking steeply up toward Stirling summit ridge

trip 29 # Spring Mountains: Wheeler Wash

Distance	Up to 5 miles, out-and-back
Hiking Time	2 to 6 hours
Elevation	+/-700 feet
Difficulty	Moderate
Trail Use	Leashed dogs, backpacking option, map and compass
Best Times	Cold to warm
Agency	U.S. Forest Service Spring Mountains National Recreation Area at (702) 515-5400; www.fs.fed.us/r4/htnf/districts/smnra
Recommended Maps	*Las Vegas* 1:100,000; *Wheeler Well* 7.5-minute
GPS Waypoints	Ovens: 36.346° N, 115.828° W
	Peak 8216: 36.361° N, 115.862° W
Vehicle	High-clearance or 4WD vehicle recommended

HIGHLIGHTS On the west slope of the Spring Mountains, you'll find solitude, forests, and some darn big ovens once used to make charcoal that fired an ore smelter near Death Valley. Remember your map and compass, as there is no trail, and hiking through the pinyon-juniper forests in these rolling hills requires focused attention on navigation. This area is part of the 69,650-acre Mt. Stirling Wilderness Study Area—it meets the criteria for wilderness designation set forth by Congress, but it's still waiting for Congress to designate it a wilderness area.

DIRECTIONS From Las Vegas, take Highway 160 west about an hour to Pahrump. Turn right (east) onto Wheeler Pass Road and follow it about 10.5 miles to an intersection, where a sign indicates a left turn to Wheeler Pass. (There are many unofficial vehicle routes and tracks entering and leaving Wheeler Pass Road. Try to stay on the main road, and don't get too upset if you take a wrong turn—it's all part of the adventure.) Turn left (north) onto an unmaintained jeep track and continue past towering rock formations toward Wheeler Pass for about 4.5 miles to the large, beehive-shaped charcoal ovens to your left (west). There is no sign and no official trailhead. Park here.

FACILITIES/TRAILHEAD The nearest facilities are in Pahrump. There are five campgrounds in the Spring Mountains, offering a total of 143 sites. Two are in Lee Canyon, two are in Kyle Canyon, and

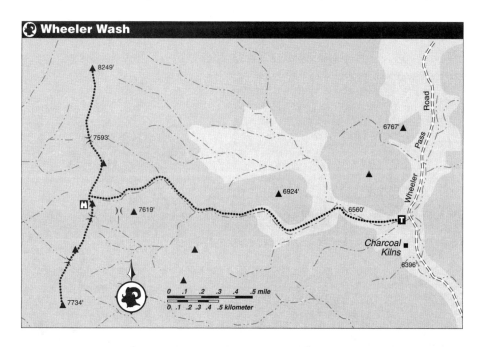

one is on Highway 158 between the two canyons. Both first-come, first-served and reservation sites are available. There are no designated campsites on the west side of the Spring Mountains, near Wheeler Wash. For more information, call (702) 515-5400. Unless otherwise posted, backcountry camping is allowed at least 100 feet from water (although I suggest camping at least 200 feet from water, as recommended by Leave No Trace and the State of Nevada). Campfires may be prohibited, depending on the season. Permits are required for camping in the Mt. Charleston Wilderness Area (register at trailheads).

Before leaving on your hike, explore the charcoal ovens built here in 1875 to reduce pinyon and juniper trees to charcoal, which in turn fired an ore smelter in Tecopa, about 60 miles away near Death Valley. They were based on the design of the Roman arch, with delicately angled bricks that support each other. Without interference, they could stand on their own for centuries. Unfortunately, vandals have decided otherwise, and the ovens have been fenced to protect them from further destruction. (The forest, on the other hand, has recovered nicely.) The Forest Service is always looking for volunteers to help rebuild and maintain them. Call the number above if you're interested.

To begin your hike, head due west into the hills through thick pinyon and juniper forest. There is no trail, and the only true destinations are nice views and solitude. The drainages climbing westerly from the ovens provide nice routes that climb about 2 miles to a ridge at about 7600 feet. From here, you can follow the ridgeline south to Peak 7734, or hike north to Peak 8249 and beyond.

In these thickly forested, rolling mountains, you can find excellent opportunities to leave it all behind. Sitting here among this solitude, it's hard to imagine the fastest-growing metropolitan area in the U.S. is only 30 miles away as the crow flies.

Here and there along the ridgelines you'll find inviting spots to camp. If you are backpacking, please do not build campfires. This forest has been waiting for an excuse to burn for decades. You don't want to be the one to start the "big one." If you need to cook, please use your camp stove.

When you've had your fill of solitude, retrace your steps to return.

The western slopes of the Spring Mountains are less visited and developed than the east.

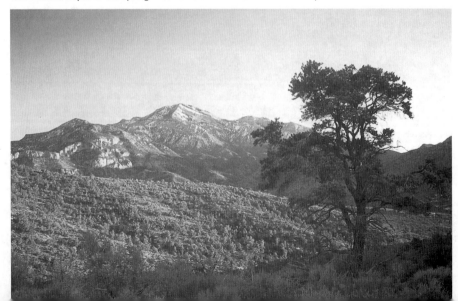

trip 30 ## Ash Meadows National Wildlife Refuge

Distance	Several short trails less than a mile each, out-and-back
Hiking Time	Varies
Elevation	2200 feet
Difficulty	Easy
Trail Use	Leashed dogs, good for kids
Best Times	Cold to warm (rare plants bloom between August and September; birds migrate between spring and fall)
Agency	U.S. Fish and Wildlife Service at (775) 372-5435; www.desertcomplex.fws.gov
Recommended Maps	Free maps available at the refuge headquarters and information kiosks in the refuge
GPS Waypoints	Headquarters: 36.253° N, 116.205° W
Vehicle	Passenger car OK

HIGHLIGHTS This ancient and beautiful oasis is home to 24 species found nowhere else on Earth. Highlights of the refuge include Point of Rocks Springs, Crystal Reservoir, Peterson Reservoir, the refuge headquarters, and Crystal Springs Boardwalk interpretive trail and Devil's Hole, which are managed by Death Valley National Park. These and other sites offer opportunities for walking, nature viewing, and picnics in the shade. Each is a short drive from the others.

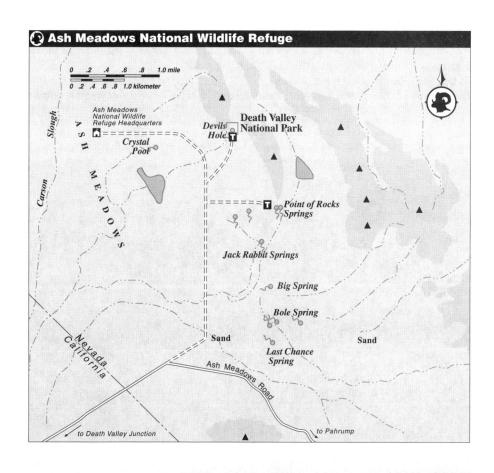

DIRECTIONS From Las Vegas, take Highway 160 west over Mountain Pass, approximately 60 miles to Pahrump. A few miles north of the main part of town, turn left (west) onto Bell Vista Road, which leads through neighborhoods and into the hills west of town. It eventually turns into Ash Meadows Road and leads to the refuge, which is on the right (north) side of the road. All roads on the refuge are unpaved but graded and OK for passenger cars. However, they may be impassable during storms. Call the refuge for current conditions.

FACILITIES/TRAILHEAD Water, restrooms, rangers, and information are available at the refuge headquarters.

In the arid Mojave Desert, water is life, and in the oasis of Ash Meadows National Wildlife Refuge, life takes rare, beautiful, and unique forms.

The 22,000-acre refuge protects spring-fed wetlands, dunes, and uplands habitat, which are home to at least 24 plant and animal species that are endemic to Southern Nevada.

Of the endemic species, 13 are listed as threatened or endangered, giving Ash Meadows a greater concentration of unique species than any other place in the U.S.

The water comes from deep aquifers that stretch for 100 miles to the northeast, coming to the surface with roughly 10,000 gallons per minute at seven major springs. Lesser flows bubble up through more than 20 smaller springs and seeps. The water here is ancient, believed to have entered the aquifers thousands of years ago. Tall reeds and groves of mesquite and ash trees provide shade for the springs in hot weather.

The four endangered species found on the refuge are all fish: the Devil's Hole pupfish, the Ash Meadows Amargosa pupfish, the Warm Springs pupfish, and the Ash Meadows speckled dace. Threatened species include one beetle, the Ash Meadows naucorid, and six plants: Ash Meadows milkvetch, spring-loving centaury plant, Ash Meadows sunray, Ash Meadows ivesia, Ash Meadows gumplant, and Ash Meadows blazing star.

Birders will be happy to know that a few pairs of endangered southwestern willow

An ancient, mysterious underground aquifer bubbles forth at Ash Meadows.

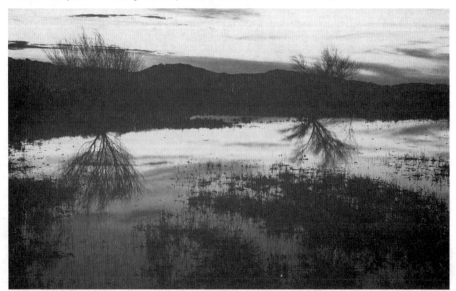

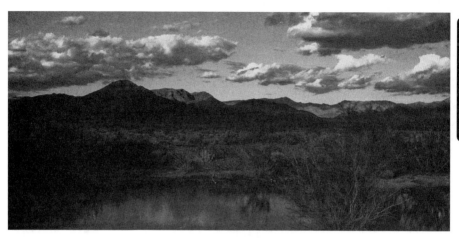

Isolated springs like those at Ash Meadows are hot spots for rare desert life.

flycatchers breed in the refuge between June and August each year. Peregrine falcons and bald eagles also stop by Ash Meadows during migration.

In the 1960s, areas of the refuge were drained and mined for peat, while water courses were altered to provide irrigation for agriculture. Refuge employees and volunteers are working to restore the habitats of Ash Meadows, returning waterways to their natural channels and removing introduced species such as crayfish and salt

cedar trees. This work and planned trail and interpretive additions mean the refuge will improve and change over the years.

Although the unique species at Ash Meadows have survived here for thousands of years and are protected by federal laws, their futures remain uncertain. As Nevada's population continues to grow, some experts fear groundwater pumping throughout the state will dry up the springs at Ash Meadows, threatening the small fish and plants that depend on them.

trip 31 **Death Valley: Grapevine Peak**

Distance	6 miles, out-and-back
Hiking Time	2 to 4 hours
Elevation	+/-2500 feet
Difficulty	Moderate
Trail Use	Backpacking option, map and compass
Best Times	Cool to hot
Agency	Death Valley National Park at (760) 786-3200; www.nps.gov/deva
Recommended Maps	*Trails Illustrated Death Valley* (#221)
GPS Waypoints	Top of Phinney Canyon: 36.954° N, 117.122° W
	Grapevine Peak: 36.965° N, 117.149° W
Vehicle	High-clearance or 4WD vehicle recommended

HIGHLIGHTS Grapevine Peak is part of the Nevada Triangle of Death Valley National Park and within the 44,000 acres of Nevada wilderness designated by the 1994 California Desert Protection Act. The view from the summit is a knockout, stretching west across Death Valley, the Cottonwood Mountains, the Saline Range, the Inyo Mountains, and all the way to the Sierra Nevada. On a climb of the peak in April, I was once met with snow, rain, and whiteout conditions, reminding me that views are never guaranteed, and that plastic maps, map-and-compass skills, and extra clothing layers are good things to have along in every season.

DIRECTIONS Although Grapevine Peak is in Death Valley National Park, access is not through the main part of the park. The only national park facility en route is the Death Valley Visitor Center in Beatty. Take Highway 95 north from Las Vegas for 115 miles to Beatty. To stop at the Death Valley Visitor Center in Beatty, turn left on Main Street and drive a quarter mile. Gas up in Beatty, then continue north on 95 for another 13.7 miles to an unsigned dirt road. Turn left (west), pass through the gate (close it behind you), then continue west past the power line and soon into the boundary of Death Valley National Park. About 12 miles from 95, veer right (north) at the fork toward Phinney Canyon. After 16 miles, the road drops into a wash. At 20 miles, about a mile before the road's summit, the road becomes too difficult for all but the hardiest high-clearance 4WD vehicles. Park before the road gets too rough, then follow the directions below to Grapevine Peak.

FACILITIES/TRAILHEAD The nearest facilities are in Beatty. Developed campsites are available at Mesquite Spring, 3 miles west of Scotty's Castle (30 sites); Stovepipe Wells (two campgrounds with a total of 204 sites); and Furnace Creek (three campgrounds with a total of 1,228 sites). Reservations are recommended for Furnace Creek Campground in the winter. Call (800) 365-2267 for reservations. Backcountry camping is allowed 2 miles away from developed areas, paved roads, day-use areas, and roadways. Please camp only on previously disturbed areas to minimize impact.

From your car, hike up the road another mile or so, into designated wilderness and to the 7500-foot saddle. From the saddle, follow the closed vehicle route northwest, then southwest as it drops into the next valley. About a quarter mile west of the saddle, at the northernmost point of the road, turn right (north) and climb about a half mile off-road to the top of the ridge. There is no trail. At the top of the ridge,

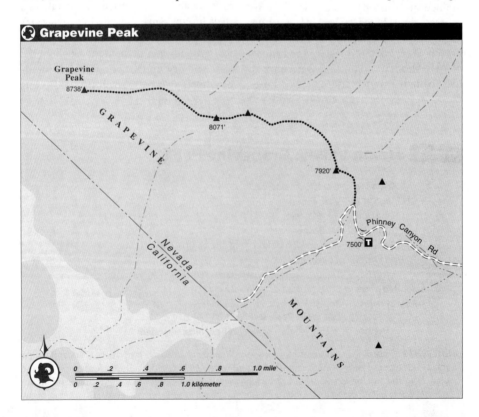

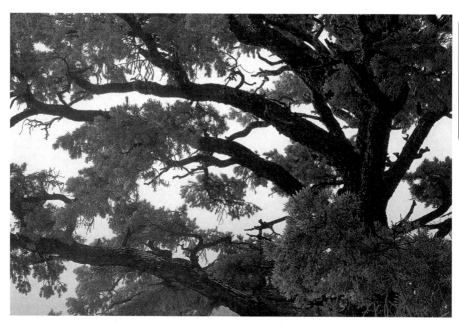

The noble pinyon pines on Grapevine Peak are rare elsewhere in the national park.

turn left (west) and follow the ridgeline to the top of Grapevine Peak.

If you're expecting dry and desolate Death Valley National Park, you'll be surprised on your approach to Grapevine Peak. Yucca and Joshua trees on the lower slopes give way to sagebrush, bitterbrush, pinyon, juniper, and ephedra as you climb higher into the mountains. As you approach the peak, keep your eyes open for pinyon pines that are grander and larger than most you'll encounter in Nevada.

Retrace your steps to return.

trip 32 Death Valley: Titus Canyon

Distance	6 miles or longer, out-and-back (from west to east)
Hiking Time	1 to 4 hours
Elevation	+6562/-5395 feet (for the drive); +/-1500 feet (for a 6-mile hike)
Difficulty	Moderate
Trail Use	Good for kids
Best Times	Cool to warm
Agency	Death Valley National Park at (760) 786-3200; www.nps.gov/deva
Recommended Maps	*Trails Illustrated Death Valley* (#221)
GPS Waypoints	Red Pass: 36.828° N, 117.032° W
	Titus Mouth Trailhead: 36.821° N, 117.173° W
Vehicle	High-clearance or 4WD vehicle recommended

HIGHLIGHTS This classic 4WD (or two-foot!) canyon should sit near the top of your must-see list. Named after Morris Titus, a prospector who disappeared in this area in 1906, Titus Canyon offers fun driving (or hiking), beautiful scenery, and extraordinary geology. From Red Pass, the Titus Canyon

Titus Canyon

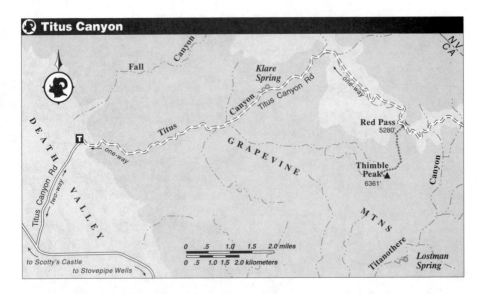

Road drops a vertical mile, at times winding through passages hundreds of feet deep but barely wide enough for your vehicle. Check with Death Valley rangers before driving this route, as it's often closed because of snow, mud, or flash floods. *Do not enter the canyon if thunderstorms threaten.*

DIRECTIONS Take Highway 95 north from Las Vegas for 115 miles to Beatty and stock up on gas and supplies. Turn left (west) on Main Street (Highway 374).

For the Titus Canyon Drive, continue west for 6 miles on Highway 374 to the Titus Canyon turnoff on the right (north). This is where the one-way, 26-mile Titus Canyon Road begins.

For the hike, drive 25 miles west from Beatty on 374 into Death Valley National Park, then turn right (north) toward Scotty's Castle and continue for 14 miles. Then turn right (east) onto Titus Canyon Road, which climbs 2.7 miles to the signed trailhead.

FACILITIES/TRAILHEAD The nearest facilities are in Beatty. No camping is allowed along the 26-mile Titus Canyon Road. Developed campsites are available at Mesquite Spring, 3 miles west of Scotty's Castle (30 sites); Stovepipe Wells (two campgrounds with a total of 204 sites); and Furnace Creek (three campgrounds with a total of 1,228 sites). Reservations are recommended for Furnace Creek Campground in the winter. Call (800) 365-2267 for reservations. Backcountry camping is allowed 2 miles away from developed areas, paved roads, day-use areas, and roadways. Please camp only on previously disturbed areas to minimize impact.

If you are hiking from the western mouth of Titus Canyon, head east from your car, following the road into the canyon. Watch for cars coming west down the canyon. The geology is fascinating along the way, but the sand and gravel are deep, making for slow hiking. Once you have traveled as far as you like, retrace your steps to return to your car, then drive west back down to Scotty's Castle.

If you are driving Titus Canyon Road, follow it from the turnoff (6 miles west of Beatty on Highway 374) for 26 miles to its end at the canyon mouth in Death Valley. At 12 miles, you reach Red Pass, the high point of your drive and the trailhead for Thimble Peak. After Red Pass, the road drops, twists, and turns until it spills out onto the top of an alluvial fan in Death Valley.

About 2.5 miles west of Red Pass, a sign on the left (south) of the road indicates the remains of Leadfield, one of the great investor scams of the early 20th century. In March 1926, promoter C. C. Julian claimed riches would flow from this district. Already under investigation for fraud in California, Julian lured 300 people to this beautiful but mineral-poor site. They built a post office and began digging for riches. Eight months later, with nothing to show for all the hard work, the people left, the post office closed, and Leadfield became a ghost town. Julian allegedly fled to Singapore to escape punishment.

At Klare Spring, 5 miles from Red Pass, you'll see a sign about native petroglyphs on the rocks. Unfortunately, the Klare petroglyphs by the road have fallen victim to easy vehicle access and low IQs. It's hard to distinguish the petroglyphs through all the graffiti. Now that these ancient and priceless clues to our past are destroyed, current and future generations will never get to experience them.

Bighorn sheep often drink from Klare Spring, so keep your eyes peeled and consider yourself lucky if you catch a glimpse of these noble and agile local residents.

In lower Titus Canyon (the end of the drive, but the beginning of the hike), rocks in the walls range from layered limestone to jumbled, jigsaw-puzzle conglomerates—all of which have been thrust up, broken, bent, shattered, and reconfigured by Earth's powerful dynamic forces.

If you're ready to explore more canyon wonders, a hiking trail heads north from the parking area at the mouth of Titus (at the end of the drive) and leads 3 miles into more beautiful formations in Fall Canyon, which parallels Titus to the north.

The admirable architecture of Scotty's Castle

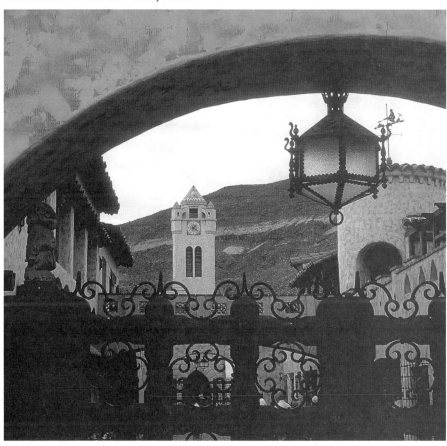

trip 33 Death Valley: Thimble Peak

Distance	3.5 miles, out-and-back
Hiking Time	2 to 4 hours
Elevation	+/-1325 feet
Difficulty	Difficult
Trail Use	Map and compass
Best Times	Cool to warm
Agency	Death Valley National Park at (760) 786-3200; www.nps.gov/deva
Recommended Maps	*Trails Illustrated Death Valley* (#221); *Thimble Peak* 7.5-minute
GPS Waypoints	Red Pass: 36.828° N, 117.032° W
	Thimble Peak: 36.811° N, 117.040° W
Vehicle	High-clearance or 4WD vehicle recommended

HIGHLIGHTS This short, steep hike from Titus Canyon leads to soaring views over the Amargosa Range and Death Valley. Thimble Peak is also near the boundary between Great Basin plant communities to the north and Mojave Desert plants to the south, so take note of the changing biodiversity on your hike. Because the road through Titus Canyon is one-way, east to west, it is necessary to drive the entire 26 miles to do this hike.

DIRECTIONS Take Highway 95 north from Las Vegas for 115 miles to Beatty and stock up on gas and supplies. Turn left (west) on Main Street/Highway 374 and continue 6 miles to the Titus Canyon turnoff on the right (north). Drive 12 miles to Red Pass, the unsigned trailhead for Thimble Peak. Park well off the road.

FACILITIES/TRAILHEAD The nearest facilities are in Beatty. No camping is allowed along 26-mile Titus Canyon Road. Developed campsites are available at Mesquite Spring, 3 miles west of Scotty's Castle (30 sites); Stovepipe Wells (two campgrounds with a total of 204 sites); and Furnace Creek (three campgrounds with a total of 1,228 sites). Reservations are recommended for Furnace Creek Campground in the winter. Call (800) 365-2267 for reservations. Undeveloped backcountry camping is allowed 2 miles away from developed areas, paved roads, day-use areas, and roadways. Please camp only on previously disturbed areas to minimize impact.

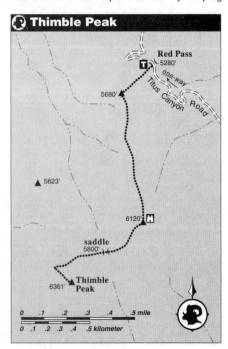

From the car, climb cross-country due south up the ridge for about a mile to point 6120 and incredible views over Titanothere Canyon to the south and into Death Valley. Hiking to this point is moderate, and a faint climbers' route guides the way. It's a good destination for those who want views without the more difficult scramble from here to Thimble Peak, which rises prominently to the southwest.

To continue to Thimble Peak, hike down southwest and across the low saddle, then climb across the northern face of Thimble, aiming for one of several navigable notches on Thimble's northwest ridge. Once on the ridge, turn left for a manageable scramble to the summit.

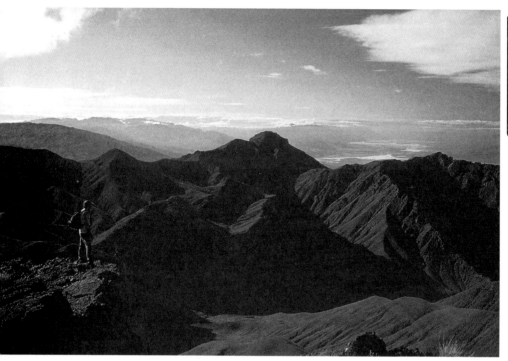

The halfway point to Thimble Peak offers accessible views to those who can't make the final steep push up it.

Although it's not the tallest peak in Death Valley National Park, Thimble is prominent in its profile, visible as a striking knob from places such as Stovepipe Wells. Its vertical southern face is made of banded limestone layers formed 240 million to 500 million years ago at the bottom of the sea. Between 240 million and 60 million years ago, the Pacific and North American continental plates began colliding, pushing up mountain ranges like the Sierra to the west.

About 30 million years ago, the plates shifted direction and began to slide past each other, stretching apart the crust between the Sierra Nevada and the Colorado Plateau. Mountain blocks lifted, creating the Grapevine Mountains, where Thimble is located.

The valleys between dropped and filled with gravel and debris washed down from the mountains. If the gravel had not filled in, Death Valley would be 5000 to 8000 feet deeper.

Thimble Peak is near the boundary between Great Basin plant communities to the north and Mojave Desert plants to the south. Look north from Thimble to see pinyon pine, juniper, and sage-covered slopes of Grapevine and Wahguyhe peaks. On Thimble itself, look for Great Basin plants that give way to the blackbrush scrub community of the Mojave. And don't forget to look at the views.

Once you've taken it all in, retrace your steps to return.

trip 34 Death Valley: Stovepipe Wells Sand Dunes

Distance	2 miles (to highest summit), out-and-back
Hiking Time	Varies
Elevation	+/-140 feet
Difficulty	Moderate
Trail Use	Good for kids, map and compass
Best Times	Cool to warm
Agency	Death Valley National Park at (760) 786-3200; www.nps.gov/deva
Recommended Maps	*Trails Illustrated Death Valley* (#221)
GPS Waypoints	Highest dune: 36.619° N, 117.113° W
Vehicle	Passenger car OK

HIGHLIGHTS Pack a picnic, strike your best Lawrence of Arabia pose, and spend a few hours exploring these shifting sand dunes in the heart of the largest national park in the Lower 48. The soft lines
of the dunes contrast beautifully with the rugged mountains ringing Death Valley. Their summits
provide a nice view of this immense landscape. Early morning and late afternoon light stretch their
shadows into a spectacular show. A full moon's even nicer.

DIRECTIONS From Las Vegas, take Highway 160 west about 60 miles to Pahrump. On the north side of
town (about 3 miles north of the light at Basin Road), turn left (west) onto Bell Vista Road and follow
it about 25 miles to Death Valley Junction. Turn right (north) onto Highway 127 for 0.2 mile, then left
(west) onto Highway 190 for about 28 miles to Furnace Creek. Continue north on 190 from Furnace
Creek for 19 miles, then turn left (west), following 190 for 7 miles to the dunes, which are 2 miles east
of Stovepipe Wells, on the north side of the road. Park along the side of the road, but make sure you
pull well off the pavement.

FACILITIES/TRAILHEAD The nearest facilities are at Stovepipe Wells, 2 miles west on Highway 190.
Developed campsites are available at Mesquite Spring, 3 miles west of Scotty's Castle (30 sites);
Stovepipe Wells (two campgrounds with a total of 204 sites); and Furnace Creek (three campgrounds
with a total of 1,228 sites). Reservations are recommended for Furnace Creek Campground in the
winter. Call (800) 365-2267 for reservations. Undeveloped backcountry camping is allowed 2 miles
away from developed areas, paved roads, day-use areas, and roadways. Please camp only on previously disturbed areas to minimize impact.

From your car, hike due north into the dune field. Remember that progress is slow in soft, deep sand. Expect to take longer hiking than you normally would on solid ground.

There's plenty here to explore: Cover-
ing 14 square miles, the Stovepipe Wells Sand Dunes rise 120 feet above the valley floor. As you hike, look for other tracks in the sand. If the wind or other humans haven't destroyed the tracks, you might be

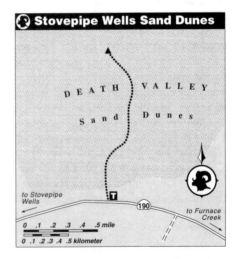

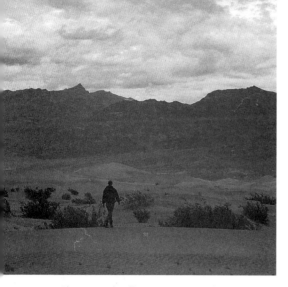

able to see evidence of coyotes, kit foxes, kangaroo rats, beetles, rabbits, lizards, and ravens. You're most likely to see the animals at dawn or dusk, if there aren't too many people causing a ruckus.

There is no trail, but a decent sense of direction should direct you back south to the road and your car if you're careful.

Please avoid walking on sensitive plants while exploring the dunes.

trip 35 Death Valley: Mosaic Canyon

Distance	Up to 5 miles, out-and-back
Hiking Time	30 minutes to 3 hours
Elevation	+/-2000 feet
Difficulty	Moderate
Trail Use	Good for kids
Best Times	Cool to warm
Agency	Death Valley National Park at (760) 786-3200; www.nps.gov/deva
Recommended Maps	*Trails Illustrated Death Valley* (#221)
GPS Waypoints	Canyon entrance: 36.570° N, 117.143° W
Vehicle	Passenger car OK

HIGHLIGHTS Mosaic Canyon is a wonderful trail for the whole family because the attractions begin almost immediately out of the parking lot. Look on the ground as you hike the first steps toward the mouth of the canyon. You'll notice breccia composed of sharp chunks of marble encased in a natural cement of minerals, then polished smooth by eons of flash floods and millions of tourist feet. However, this is **not** the place to be in a flash flood. *When thunderstorms are active anywhere in the region, hike somewhere else.*

DIRECTIONS From Las Vegas, take Highway 160 west about 60 miles to Pahrump. On the north side of town (about 3 miles north of the light at Basin Road), turn left (west) onto Bell Vista Road and follow it about 25 miles to Death Valley Junction. Turn right (north) onto Highway 127 for 0.2 mile, then left (west) onto Highway 190 for about 28 miles to Furnace Creek. Continue north on 190 from Furnace Creek for 19 miles, then turn left (west), following 190 for 9 miles to Stovepipe Wells. From Stovepipe Wells, drive 0.15 mile west to signed MOSAIC CANYON ROAD. Turn left (south) and drive 2 miles to the trailhead on the north slope of Tucki Mountain.

FACILITIES/TRAILHEAD The nearest facilities are 2.15 miles from the trailhead at Stovepipe Wells. Developed campsites are available at Mesquite Spring, 3 miles west of Scotty's Castle (30 sites); Stovepipe Wells (two campgrounds with a total of 204 sites); and Furnace Creek (three campgrounds with a total of 1,228 sites). Reservations are recommended for Furnace Creek Campground in the winter. Call (800) 365-2267 for reservations. Undeveloped backcountry camping is allowed 2 miles away from developed areas, paved roads, day-use areas, and roadways. Please camp only on previously disturbed areas to minimize impact.

The trail leads south up the wash and into Mosaic Canyon, which twists and turns as a narrow slot south and then east. As soon as you enter the canyon, you'll discover its treasures. You'll find yourself following a narrow slot of beautifully polished marble. The rocks around you began as many as 900 million years ago as sediments settling at the bottom of the sea. Buried deeper and deeper by additional sediments, the rock ended up deep within the Earth, where extreme heat and pressure metamorphosed it into marble.

After a quarter mile, the canyon widens and veers south toward the heart of Tucki Mountain, formed when continental plates crashed together. Cracks in the rock allowed water to seep through, eventually carving out this narrow twisting canyon. Along the way, look for walls of conglomerate, where ages-old, storm-washed rubble piled high, only to be eroded away again, leaving walls decorated with embedded rocks of all shapes, colors, and sizes.

About 1.2 miles from the trailhead, the canyon narrows again. When you reach the point where the canyon is blocked by rockfall, look for a route to scramble up to the left (east). More scrambling over smooth rock is necessary to continue farther, until travel is blocked by a 30-foot waterfall.

Retrace your steps to return.

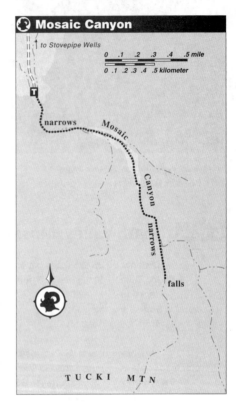

trip 36 Death Valley: Telescope Peak

Distance	12 miles, out-and-back
Hiking Time	Long day or overnight
Elevation	+/-3200 feet
Difficulty	Moderate to difficult
Trail Use	Backpacking option
Best Times	May or June until the first snow in fall
Agency	Death Valley National Park at (760) 786-3200; www.nps.gov/deva
Recommended Maps	*Trails Illustrated Death Valley* (#221)
GPS Waypoints	Trailhead: 36.230° N, 117.068° W
	Peak: 36.369° N, 117.089° W
Vehicle	High-clearance recommended
Note	Water is unavailable on this hike. Carry all you'll need (at least 1 gallon per person per day).

HIGHLIGHTS Although farther than my "couple hours' drive from Vegas" rule, the hike up Telescope Peak is such a classic, rewarding hike that it's worth the extra hour's drive. Rising to 11,049 feet, Telescope Peak is the highest point of the Panamint Range, and the tallest peak in Death Valley. It offers amazing views that stretch from Mt. Charleston to the High Sierra and across Death Valley National Park. Ancient bristlecone pine trees provide stately company on the highest reaches of the peak.

DIRECTIONS From Las Vegas, take Highway 160 west about 60 miles to Pahrump. On the north side of town (about 3 miles north of the stoplight at Basin Road), turn left (west) onto Bell Vista Road and follow it about 25 miles to Death Valley Junction. Turn right (north) onto Highway 127, then quickly left (west) onto Highway 190 for about 28 miles to Furnace Creek. Continue north on 190 from Furnace Creek for 19 miles, then turn left (west), following 190 for 9 miles to Stovepipe Wells. From Stovepipe Wells, drive 11 miles west, then turn left (south) on the Emigrant Canyon Road and follow it 21 miles to the Wildrose Canyon Road. Turn left (east) and drive 7 miles to the Wildrose Charcoal Kilns.

At this point, the road becomes steep and rough for the final 2 miles to the trailhead. High-clearance 4WD is now recommended, but careful negotiation with a passenger car might be possible, depending on road conditions, your vehicle's clearance, and your driving skills. If you're in a passenger car and can't make the final mile, you can park or camp at Thorndike Campground, a mile from the trailhead, and hike from there.

The view of the rugged canyons of the Panamint Range reward those who reach Telescope's summit.

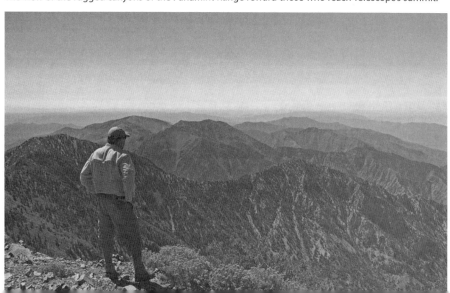

Telescope Peak

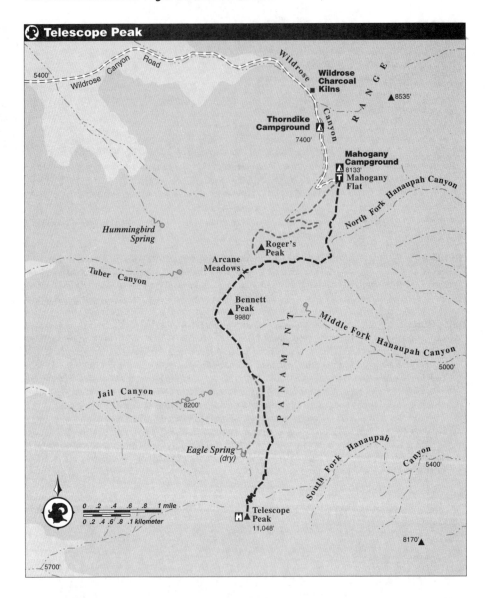

FACILITIES/TRAILHEAD The trailhead is at Mahogany Flat Campground, which doesn't have water but offers pit toilets, fire pits, and picnic tables. Thorndike Campground offers similar accommodations. Wildrose (9 miles from the trailhead) offers 30 sites and water from April through November. Emigrant Campground (11 miles west of Stovepipe Wells) has water and 10 sites. The nearest full facilities are 41 miles from the trailhead at Stovepipe Wells. Other campgrounds in Death Valley are at Mesquite Spring, 3 miles west of Scotty's Castle (30 sites); Stovepipe Wells (two campgrounds with a total of 204 sites); and Furnace Creek (three campgrounds with a total of 1,228 sites). Reservations are recommended for Furnace Creek Campground in the winter. Call (800) 365-2267 for reservations. Undeveloped backcountry camping is allowed 2 miles away from developed areas, paved roads, day-use areas, and roadways. Please camp only on previously disturbed areas to minimize impact.

Thanks to the adiabatic lapse rate (the tendency of air to cool about 5°F for every thousand-foot gain in elevation), summer heat is not a major factor when climbing Telescope Peak. On my last trip to the peak, the midday temperature at Furnace Creek was 105°F. An hour later, at the 8,133-foot trailhead, the temperature was a cool 66°F. But don't write off sun and heat entirely, because much of the trail is exposed to fierce, high-altitude sun that requires diligent countermeasures. And of course, for high-elevation locations like these, high winds and cold temperatures will probably also factor in, so be prepared for everything. Snow on the trail will be a factor in spring and early summer, making the north-facing and higher slopes difficult, if not dangerous to hike (hikers have slid to their deaths on the steep, icy, higher slopes of Telescope). Lightning can also be a factor, so avoid exposed ridges when thunderstorms threaten.

The hike begins at the south end of Mahogany Campground, skirting to the east, then south of Roger's Peak, where a communication facility sits. After 2 miles, it gains the crest of the Panamints and turns south, following the crest south to Telescope Peak. The hike begins among pinyon, juniper, and mountain mahogany trees. Limber pines are your companions as you climb higher. You enter the bristlecone zone in the final couple miles to the summit. Once you reach the crest, your view stretches from Mt. Charleston to the High Sierra. But the best drama waits at the summit, where you can gaze at Mt. Whitney, the highest point in the Lower 48, then turn your head and look down 11,331 feet to Badwater Basin, the lowest point in the Western Hemisphere. Only two other peaks in North America offer more vertical relief: Denali and Mount Rainier. The view south across the rugged peaks and canyons of the Panamints isn't so bad, either.

Fit, motivated hikers can make it to the peak and back in one long day (start at first light), but I prefer backpacking to maximize enjoyment and minimize comparisons to the Bataan Death March.

For backpackers, the first available campsites wait at the crest, 2 miles up the trail. Even better sites sit among the trees another half mile farther south, as well as here and there along the crest to the summit. The peak itself has at least two places where you can bivouac and enjoy summit sunset and sunrise—better than TV any day.

Retrace your steps to return.

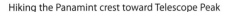

Hiking the Panamint crest toward Telescope Peak

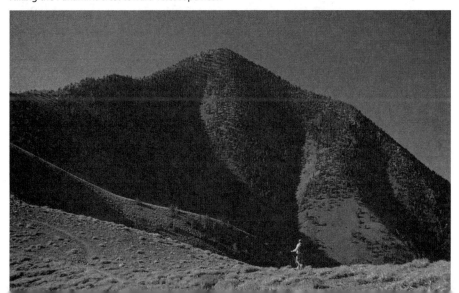

Wildrose Charcoal Kilns

A pleasant history lesson waits only 2 miles from the trailhead to Telescope Peak, at the Wildrose Charcoal Kilns. Completed in 1877, these 10 kilns employed 40 workers, who used them to produce charcoal for the silver-lead smelters in the Argus Range, 25 miles away. They operated for only 2 years before the mine closed, shutting down the kilns. Because of their short life span and remote location, they are considered among the best-preserved charcoal kilns in the West.

trip 37 Death Valley: Golden Canyon

Distance	3 miles, out-and-back
Hiking Time	1 to 2 hours
Elevation	+/-500 feet
Difficulty	Moderate
Trail Use	Good for kids
Best Times	Cold to warm
Agency	Death Valley National Park at (760) 786-3200; www.nps.gov/deva
Recommended Maps	*Trails Illustrated Death Valley* (#221)
GPS Waypoints	Red Cathedral: 36.426° N, 116.827° W
Vehicle	Passenger car OK

HIGHLIGHTS This self-guided interpretive hike explores colorful geologic history. Layers in the canyon walls tell of mountain ranges that have long since washed away and of an ancient lake that deposited layer after layer of mud and clay on its bottom. Millions of years of earthquakes have pushed these formations up, while erosion carved them away, leaving the visual spectacle you see around you. For more detail, pick up one of the interpretive brochures available at the trailhead. *Do not, however, visit this area when thunderstorms are active anywhere in the region, or you might get caught in a flash flood.*

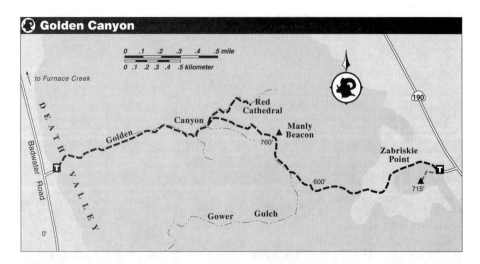

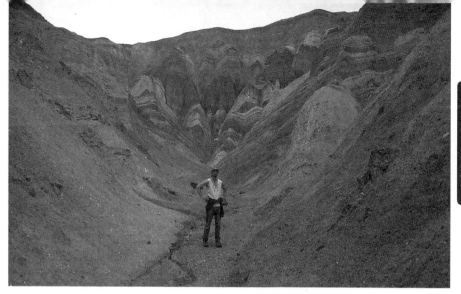

Artists have tried to capture the color and form of Death Valley geology.

DIRECTIONS From Las Vegas, take Highway 160 west about 60 miles to Pahrump. On the north side of town (about 3 miles north of the stoplight at Basin Road), turn left (west) onto Bell Vista Road and follow it about 25 miles to Death Valley Junction. Turn right (north) onto Highway 127 for 0.2 mile, then left (west) onto Highway 190 for about 28 miles to Furnace Creek. Turn left (south) onto Badwater Road, following it south for 2 miles to the signed turnoff to Golden Canyon on the left (east) side of the road. The access road climbs east for less than a mile to the trailhead.

FACILITIES/TRAILHEAD Pit toilets are available at the trailhead. Other facilities are available at Furnace Creek. Developed campsites are available at Mesquite Spring, 3 miles west of Scotty's Castle (30 sites); Stovepipe Wells (two campgrounds with a total of 204 sites); and Furnace Creek (three campgrounds with a total of 1,228 sites). Reservations are recommended for Furnace Creek Campground in the winter. Call (800) 365-2267 for reservations. Undeveloped backcountry camping is allowed 2 miles away from developed areas, paved roads, day-use areas, and roadways. Please camp only on previously disturbed areas to minimize impact.

From the trailhead, the trail heads east and immediately enters Golden Canyon. After a mile and a half, the Golden Canyon trail ends at Red Cathedral, an impressive wall of iron-stained rock.

Located below Zabriskie Point and near the Artist's Palette in the Amargosa Range, Golden Canyon is not only beautiful, it offers a glimpse at what this area was like before Death Valley was created.

The trailhead itself sits on the top of an alluvial fan rising 150 feet from the valley floor. When rain-caused flash floods wash through the Golden Canyon and other canyons around the park, they carry rocks and other debris to the fan beyond the canyon's mouth.

The short section of pavement a few hundred yards in the canyon is also a testament to the power of flash floods. Until 1976, cars drove into Golden Canyon, but four days of rain washed away the road, adding asphalt to the accumulating alluvium below the canyon mouth.

A half mile before the end of the trail at Red Cathedral, a sign on the right (south) marks the 2-mile trail to Zabriskie Point, on which you can further explore colored canyon and badlands. Ambitious hikers can retrace their steps to Golden Canyon from Zabriskie Point or arrange a car shuttle or pickup. By car, Zabriskie Point is 4 miles north, then east of the Golden Canyon Trailhead, via Badwater Road and Highway 190.

trip 38 Death Valley: Salt Creek Interpretive Trail

Hiking Time	Up to 1 hour
Elevation	-248 feet (below sea level)
Difficulty	Easy
Trail Use	Good for kids
Best Times	Cool to warm
Agency	Death Valley National Park at (760) 786-3200; www.nps.gov/deva
Recommended Maps	Free *Death Valley National Park* map; *Trails Illustrated Death Valley* (#221)
GPS Waypoint	Picnic Area: 36.354° N, 116.594° W
Vehicle	Passenger car OK

HIGHLIGHTS Death Valley National Park is the driest place in the U.S., but that doesn't mean there's no water. A few springs like the one at Salt Creek bubble forth here and there in the valley, and where there's water, there's life. Take this boardwalk stroll along a perennial stream and look for the endangered pupfish. In winter and spring, the springs stretch into ribbons of creeks, and the pupfish populate these ample waters by the millions. In the peak of summer, however, the water retreats to the source of the springs. At times like these, the pupfish population dwindles to only a few hundred members.

DIRECTIONS From Las Vegas, take Highway 160 west about 60 miles to Pahrump. On the north side of town (about 3 miles north of the light at Basin Road), turn left (west) onto Bell Vista Road, and follow it about 25 miles to Death Valley Junction. Turn right (north) onto Highway 127 for 0.2 mile, then left (west) onto Highway 190 for about 28 miles to Furnace Creek. Continue north on 190 from Furnace Creek for 13.5 miles (veering left, west, at Beatty Junction). Turn left (west), following the sign to SALT CREEK INTERPRETIVE TRAIL for 1 mile to the trailhead.

FACILITIES/TRAILHEAD Restrooms are available at the trailhead. Developed campsites are available at Mesquite Spring, 3 miles west of Scotty's Castle (30 sites); Stovepipe Wells (two campgrounds with a total of 204 sites); and Furnace Creek (three campgrounds with a total of 1,228 sites). Reservations are recommended for Furnace Creek Campground in the winter. Call (800) 365-2267 for reservations. Undeveloped backcountry camping is allowed 2 miles away from developed areas, paved roads, day-use areas, and roadways. Please camp only on previously disturbed areas to minimize impact.

Follow the boardwalk northwest from the parking area along the creek, then circle back to your car.

Look closely as you walk, and you'll see the flash of Salt Creek pupfish. These two-inch fish, navigating the shallow water of Salt Creek and facing the extreme heat of the Death Valley sun, seem as though they would barely last through summer. Although they are an endangered species, they have endured at this place for more than 10,000 years.

During the last ice age, between 70,000 and 10,000 years ago, a great lake fed by ample rain and runoff from glaciers high in

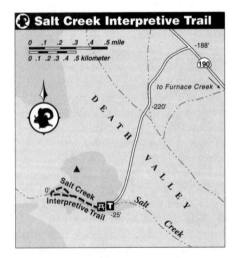

Salt Creek Interpretive Trail

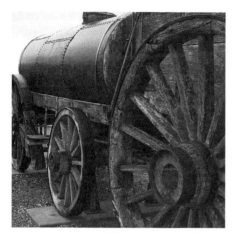

A locomotive at Harmony Borax Works near Salt Creek

the Sierra Nevada to the west filled what we now call Death Valley.

As the climate changed, the weather warmed, and the great lake disappeared, the pupfish survived only where springs persisted. Separated by miles of searing desert heat, the pupfish living in these isolated springs and pools evolved into nine distinct species, each of which is on the endangered species list. The Salt Creek pupfish is endemic—it lives in this creek and nowhere else.

trip 39 Death Valley: Badwater Basin

Distance	2 miles, out-and-back
Hiking Time	Up to 1 hour
Elevation	-282 feet (below sea level)
Difficulty	Easy
Trail Use	Good for kids
Best Times	October to April
Agency	Death Valley National Park at (760) 786-3200; www.nps.gov/deva
Recommended Maps	Free *Death Valley National Park* map; *Trails Illustrated Death Valley* (#221)
GPS Waypoints	Badwater Basin: 36.229° N, 116.466° W
Vehicle	Passenger car OK

HIGHLIGHTS This lowest, driest, and hottest place in the Western Hemisphere is home to endangered fish and an amazing sense of space and scale.

DIRECTIONS From Las Vegas, take Highway 160 west about 60 miles to Pahrump. On the north side of town (about 3 miles north of the stoplight at Basin Road), turn left (west) onto Bell Vista Road, and follow it about 25 miles to Death Valley Junction. Turn right (north) onto Highway 127 for 0.2 mile, then left (west) onto Highway 190 for about 28 miles to Furnace Creek. Turn left (south) onto Badwater Road and drive 17 miles to the signed Badwater Basin parking area on the right (west) side of the road.

FACILITIES/TRAILHEAD Restrooms and information are available at the trailhead. Developed campsites are available at Mesquite Spring, 3 miles west of Scotty's Castle (30 sites); Stovepipe Wells (two campgrounds with a total of 204 sites); and Furnace Creek (three campgrounds with a total of 1,228 sites). Reservations are recommended for Furnace Creek Campground in the winter. Call (800) 365-2267 for reservations. Undeveloped backcountry camping is allowed 2 miles away from developed areas, paved roads, day-use areas, and roadways. Please camp only on previously disturbed areas to minimize impact.

Follow the trail west, beyond the boardwalk, out onto the salt flats. After a few minutes, the trail splits into two, and both paths continue only a short distance farther. Follow one of them to the end and enjoy the extreme sense of space it provides. Also notice the pressure ridges, cracks, and formations in the salt around you, created by the evaporation of water. Find a place where no one has walked and look closer still at salt formations to appreciate the elegance and detail of their structure.

Now stand up and look to the west, to Telescope Peak rising 11,331 vertical feet above the valley floor. The extremes of scale can be dizzying. Although you can't see it from Badwater, Mt. Whitney—at 14,491 feet, the highest point in the Lower 48—is only 135 miles to the west.

To the east, the Black Mountains rise steeply behind the parking lot and road, exposing some of the park's oldest rocks. As many as 1.8 billion years ago, extreme heat and pressure metamorphosed volcanic and sedimentary rocks deep in the Earth. Today, this contorted gneiss is nearly unrecognizable from its original form.

While you're looking at the ancient rocks in the cliff face, notice the sign indicating sea level high above. Let's hope the mountains don't open up and let the sea in while you're standing here.

Although Death Valley is the driest place in the country, Badwater is not dry. Located at the bottom of the large basin that is Death Valley, a shallow lake often forms after it rains in Badwater. The salt pond by the parking area never completely dries out, and it hosts an endangered snail, despite containing water four times saltier than the sea.

It is also hotter than most places on Earth. On July 10, 1913, Badwater experienced the highest temperature ever recorded in the U.S., a sizzling 134°F (the highest temperature ever recorded on Earth, 136°F, occurred in Libya on September 13, 1922). Low elevation contributes to the brutal heat at Badwater, but the high mountains on each side of the valley help by recirculating the air and preventing it from dissipating at night. You didn't choose to visit in July or August, did you?

Before you get too hot, retrace your steps to your car.

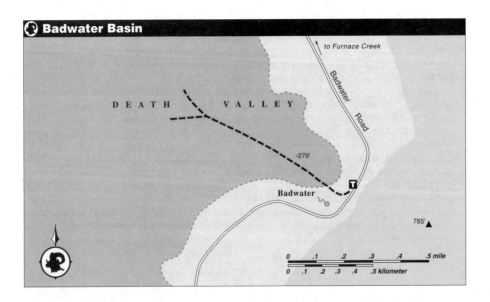

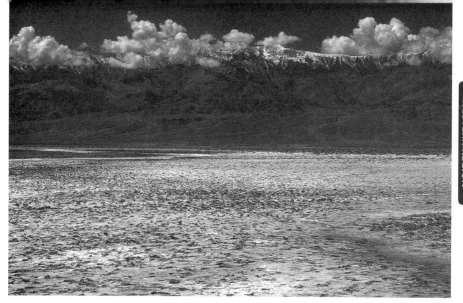

Telescope Peak rises 11,331 feet above Badwater Basin.

trip 40 # Death Valley: Sidewinder Canyon

Distance	5 miles, out-and-back or loop
Hiking Time	2 to 4 hours
Elevation	+/-1500 feet
Difficulty	Moderate to difficult
Trail Use	Map and compass
Best Times	Cool to warm
Agency	Death Valley National Park at (760) 786-3200; www.nps.gov/deva
Recommended Maps	*Trails Illustrated Death Valley* (#221); *Gold Valley, CA* 7.5-minute
GPS Waypoints	Canyon mouth: 36.056° N, 116.743° W
Vehicle	Passenger car OK

HIGHLIGHTS This trip takes you through a surprising and remote labyrinth of slot canyons in the Black Mountains of Death Valley. Eons ago, the many rocks in the walls of the canyon were part of the Black Mountains higher up, until they were washed down and deposited in this alluvial fan by recurring flash floods. Over time, minerals in the deposits set the rock like concrete, forming the hard, cobbled conglomerate. More recent floods in turn carved into the alluvium, forming these canyons. Higher in the main canyon, the cobble gives way to metamorphic rock of the Black Mountains that is hundreds of millions of years old. This is not the place to be during a flash flood. *Please stay out of tight canyons and washes when thunderstorms are active anywhere in the area.*

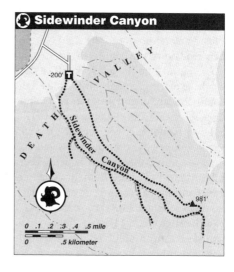

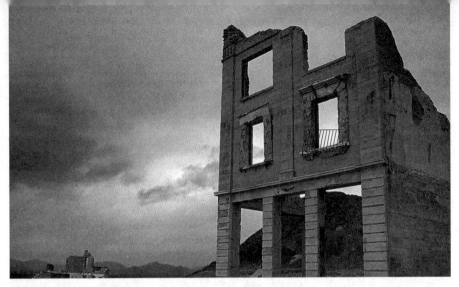

Rhyolite, west of Beatty, is one of the best-preserved and picturesque ghost towns of the region.

DIRECTIONS From Las Vegas, take Highway 160 west about 60 miles to Pahrump. On the north side of town (about 3 miles north of the light at Basin Road), turn left (west) onto Bell Vista Road, and follow it about 25 miles to Death Valley Junction. Turn right (north) onto Highway 127 for 0.2 mile, then turn left (west) onto Highway 190 for about 28 miles to Furnace Creek. Turn left (south) onto Badwater Road and drive 31 miles (14 miles south of the Badwater Basin parking area). Then turn left (southeast) onto an unsigned dirt road. At the T intersection a half mile later, turn right (south) and park by the gravel pit at the end.

FACILITIES/TRAILHEAD The nearest restrooms are at Badwater Basin. Developed campsites are available at Mesquite Spring, 3 miles west of Scotty's Castle (30 sites); at Stovepipe Wells (two campgrounds with a total of 204 sites); and at Furnace Creek (three campgrounds with a total of 1,228 sites). Reservations are recommended for Furnace Creek Campground in the winter (call 800-365-2267). Undeveloped backcountry camping is allowed 2 miles from developed areas, paved roads, day-use areas, and roadways. Please camp only on previously disturbed areas to minimize impact.

From the car, hike 0.3 mile due south, up the alluvial fan, and into the mouth of the shallow canyon on your left (southeast). There is no trail. After 0.7 mile, the canyon splits. Explore the slot to the right (south), then head down the left (north) fork.

As you hike up the left fork, other slots worth exploring merge from the right (south). Be careful exploring the dark, winding passageways and climbing up waterfalls and over boulders. If you get hurt, it could be a long time before anyone finds you.

At 1.7 miles, the canyon widens, veers right (south) and climbs from the conglomerate and into the steep rock of the Black Mountains. Scrambling skills are necessary to explore this section, but you are rewarded with steep canyon walls and jumbled boulders for another half mile or so. Sidewinder

Canyon is one of my favorite spots in Death Valley. No signs. No crowds. No warning of what beauty awaits those who venture onto routes less traveled.

To make an enjoyable loop, return to the wide, conglomerate section of the canyon. The north wall of this section is only about 50 feet high. Find a good place to scramble up out of the canyon and onto the ridge above (the easiest route I found was about 150 yards downstream, to the west). Your perch on the top of this low ridge offers a nice view of Death Valley sweeping off to the north. Follow the ridge and washes down to the northwest and back to the parking area, which should be easily visible after a few minutes of walking. If you don't choose this loop, return the way you came.

WESTERN REGION

trip 41 Death Valley: Zabriskie Point

Distance	0.25 mile, out-and-back
Hiking Time	30 minutes to 1 hour
Elevation	+/-73 feet (+216/-956 feet for Gold Canyon)
Difficulty	Moderate
Trail Use	Good for kids
Best Times	Cold to warm
Agency	Death Valley National Park at (760) 786-3200; www.nps.gov/deva
Recommended Maps	Free *Death Valley National Park* map; *Trails Illustrated Death Valley* (#221)
GPS Waypoints	Zabriskie entrance: 36.420° N, 116.808° W
Vehicle	Passenger car OK

HIGHLIGHTS Few places on this planet play with color, light, and shadow the way the colorful badlands of Zabriskie Point do in early morning and late afternoon. Millions of people have watched the shadows stretch and colors shift as the sun paints its light across the landscape. More than a few artists have struggled to capture its magic. You can catch its magic, too, after a short walk to this overlook.

DIRECTIONS From Las Vegas, take Highway 160 west about 60 miles to Pahrump. On the north side of town (about 3 miles north of the light at Basin Road), turn left (west) onto Bell Vista Road, and follow it about 25 miles to Death Valley Junction. Turn right (north) onto Highway 127 for 0.2 mile, then turn left (west) onto Highway 190 for about 28 miles toward Furnace Creek. Zabriskie Viewpoint is about 5 miles east of Furnace Creek on Highway 190.

FACILITIES/TRAILHEAD Restrooms are available here and at Furnace Creek. Developed campsites are available at Mesquite Spring, 3 miles west of Scotty's Castle (30 sites); Stovepipe Wells (two campgrounds with a total of 204 sites); and Furnace Creek (three campgrounds with a total of 1,228 sites). Reservations are recommended for Furnace Creek Campground in the winter. Call (800) 365-2267 for reservations. Undeveloped backcountry camping is allowed 2 miles away from developed areas, paved roads, and day-use areas and roadways. Please camp only on previously disturbed areas to minimize impact.

Although most people enjoy Zabriskie from the parking lot and the quarter-mile walk to the overlook, hikers who want more of a challenging, intimate encounter with these badlands continue 2 miles down to Golden Canyon. Avoid the hike back by arranging a vehicle shuttle or someone to pick you up at the Golden Canyon Trailhead, which is west on Highway 190 and then 2 miles south on Badwater Road.

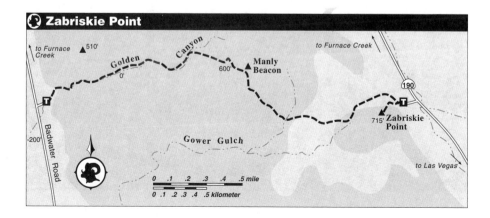

The spectacle of color here began about 6 million years ago, when this area was underneath a large, calm lake. Sediments settled into mud and clay, and, over millions of years, they were covered by even more layers, until they were compacted and gently cemented into mudstone.

Eventually, tectonic forces pushed them up into mountains. Water does not penetrate this mudstone easily, rendering this landscape practically devoid of plant life. However, it does erode quickly. Over the millennia, rainfall has created and deepened the grooves and rills you see at Zabriskie. This process continues today, shaping this area into something that will look very different in the future.

The point is named for Christian Brevoort Zabriskie, manager of the Pacific Coast Borax Company, which owned tracts of land in Death Valley. He turned to tourism after his mining operations failed to turn a profit.

The lines and colors of Zabriskie Point can grow magical early and late in the day.

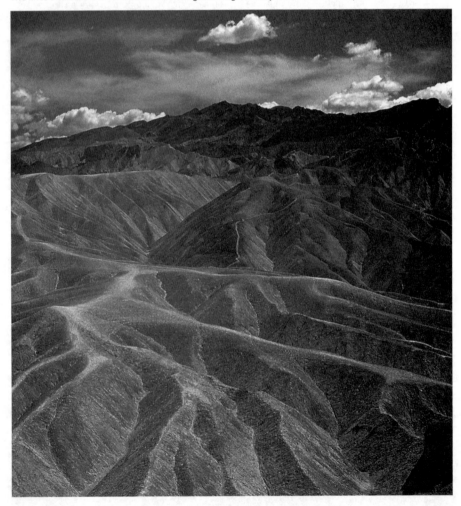

WESTERN REGION

trip 42 Death Valley: Dante's View

Distance	0.5 mile, out-and-back
Hiking Time	30 minutes to 1 hour
Elevation	5460 feet; +/-262 feet (for Dante's Peak)
Difficulty	Easy (moderate for Dante's Peak)
Trail Use	Good for kids
Best Times	Cold to warm
Agency	Death Valley National Park at (760) 786-3200; www.nps.gov/deva
Recommended Maps	*Trails Illustrated Death Valley* (#221)
GPS Waypoints	Dante's Peak: 36.226° N, 116.725° W
Vehicle	Passenger car OK

HIGHLIGHTS Take this scenic drive to a breathtaking view over Death Valley, with an optional short hike up Dante's Peak. Although it's neither a long hike, nor the most secluded part of the park, Dante's View is a must-see destination by any measure. Dante's Peak offers a relative escape from the crowds and vehicle noise at the Dante's View parking area below.

DIRECTIONS From Las Vegas, take Highway 160 west about 60 miles to Pahrump. From the north side of town (about 3 miles north of the stoplight at Basin Road), turn left (west) onto Bell Vista Road, and follow it about 25 miles to Death Valley Junction. Turn right (north) onto Highway 127 for 0.2 mile, then left (west) on Highway 190 for about 17.5 miles to the Dante's View turnoff on the left (south) side of the road. Follow the road 13 miles as it climbs to the parking area. *The final few miles are steep with tight turns. Large RVs and trailers are prohibited and must be left at parking areas below.*

FACILITIES/TRAILHEAD Restrooms and information are available here. Developed campsites are available at Mesquite Spring, 3 miles west of Scotty's Castle (30 sites); Stovepipe Wells (two campgrounds with a total of 204 sites); and Furnace Creek (three campgrounds with a total of 1,228 sites). Reservations are recommended for Furnace Creek Campground in the winter. Call (800) 365-2267 for reservations. Undeveloped backcountry camping is allowed 2 miles away from developed areas, paved roads, day-use areas, and roadways. Please camp only on previously disturbed areas to minimize impact.

S itting at Dante's View, you almost know what it's like to fly. The view is epic and deserves the comparison to the classic saga Dante's *Inferno*. From the parking area, the Black Mountains plummet a vertical mile to Badwater Basin, which, at 282 feet below sea level, is the lowest, hottest, and driest spot in the Western Hemisphere.

Across Death Valley to the west, Telescope Peak rises 11,331 feet above the valley floor. To the north and south, Death Valley itself stretches for 130 miles, painted with ribbons of water and salt across the valley floor. On a clear day, look for snowcapped peaks of the Sierra Nevada more than 135 miles to the northwest.

Dante's View is not the high point of this ridgeline. Dante's Peak waits a short hike north, where you will be able to enjoy the

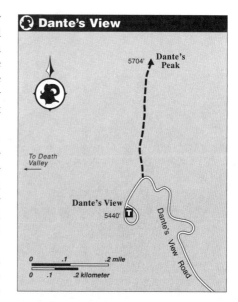

Dante's View

5704' Dante's Peak

To Death Valley

Dante's View 5440'

Dante's View Road

0   .1   .2 mile
0   .1   .2 kilometer

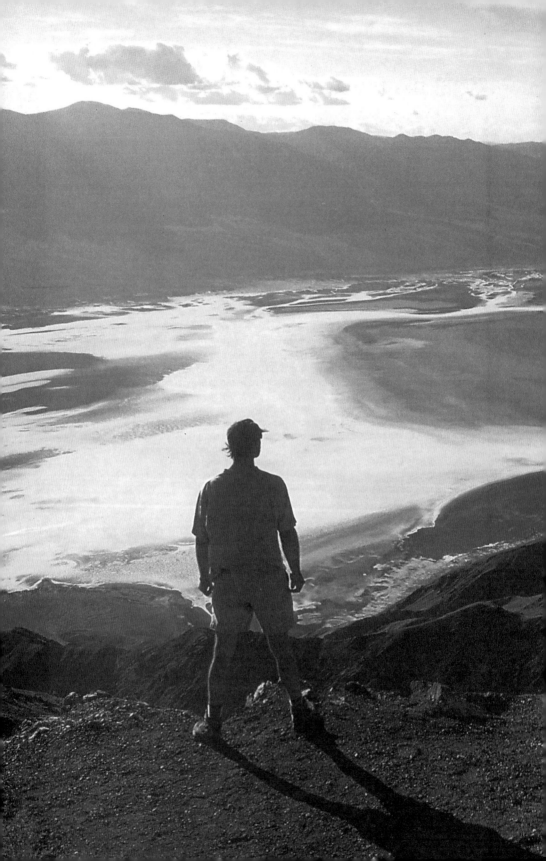

view with relative solitude. To bag Dante's Peak, walk back down the road less than 0.1 mile, where a use trail heads up the ridge to the left (west) of the road about 0.4 mile to the top. Along the way, detour to a rocky promontory to the west, for a view straight down to the valley below.

Once on Dante's Peak, you have to decide which small knob is the true summit. The benchmarks have the answer, but don't worry if you can't figure it out. The difference is mere inches.

The vistas from Dante's View were created by great geologic forces some 30 million years ago, when the North American and Pacific continental plates began sliding past each other and pulling apart what is now the Great Basin. Sections of the North American plate shifted and tilted, creating both the mountains and the valleys between them.

Over the millennia, erosion filled the valleys with gravel, sediment, and other debris washed down from the mountains above. Were it not for the gravel filling Death Valley far below, the valley bottom would be another 5000 to 8000 feet lower.

After you've taken in the view—or watched the sun set—retrace your steps to return.

The view from Dante's Peak encompasses most of the 130-mile-long Death Valley.

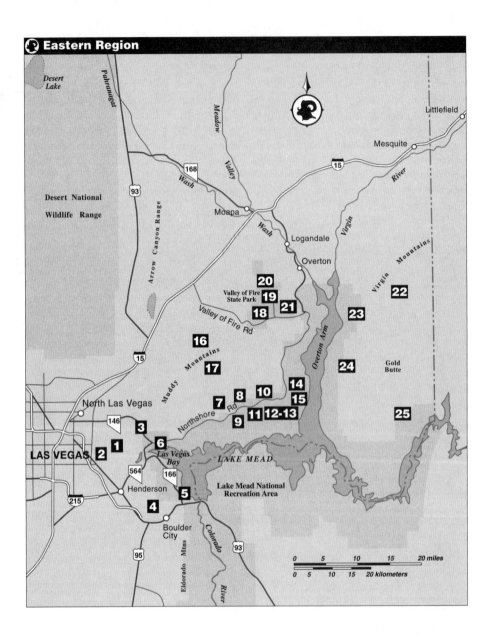

Desert Lake

Pahranagat

Meadow Valley Wash

168

93

Desert National Wildlife Range

Arrow Canyon Range

Moapa

Wash

Logandale

Overton

Virgin River

Mesquite

Littlefield

15

Virgin Mountains

Valley of Fire State Park

20
19
18 21

Valley of Fire Rd

16

Muddy Mountains

17

15

North Las Vegas

146

3

LAS VEGAS 2 1

Northshore Rd

7 8 10

9 11 12-13

14
15

Overton Arm

23

22

24

Gold Butte

25

6

Las Vegas Bay

LAKE MEAD

564

166

Henderson

5

215

4

95

Boulder City

Eldorado Mtns

Colorado River

93

Lake Mead National Recreation Area

0   5   10   15   20 miles
0   5   10   15   20 kilometers

chapter 2

Eastern Region
INCLUDING LAKE MEAD, VALLEY OF FIRE, & GOLD BUTTE

East of Las Vegas (which I define as east of Interstate 15 and north of Highway 93, through Boulder City), you'll find some of the region's most colorful, magical, and magnificent natural wonders, including Lake Mead National Recreation Area and Valley of Fire State Park. This section leads you to the most popular destinations in these parks, as well as a few places in these parks and elsewhere that the crowds have yet to discover. Described below are some of the wonders of this region, including Lake Mead National Recreation Area, the Valley of Fire State Park, and Gold Butte.

Lake Mead National Recreation Area
After the completion of Hoover (then Boulder) Dam in 1936, the Colorado River filled the river canyons for 115 miles upstream to the mouth of the Grand Canyon. Agreements between the National Park Service and the Bureau of Reclamation in the 1930s and '40s established the Lake Mead National Recreation Area (originally called the Boulder Dam National Recreation Area), the nation's first national recreation area.

Today, Lakes Mead and Mohave (the next lake downstream, formed by Davis Dam above Laughlin, Nevada) and their 300 square miles of water and 1,000 miles of shoreline attract 9 million visitors each year—nearly triple the number of visitors to Grand Canyon National Park. The majority flock to Hoover Dam or to the water to take advantage of boating, fishing, and wet fun in hot weather. But Lake Mead National Recreation Area is more than just a lake. Few realize that water makes up only about 13 percent of the area, leaving more than

1.3 million acres of wild, rugged beauty and solitude to explore.

Dramatic, colorful geology is the overwhelming attraction of this arid landscape. The rocks exposed in the area date back nearly 2 billion years, representing every major period of the Earth's formation. Their placement relative to each other tells us about the events that have shaped the planet until now.

Although they seem scarce at first glance, the plants and animals here are diverse and have developed fascinating strategies to survive in this harsh landscape. Look closely (although not too closely at rattlesnakes!), and you'll appreciate their beauty.

If you're looking for a scenic drive to fill an afternoon, take Lake Mead Blvd. east from North Las Vegas, turn left (east) and follow Northshore Road east for 43 miles. Then turn left (west) and drive through Valley of Fire to I-15, where a left (south) turn will lead you back to Vegas. Three to four hours gives you time to make this beautiful drive, with a few stops along the way.

Valley of Fire State Park
Dedicated in 1935, Valley of Fire is Nevada's oldest state park, and it has grown to comprise more than 40,000 acres. Like Red Rock Canyon National Recreation Area west of Las Vegas, geology takes center stage here, where you'll find a wonderland of colorful, sculpted sandstone, ancient petroglyphs, and vibrant desert life. Also like Red Rock Canyon, Valley of Fire is a must-see for everyone in Las Vegas.

Comparisons between these two natural attractions are understandable because both offer similar geologic formations. Between 65 million and 250 million years ago, what is now the Mojave Desert lifted from the seas, and a great desert of sand dunes formed across the landscape. These dunes have since cemented into stone. Collisions between continental plates then lifted and shifted many of these old rocks. South of the visitor center, you can look at the Arrowhead Fault, where 500-million-year-old seabed limestone rests against much younger sandstones. The Arrowhead Fault is related to the Keystone Thrust Fault in Red Rock Canyon.

Weather and time have eroded these stones into twisting canyons, majestic arches, sheer walls, rippled domes, and improbable pinnacles. Iron, magnesium, and other minerals in the rock have dyed the stone into its palette of fiery hues. If Red Rock Canyon is known for its steep towering canyons, Valley of Fire is a sculpture garden of shape and color. Erosion continues today, sculpting the landscape even further, and making the wonderful rock formations you see a snapshot in geologic time.

Archaeological evidence shows that humans have lived in Valley of Fire for at least 4,000 years. Among the first arrivals were "Desert Archaic" peoples. Sometime around 300 B.C., other peoples began settling in the area, including the Ancestral Puebloan, Yuman, and Southern Paiute. All of these groups left behind mysterious petroglyphs and other artifacts that tell us of their lives. The artifacts they left are fragile, irreplaceable, and protected by state and federal laws. Please do not disturb these artifacts. Leave them as you find them so others may enjoy them, too.

Although they are difficult to see in this harsh landscape, a variety of animals have found ways to survive here. You have a good chance of seeing lizards, ravens, antelope, ground squirrels, coyotes, black-tailed jackrabbits, and maybe a roadrunner. If you're really lucky, you might glimpse a desert tortoise, kit fox, a herd of bighorn sheep, or an eagle soaring overhead. Please enjoy animals from a distance, and do not feed them. This is their home, and they have the best chance of surviving in this harsh climate if we leave them alone and let them use skills and instincts they have evolved over millennia.

Travelers with only a few hours to spend here will be happy to know that the park's two main roads offer a feast for the eyes, and every destination mentioned in this book is accessible via a short hike. More intrepid, prepared backcountry explorers can find pockets of solitude and adventure that make Valley of Fire seem a million miles, or a million years, from the bright lights of Las Vegas.

Gold Butte

Surrounded by the Virgin River and the Overton Arm of Lake Mead to the west, Lake Mead to the south, Arizona to the east, and the Virgin Mountains to the north, the 300,000-acre region known as Gold Butte offers wondrous geology, intriguing history, remote, undeveloped camping opportunities, and timeless solitude.

For thousands of years, various peoples have lived in this region, including the Fremont, Ancestral Puebloan, Patayan, and Southern Paiute. Petroglyphs on sandstone walls throughout the area hint at humans' presence over the centuries. These and all other artifacts are protected by numerous state and federal laws, so please respect them from a distance.

In 1905, Gold was discovered in the area, and soon the town of Gold Butte boasted many homes, a post office, and a school. By 1911, most of the mining had ceased, and the houses had been moved to nearby St. Thomas, on the banks of the Virgin River. Today, little remains of the town, save a few rusting pieces of machinery and a foundation or two.

The 62-mile Gold Butte Back Country Byway provides an excellent opportunity for a (long) day trip or a weekend car-camp expedition. The main road between Whitney Pockets and the old town site of Gold Butte is a well-graded dirt road, accessible to any vehicle. The western portion of the byway, between Devil's Throat and Gold Butte, requires a high-clearance 4WD vehicle. The Gold Butte region has become a favorite place for off-road vehicle enthusiasts to drive every which way, with nary a care for the sensitive soils, wildlife, archaeological resources, beautiful views, or enjoyment of other visitors. Please help keep Gold Butte beautiful and pristine by staying on designated routes.

There are absolutely no services in Gold Butte. Top off your tank in Glendale or Mesquite, stock your vehicle with all provisions and emergency gear you might need (see more on safe desert driving, page 20), please stick to designated routes, and get ready to feel a thousand miles, or a thousand years, from Las Vegas.

Eastern Region

Landscapes east of Las Vegas prove that desolation can be beautiful.

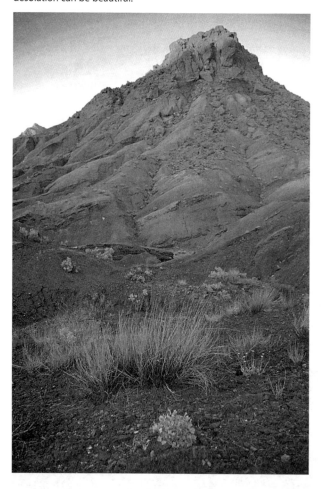

trip 1 Wetlands Park Nature Preserve

Distance	Up to 7 miles (several trails), loop
Hiking Time	30 minutes to 2 hours
Elevation	1620 feet
Difficulty	Easy
Trail Use	Leashed dogs, good for kids
Best Times	Cool to warm
Agency	Wetlands Park at (702) 455-7522; www.accessclarkcounty.com/depts/parks/locations/pages/Wetlands.aspx
Recommended Maps	Free map available at visitor center
GPS Waypoints	Visitor center: 36.101° N, 115.022° W
Vehicle	Passenger car OK

HIGHLIGHTS Clark County Wetlands Park is a perfect place to grab some fresh air and exercise during a busy weekend in Vegas. Located on the Las Vegas Wash between town and Lake Mead, Wetlands Park is a work in progress to restore some of the wetlands for the birds and animals historically associated with this area.

DIRECTIONS From Las Vegas, take Tropicana Ave. east. About 1.5 miles east of Boulder Highway, when the road veers right (southeast) and changes names from Tropicana to Rebel Road (which heads toward Sam Boyd Stadium), turn left onto Wetlands Park Lane to reach the nature preserve and visitor center.

FACILITIES/TRAILHEAD Restrooms and information signs are available at the trailhead.

The park is open dawn to dusk every day, and the visitor center is open 10 A.M. to 4 P.M. every day. There is no charge to enter. To protect birds and other wildlife, pets (on leash) and bicycles are allowed only on the Duck Creek Trail. The park is constantly developing trails and other features, so check with the visitor center for updates.

For thousands of years, Las Vegas Wash has nourished birds, animals, and people as it channeled runoff from natural springs, mountains, and storms. Ever-growing Las

Wetlands Park brings a splash of life and color to Las Vegas.

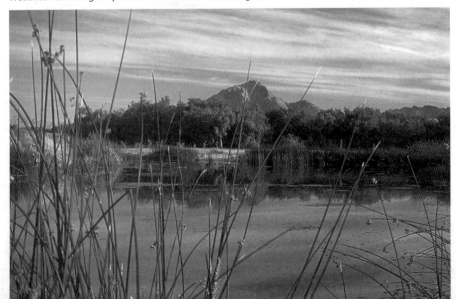

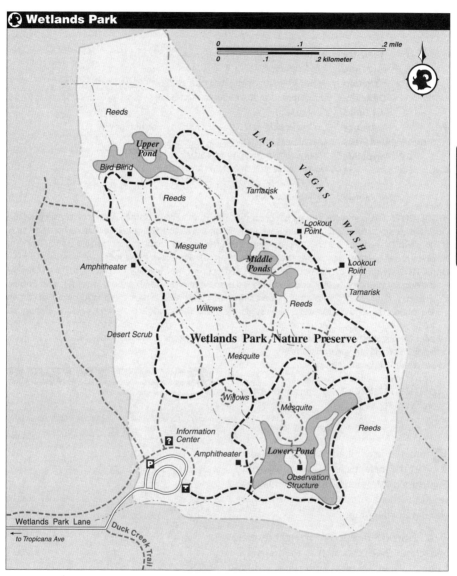

Vegas adds to this flow with runoff from sprinklers, fountains, swimming pools, and city streets. The increased flow has eroded the banks of the wash and polluted Lake Mead with a city's worth of chemicals ranging from antifreeze to fertilizers.

To stem the erosion, slow the runoff, and purify the water, the park features a series of dams and other water-calming features. Not only is this a nice place to watch wildlife and take a stroll, the resulting ponds and marshes prevent fast water from eroding the marsh. They also filter pollutants from the water, making everyone downstream a little healthier.

trip 2 **Frenchman Mountain**

Distance	2.4 miles or 4 miles, out-and-back
Hiking Time	2 to 5 hours
Elevation	+/-1413 feet (to North Summit); +/-2300 feet (to South Summit)
Difficulty	Difficult (option A); moderate (option B)
Best Times	Cool to warm
Agency	Las Vegas BLM at (702) 515-5000; www.nv.blm.gov/vegas
Recommended Maps	*Lake Mead* 1:100,000
GPS Waypoints	Trailhead: 36.199° N, 114.987° W
	North Summit: 36.188° N, 114.997° W
	South Summit: 36.179° N, 114.996° W
Vehicle	Passenger car OK

HIGHLIGHTS Frenchman Mountain is a great place to bring a picnic dinner, watch the sunset over the distant Spring Mountains and Red Rock Canyon, then watch the lights of Vegas carpet the valley floor, which seems to start right at your feet. Don't forget your headlamp for the hike down. Trekking poles are also recommended, as the many rocks on the way down make for slippery travel.

DIRECTIONS From I-15 on the north end of Las Vegas, take Lake Mead Blvd. east toward Lake Mead. At the edge of town, the houses end, and the road narrows from five lanes to two. Travel 1.3 miles farther, then turn right (south) onto an unsigned, unpaved gravel road, which climbs south up Frenchman Mountain. (The road is a quarter mile west of Lake Mead Blvd.'s saddle between Frenchman Mountain to the south and Sunrise Mountain to the north.) Drive a quarter mile or so on the unpaved road, then park. Do not attempt to drive up the mountain. It's one of the steeper, rockier roads west of the Mississippi, and it will get you into trouble.

Note: Vandalism is prevalent in this area. Do not leave valuables in your car.

FACILITIES/TRAILHEAD The nearest facilities are in Las Vegas.

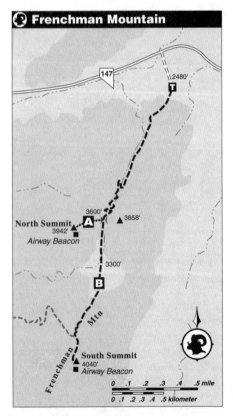

From the car, hike south up the road, past the metal gate, and up, up, up onto Frenchman Mountain. After 1 mile, you reach the north summit of the road, where you have two options:

A. North Summit: Turn right (west), and climb 200 vertical feet to the north summit. There is only a faint route and the terrain is difficult, but it is the most direct route to a view. Do not climb straight up. Instead, aim west-southwest toward the wooden platform and power poles, which are on the true summit.

B. South Summit: Continue south on the road, down across the saddle, then up an even steeper section to the south summit. The advantages to the longer walk to the south summit are an easier route along road (which is steep as heck) and a better view of Rainbow Gardens and Lake Las Vegas.

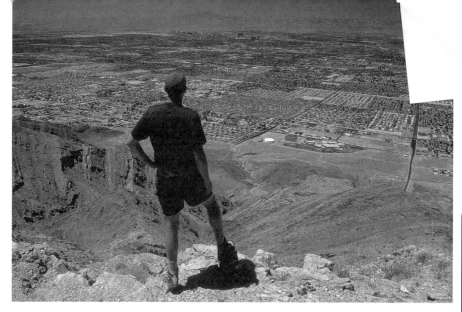

From the top of Frenchman Mountain, Las Vegas stretches like a carpet at your feet.

Frenchman Mountain is one of the most accessible peaks to Las Vegas. Unfortunately, litter and vandalism at the trailhead mar the mountain's stunning geology and sweeping views over the Las Vegas Valley.

Geologically, the many layers, ridges, and colors of Frenchman Mountain and Rainbow Gardens to the east are reminiscent of the Grand Canyon. In fact, they are the same layers. They're simply tilted back and arranged horizontally rather than stacked on top of each other. Older layers at the western base of Frenchman date back 1.7 billion years. Younger layers are to the east, near Lake Mead.

Once you have taken in the view, retrace your steps to return.

The Great Unconformity: A Small Step for Man, A Giant Leap for Geology

The Great Unconformity lies at the western base of Frenchman Mountain, a quarter mile east of the last houses and the point where Lake Mead Blvd. narrows from five lanes to two. Look for an interpretive display on the right (south) side of the Lake Mead Blvd. In May 2004, the sign was vandalized into illegibility, but the geology remains.

To the right of the display lies 1.7-million-year-old Precambrian granite and schist. Formed deep within a long-gone mountain range, it eroded over hundreds of millions of years until it became exposed some 550 million years ago. Then sea levels rose, and sands settling on the sea bottom buried the granite and schist. The sandy sediments created what is now 545-million-year-old Tapeats sandstone, to the left side of the display.

The line between the two represents 1.2 billion years. Millions of years of shifting, faulting, sliding, tilting, and eroding later, it appears in a road cut on the outskirts of Vegas. If you want to see the Great Unconformity elsewhere, you'll have to hike down to the bottom of the Grand Canyon, 50 miles to the east. (For a detailed lesson on this great geologic feature, check out http://geoscience.unlv.edu/pub/rowland/Virtual/geology.html.)

trip 3 Lava Butte & Rainbow Gardens

Distance	1.5 miles, out-and-back
Hiking Time	2 to 3 hours
Elevation	+/-950 feet
Difficulty	Difficult
Trail Use	Leashed dogs, map and compass
Best Times	Cool to warm
Agency	Las Vegas BLM at (702) 515-5000; www.nv.blm.gov/vegas
Recommended Maps	*Lake Mead* 1:100,000; *Frenchman Mountain* 7.5-minute
GPS Waypoints	Lava Butte summit: 36.148° N, 114.936° W
Vehicle	High-clearance or 4WD vehicle recommended

HIGHLIGHTS This hike will reward you with a cameo of Grand Canyon geology and a spectacular view between Las Vegas and Lake Mead.

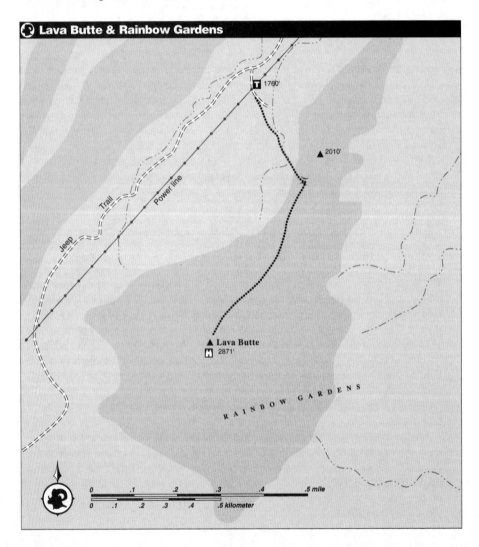

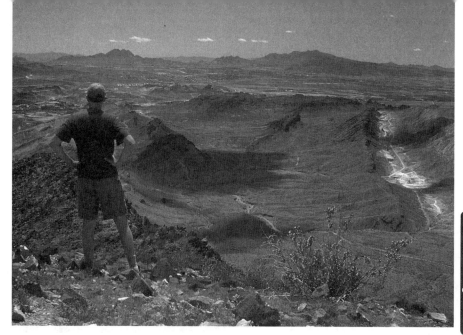

Rainbow Gardens and the Las Vegas Valley from Lava Butte

DIRECTIONS From North Las Vegas, follow Lake Mead Blvd. east toward Lake Mead. Roughly 4.4 miles east of the road's summit (about 12.5 miles east of I-15) on the north side of Frenchman Mountain, turn right (south) onto the unpaved and unsigned power line road. Continue following the power line south for 2 miles. When the power line begins to climb the canyon to the right (west) of Lava Butte, find a good place to park (I parked on a side spur accessing tower number 292-4).

FACILITIES/TRAILHEAD The nearest facilities are in Las Vegas.

From the car, hike east up and onto the north ridge of Lava Butte. Once on the ridge, turn right (south) and follow the ridge to the top. There is no true trail, and the going is steep and rocky. A faint climbers' route weaves up the ridge, but finding it is not crucial, because the going is rough no matter what.

The same geologic layers that make the Grand Canyon so spectacular are also exposed in Rainbow Gardens. Instead of standing as striped cliffs, they stretch across the landscape, comprising the numerous, multicolored north-south ridges surrounding Lava Butte between Las Vegas and Lake Mead.

Exposed rocks in this region date back more than a billion years, representing every major era of the planet's development. The oldest exposed rocks are to the west in and around Frenchman Mountain, including the 1.8-billion-year-old Vishnu schist, the oldest rock exposed in North America (it is also exposed at the bottom of the Grand Canyon). The youngest are to the east, toward Lake Mead.

Lave Butte itself is about 13 million years old and formed when fresh lava forced itself between the older, adjacent layers. As with many rocks in the Lake Mead region, tectonic activity has moved this rock tens of miles to the west from where it first spewed from the Earth.

In addition to the colorful geologic patterns and colors visible from Lava Butte's summit, the view sweeps clockwise from the Muddy Mountains to the north; across Lake Mead to the River Mountains, Lake Las Vegas, Henderson, and the North McCullough Mountains to the south; then westward to Las Vegas, with Red Rock Canyon and the Spring Mountains (capped by Mt. Charleston) peeking over the shoulder of Frenchman Mountain.

Enjoy this view, then retrace your steps to return to your car.

trip 4 Lake Mead: River Mountains Trail

Distance	2.5 miles or 5 miles, out-and-back
Hiking Time	2 to 5 hours
Elevation	+/-300 feet (option A); +/-1100 feet (option B)
Difficulty	Moderate
Trail Use	Leashed dogs, mountain biking allowed (see www.bootlegcanyon.com)
Best Times	Cool to warm
Agency	Boulder City Department of Parks and Recreation at (702) 293-9256 or Lake Mead National Recreation Area at (702) 293-8990; www.nps.gov/lame
Recommended Maps	*Boulder Beach* and *Boulder City* 7.5-minute
GPS Waypoints	Red Mountain: 35.995° N, 114.861° W Black Mountain: 36.006° N, 114.852° W
Vehicle	High-clearance or 4WD vehicle recommended (option A); passenger car OK (option B)

HIGHLIGHTS Locals call it Radar Mountain after the communications display near the summit. Mountain bikers from around the world come to ride the technical trails at what they call Bootleg Canyon. Hikers, who call this area the River Mountains, will enjoy diverse plants, colorful geology, and wonderful views of Lake Mead and Las Vegas. No matter what you call it, you'll enjoy this hike to the summits of Red and Black mountains between Boulder City and Henderson. If you visit in the afternoon, you can watch the sunset over Lake Mead and Las Vegas.

DIRECTIONS There are two trailheads to access trails in the River Mountains:

A. Red and Black mountains: For the shorter and easier route, take Highway 93 south from Las Vegas to Boulder City. As you enter Boulder City, at 0.7 mile east of Veterans Memorial Drive, turn left (north) onto Yucca Street, and follow it for about 3 miles: past the end of the pavement, past the main mountain biking parking area, up the canyon, and to the unsigned upper parking area before the gate to the communications facility. Park there.

B. River Mountains Trail: For a longer, more difficult, and more scenic climb to the same summits mentioned above, continue east on 93 into Boulder City to the intersection of Nevada Highway and Buchanan Blvd./ Highway 93. Turn left on Buchanan/93, toward Hoover Dam. At 0.7 mile east of this intersection, turn left (north) into the signed parking area for the River Mountains Trail.

FACILITIES/TRAILHEAD Restrooms and information are available at the mountain biking parking area 1 mile past the end of the pavement on the way to the option B trailhead. Restrooms and information are available at the trailhead for option B. Other services are available at Alan Bible Visitor Center and at marinas along Lake Mead between Hemenway and Overton. There are six National Park Service campgrounds in the Nevada portion of Lake Mead National Recreation Area, between Cottonwood Cove (south of Las Vegas and east of Searchlight) and Echo Bay (east of the Valley of Fire State Park), offering more than 600 sites for RVs, cars, and tents. They offer running water, dump stations, picnic tables, barbecue grills, and shade. Backcountry camping is allowed throughout Lake Mead and along the lakeshore, except in developed, restricted, or ecologically sensitive areas. Backpacking and horseback camping is prohibited within 500 feet of any paved road, within 100 feet of any spring or watering device, or in areas signed NO CAMPING. Vehicle camping is allowed only in designated spots.

Follow the instructions below for your desired route into the River Mountains.

A. From the upper parking area, near the gate to the communications facility, an unsigned trail climbs south less than a half mile to the summit of Red Mountain. With the communications facility looming to the west, the view stretches south and clockwise, over Boulder City to the Eldorado Mountains, and across the Eldorado Valley to the South and North McCullough mountains. Another unsigned trail leads

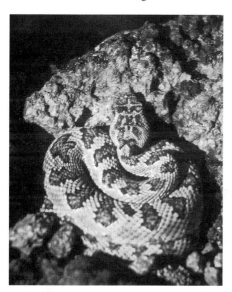

Rattlesnakes won't bother you if you don't bother them.

north from the parking area, across a saddle to the summit of Black Mountain. The view here stretches beautifully over Lake Mead to the north and east, and to the Vegas Valley to the west. Both trails are well-used and easy to find, and both peaks are less than a mile from your car. Return the way you came.

B. From the River Mountains Trailhead, follow the trail north along a cement drain between houses, then along an old railroad grade, and finally up-canyon for about 2 miles to the saddle between Red and Black mountains, near the parking area for option A. Choose right to climb Black Mountain or left to climb Red Mountain. Or better yet, do both before heading back down the way you came.

Between 15 million and 12 million years ago, the River Mountains were volcanoes spewing lava onto the landscape. Since that time, Earth movements have been tilted, cut by faults, and eroded into a jigsaw pattern that makes the original volcanoes hard to recognize. An abundance of manganese gives Black Mountain its dark hue, while iron gives color to Red Mountain.

The River Mountains are home to bighorn sheep and desert tortoises, both of which have the right of way. If you're lucky enough to meet either on the trail, please wait for them to move on at their own pace.

trip 5 Lake Mead: Railroad Tunnel Trail

Distance	Up to 7 miles, out-and-back
Hiking Time	1 to 3 hours
Elevation	+/-500 feet
Difficulty	Easy
Trail Use	Leashed dogs, good for kids, mountain biking allowed
Best Times	Cold to warm
Agency	Lake Mead National Recreation Area at (702) 293-8907; www.nps.gov/lame
Recommended Maps	Free map available at visitor center
GPS Waypoints	First tunnel: 36.017° N, 114.774° W
Vehicle	Passenger car OK

HIGHLIGHTS This trip takes you on a pleasant stroll through history high over Lake Mead to Hoover Dam. In 1931, work began on what was then called Boulder Dam, in an effort to ease flooding in California's fertile Imperial Valley. More than 30 miles of rail lines were built to haul materials needed to build the dam. Today, this short segment remains as a reminder of the work the dam required. In 2001, the Park Service began restoring the long-neglected and crumbling tunnels.

DIRECTIONS From Las Vegas, take Highway 93 south to Boulder City. Stay on 93 as it turns left (north). Drive about a quarter mile past Alan Bible Visitor Center on your right to the signed trailhead parking lot on the right (south) side of the road.

FACILITIES/TRAILHEAD Restrooms and information are available at the Alan Bible Visitor Center and at marinas along Lake Mead between Hemenway and Overton. There are six National Park Service campgrounds in the Nevada portion of Lake Mead National Recreation Area, between Cottonwood Cove (south of Las Vegas and east of Searchlight) and Echo Bay (east of the Valley of Fire State Park), offering more than 600 sites for RVs, cars, and tents. They offer running water, dump stations, picnic tables, barbecue grills, and shade. Backcountry camping is allowed throughout Lake Mead and along the lakeshore, except in developed, restricted, or ecologically sensitive areas. Backpacking and horseback camping is prohibited within 500 feet of any paved road, within 100 feet of any spring or watering device, or in areas signed NO CAMPING. Vehicle camping is allowed only in designated spots.

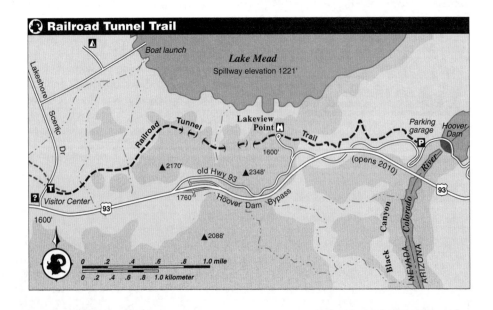

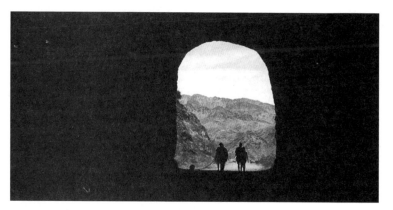

Five historic railroad tunnels offer luxurious shade.

From the parking area, the trail winds south, then east for 2.5 miles through five tunnels. It takes you through the River Mountains approximately 500 feet over Lake Mead, affording hikers sweeping views over Hemenway Harbor, north to the Black and Muddy mountains on the lake's north shore, and east to Fortification Hill and Mt. Wilson on the Arizona side of the lake.

Along the way, you might be lucky enough to spot bighorn sheep, ravens, antelope, ground squirrels, and maybe even rattlesnakes (remember, they won't bother you if you don't bother them). The multicolored rocks above and below the trail hint at the region's complex and beautiful geology. In spring, wildflowers alongside the trail prove that this is more than a desolate landscape. In summer, the tunnels provide welcome shade and reminders of the work it took to build one of the world's great engineering wonders.

The trail follows these old rail lines all the way to Hoover Dam. The trail is mostly flat until the fifth tunnel, then it drops 500 feet to the parking garage at Hoover Dam. Whenever you're ready to turn around, retrace your steps to return.

trip 6 Lake Mead: Wetlands Trail

Distance	1.25 miles, loop
Hiking Time	30 minutes to 1 hour
Elevation	+/-90 feet
Difficulty	Moderate
Trail Use	Leashed dogs, good for kids
Best Times	Cold to warm
Agency	Lake Mead National Recreation Area at (702) 293-8907; www.nps.gov/lame
Recommended Maps	Free map available at visitor center
GPS Waypoints	Parking area: 36.124° N, 114.903° W
Vehicle	Passenger car OK

HIGHLIGHTS This short walk takes you down to the life along Las Vegas Wash.

DIRECTIONS From Las Vegas, take I-15 south to Highway 215 east. From Highway 215 east in Henderson, continue east on Lake Mead Drive/Highway 146, which leads directly to the entrance station for Lake Mead NRA. Immediately east of the entrance station, turn left (north) onto Northshore Road. The unsigned parking area is on the right (east) side of Northshore Road at mile marker 1.2.

FACILITIES/TRAILHEAD There are restrooms at the trailhead. The closest other facilities are at Boulder Beach Marina a few miles south on Lakeshore Scenic Drive. More restrooms and information are available at the Alan Bible Visitor Center and at marinas along Lake Mead between Hemenway and Overton. There are six National Park Service campgrounds in the Nevada portion of Lake Mead NRA, between Cottonwood Cove (south of Las Vegas and east of Searchlight) and Echo Bay (east of the Valley of Fire State Park), offering more than 600 sites for RVs, cars, and tents. They offer running water, dump stations, picnic tables, barbecue grills, and shade. Backcountry camping is allowed throughout Lake Mead and along the lakeshore, except in developed, restricted, or ecologically sensitive areas. Backpacking and horseback camping is prohibited within 500 feet of any paved road, within 100 feet of any spring or watering device, or in areas signed NO CAMPING. Vehicle camping is allowed only in designated spots.

From the parking area, follow the trail east across the flats. After 0.3 mile, the trail descends to Las Vegas Wash and the creek running through it.

It's amazing to see what water can do to a landscape. Along the first part of the trail, 100 feet above the wash, only stalwart creosote bushes grow. At the water's edge, however, you'll find grasses, reeds, and bushes in abundance.

For thousands of years, Las Vegas Wash has nourished birds, animals, and people as it channeled runoff from natural springs, distant mountains, and storms. Ever-growing Las Vegas adds to this flow with runoff from sprinklers, fountains, swimming pools,

city streets, and Lake Las Vegas immediately upstream on the other side of the road.

Although the water might seem inviting, it has been polluted by a city's worth of antifreeze, fertilizers, and other chemicals. Resist the temptation to jump in, splash about, or let your dog do the same. Do not drink the water.

Pollution hasn't kept birds and other wildlife away, however. You have the best chance of seeing them in early morning or late afternoon, when birds and animals are more active.

To return to your car, follow the trail as it loops back to the parking lot along the wash just north of Las Vegas Wash.

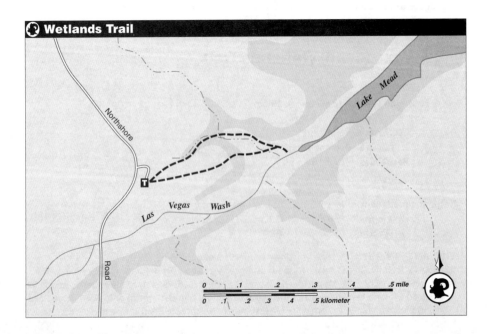

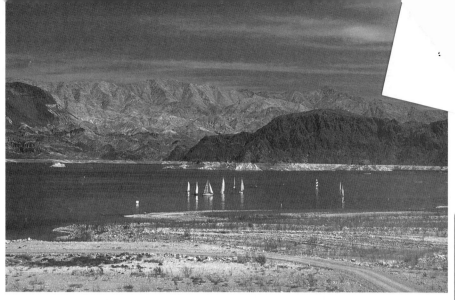

When full, Lake Mead holds enough water to cover Pennsylvania with nearly a foot of water.

trip 7 Lake Mead: Anniversary Narrows

Distance	2.5 or 5 miles, out-and-back
Hiking Time	3 to 5 hours
Elevation	+/-400 feet
Difficulty	Moderate
Trail Use	Leashed dogs, good for kids, backpacking option, map and compass
Best Times	Cold to warm
Agency	BLM Las Vegas at (702) 515-5000; www.nv.blm.gov/vegas
Recommended Maps	*Lake Mead* 1:100,000; *Calville Bay* 7.5-minute
GPS Waypoints	Calville Wash North Road: 36°196′ N, 114°687′ W Narrows: 36.221° N, 114.701° W
Vehicle	High-clearance or 4WD vehicle recommended, but passenger car may work

HIGHLIGHTS Anniversary Narrows is as beautiful a slot canyon as any other on Earth. It's not very long, but it is definitely worth the trip. The tilted sedimentary rock layers paint beautiful lines throughout the canyon. The abandoned borax mine along the way adds a taste of history. Anniversary Narrows is in the 48,000-acre Muddy Mountains Wilderness Area, designated by Congress in 2002. This is *not* the place to be during a flash flood. Hike somewhere else when thunderstorms are active anywhere in the sky.

DIRECTIONS There are two ways to drive to this hike from Las Vegas: From I-15 at North Las Vegas, take Lake Mead Blvd. east for about 14 miles to the entrance station for Lake Mead National Recreation Area. About 2 miles past (east of) the entrance station, turn left (east) onto Northshore Road. From Henderson and Hwy. 215 south, travel east on Lake Mead Drive for 7 miles. Soon after the entrance station to Lake Mead, turn left (north) onto Hwy. 167 (Northshore Road) and follow it north then east. At mile marker 16 on Northshore Road, turn left (north) onto the unpaved Calville Wash North Road. Low-clearance cars can park at 0.2 mile, adding 2.6 miles (round-trip) to the hike. High-clearance vehicles can take the left fork and follow the route as it meanders another 2 miles to the unsigned parking area on the bench above and just before Lovell Wash. Park here.

FACILITIES/TRAILHEAD There is no official trailhead/parking area for this hike. The closest restrooms are in Calville Bay at Mile 11 on Northshore Road. More restrooms and information are available at the Alan Bible Visitor Center and at marinas along Lake Mead between Hemenway and Overton.

There are six National Park Service campgrounds in the Nevada portion of Lake Mead National Recreation Area, between Cottonwood Cove (south of Las Vegas and east of Searchlight) and Echo Bay (east of the Valley of Fire State Park), offering more than 600 sites for RVs, cars, and tents. They offer running water, dump stations, picnic tables, barbecue grills, and shade. Backcountry camping is allowed throughout Lake Mead and along the lakeshore, except in developed, restricted, or ecologically sensitive areas. Backpacking and horseback camping is prohibited within 500 feet of any paved road, within 100 feet of any spring or watering device, or in areas signed NO CAMPING. Vehicle camping is allowed only in designated spots.

If you parked your passenger car below, follow the left fork (see the directions for high-clearance cars, above) to Lovell Wash, then continue with these directions. Enter Lovell Wash, then turn right (northeast), and follow it upstream, past the old borax mine ruins, for 1 mile to the mouth of Anniversary Narrows, which are about a quarter mile long. Although the terrain is gentle, the deep sand of the wash justifies the moderate difficulty rating for this hike.

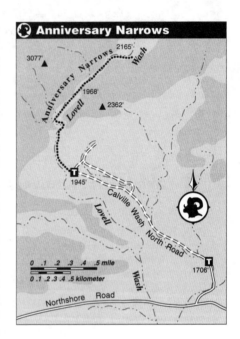

The narrows are located at the bottom of Lovell Wash, which drains out of the Muddy Mountains to the north. Borax, a cleaning agent, was discovered here in 1921. Over the next seven years, the mine produced 200,000 tons. There are several entrances and old railcar tunnels that invite exploration. Please keep in mind that these structures were shaky when they were built 80 years ago. Decades of rot, wind, rain, and rust have made them less stable. There might also be odorless-but-deadly gasses waiting for you in the tunnels. Please stay out of all mine tunnels and structures.

If you're backpacking, there is a nice campsite just beyond the mine, above the dam on the far side of the wash. There are also many nice places in the canyon beyond the narrows. Please avoid camping near water. Please do not camp in Lovell Wash or in the narrows. Not only is there a flash-flood risk during storms, but your presence will prevent wildlife from walking through on their regular commute to life-giving water at Lake Mead.

Retrace your steps to return.

Got Caliche?

Hiking across rocky ground, you may notice a white crust called caliche (ka-LEE-chee) on the bottom of many rocks. Calcium carbonate and other chemicals in the soil and in airborne dust react with rainwater to form a natural cement. Over the years, caliche can develop as a thick and durable concrete-like layer in the soil and on the bottom of many rocks.

Anniversary Narrows is one of the great treasures waiting outside Las Vegas.

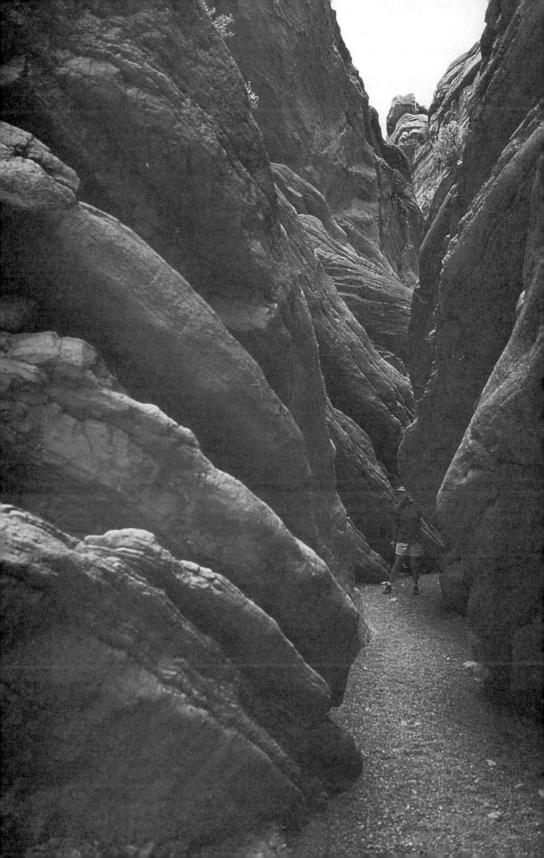

trip 8 **Lake Mead: Bowl of Fire**

Distance	2 miles, out-and-back; 3.7 miles, loop
Hiking Time	2 to 4 hours
Elevation	+/-190 feet (out-and-back); +/-400 feet (loop)
Difficulty	Moderate
Trail Use	Leashed dogs, backpacking option, map and compass
Best Times	Cool to warm
Agency	Lake Mead National Recreation Area at (702) 293-8907; www.nps.gov/lame
Recommended Maps	*Lake Mead* 1:100,000; *Muddy Peak* and *Calville Bay* 7.5-minute
GPS Waypoints	Bowl of Fire entrance: 36.222° N, 114.668° W
Vehicle	Passenger car OK

HIGHLIGHTS This hike leads to solitude, geologic wonders, and views of classic desert beauty. This isolated and fragile landscape is part of the 48,000-acre Muddy Mountains Wilderness Area. Please hike in washes or on rocks whenever possible to avoid damaging the fragile cryptobiotic soils.

DIRECTIONS There are two ways to drive to this hike from Las Vegas: From I-15 at North Las Vegas, take Lake Mead Blvd. east for about 14 miles to the entrance station for Lake Mead National Recreation Area. About 2 miles past (east of) the entrance station, turn left (east) onto Northshore Road. From Henderson and Hwy. 215 south, travel east on Lake Mead Drive for 7 miles. Soon after the entrance station to Lake Mead, turn left (north) onto Hwy. 167. (Northshore Road) and follow this as it leads north then east. Between mile markers 18 and 19, park at the roadside trashcan pullout on the left (north) side of road. Bowl of Fire is to the northwest, but your view is blocked by the low ridge immediately northwest of your car.

FACILITIES/TRAILHEAD The closest restrooms are in Calville Bay at mile 11 on Northshore Road. More restrooms and information are available at the Alan Bible Visitor Center and at marinas along Lake Mead between Hemenway and Overton. There are six National Park Service campgrounds in the Nevada portion of Lake Mead National Recreation Area, between Cottonwood Cove (south of Las Vegas and east of Searchlight) and Echo Bay (east of the Valley of Fire State Park), offering more than 600 sites for RVs, cars, and tents. They offer running water, dump stations, picnic tables, barbecue grills, and shade. Backcountry camping is allowed throughout Lake Mead and along the lakeshore, except in developed, restricted, or ecologically sensitive areas. Backpack/horseback camping is prohibited within 500 feet of any paved road, within 100 feet of any spring or watering device, or in areas signed NO CAMPING. Vehicle camping is allowed only in designated spots.

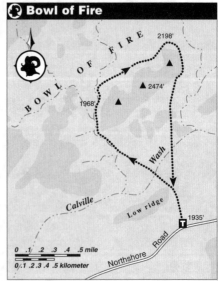

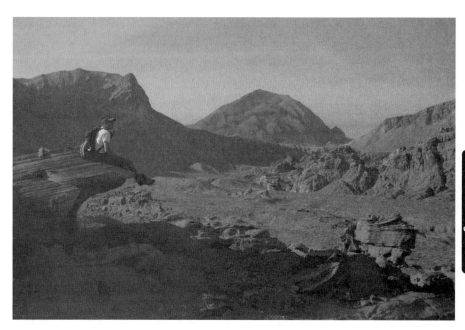

Bowl of Fire's geology is dazzlingly phantasmagoric . . . cue the dinosaurs.

From the car, hike north-northwest through a creosote-blackbrush plant community until you can cross the eastern terminus of the low ridge, about a half mile away. There is no trail, so bring a map and compass and use your route-finding skills. At the ridge, veer to the northwest toward the red rock formations. As you near Bowl of Fire, your route merges with a tributary of Calville Wash. Drop into the wash and follow it north to your destination. You have to scramble up a short, but difficult, waterfall to enter Bowl of Fire.

Once there, your route depends on your curiosity and inspiration. You don't have to look up and around to appreciate the geologic wonders of this region. Simply watching the many colorful rocks at your feet will tell you of the area's complexity and beauty. When you do look up and around, you'll be positively smitten.

Despite the area's name, fire and volcanics had nothing to do with this area's formation. The bright rocks around you are petrified sand dunes from the age of the dinosaurs between 65 million and 250 million years ago. Oxidized iron in the rock creates the bright reds and oranges. Called Aztec sandstone locally, these are the same rock formations as at Valley of Fire and Red Rock Canyon. The lighter buff-colored rock is limestone dating back as many as 500 million years. In some places, thrust-faulting has pushed this much older rock up and over the younger sandstone.

To return, retrace your steps, or make a loop by hiking northeast through Bowl of Fire for a mile, circumnavigating the ridge to your right, to the next low saddle on your right (south), then hike due south to your car, which should be visible along Northshore Road.

trip 9 Lake Mead: Hamblin Mountain

Distance	7 miles, out-and-back
Hiking Time	4 to 5 hours
Elevation	+/-1400 feet
Difficulty	Moderate to difficult
Trail Use	Leashed dogs, backpacking option, compass strongly encouraged
Best Times	Cool to warm
Agency	Lake Mead National Recreation Area at (702) 293-8907; www.nps.gov/lame
Recommended Maps	*Lake Mead* 1:100,000; *Calville Bay* 7.5-minute
GPS Waypoints	Parking: 36.210° N, 114.656° W
	Crossroads at colorful butte: 36.194° N, 114.634° W
	Summit: 36.178° N, 114.643° W
Vehicle	Passenger car OK

HIGHLIGHTS Solitude, geological wonder, and amazing views of the Black Mountains and Lake Mead all wait in this magical landscape only an hour from the Strip. You'll feel worlds away as you hike to

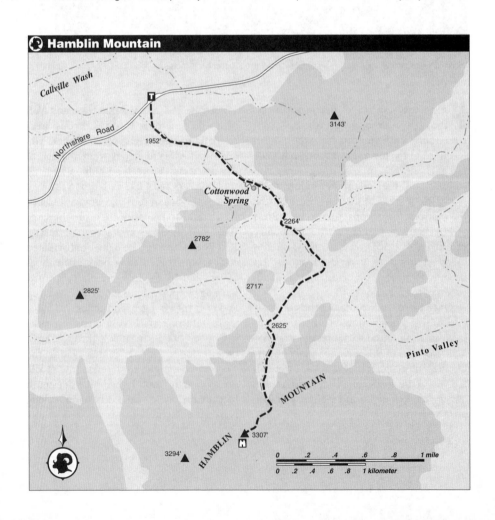

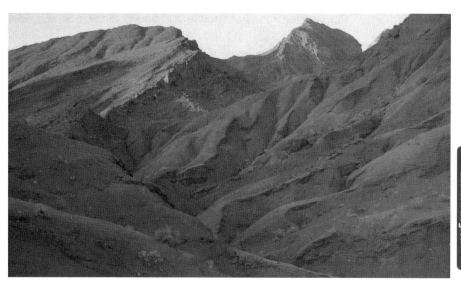

Morning or afternoon light can paint Lake Mead's landscapes with inspiring shadows and colors.

this soaring, rugged peak. Hamblin Mountain is part of the 39,000-acre Pinto Valley Wilderness Area. Please hike in washes or on rocks whenever possible to avoid damaging the fragile living soils.

DIRECTIONS There are two ways to drive to this hike from Las Vegas: From I-15 at North Las Vegas, take Lake Mead Blvd. east for about 14 miles to the entrance station for Lake Mead National Recreation Area. About 2 miles past (east of) the entrance station, turn left (east) onto Northshore Road. From Henderson and Hwy. 215 south, travel east on Lake Mead Drive. After about 7 miles, turn left (north) onto Hwy 167 (Northshore Road) and follow this as it leads north then east to the parking area. Park at the unsigned pullout on the left (north) side of Northshore Road 0.2 mile after mile marker 18.

FACILITIES/TRAILHEAD The closest restrooms are in Calville Bay at mile 11 on Northshore Road. More restrooms and information are available at the Alan Bible Visitor Center and at marinas along Lake Mead between Hemenway and Overton. There are six National Park Service campgrounds in the Nevada portion of Lake Mead National Recreation Area, between Cottonwood Cove (south of Las Vegas and east of Searchlight) and Echo Bay (east of the Valley of Fire State Park), offering more than 600 sites for RVs, cars, and tents. They offer running water, dump stations, picnic tables, barbecue grills, and shade. Backcountry camping is allowed throughout Lake Mead and along the lakeshore, except in developed, restricted, or ecologically sensitive areas. Backpack/horseback camping is prohibited within 500 feet of any paved road, within 100 feet of any spring or watering device, or in areas signed NO CAMPING. Vehicle camping is allowed only in designated spots.

NOTE Hamblin Mountain is not visible from your car (however, it is visible from Northshore Road to the west, just east of a small summit at mile marker 15). The unsigned route also follows unnamed, meandering, and disorienting washes and ridges. I have a good sense of direction, and I needed to refer to my compass regularly to stay on track. I *strongly* recommend a compass for this trip.

On the west side of the pullout, look south across Northshore Road for an unsigned trail climbing the bank. Cross the street (carefully—you're on a blind corner) and follow the trail south across a relatively flat table to the edge of the wash that drains from the southeast. Follow the trail as it drops into the wash, then turn left (south-east), following the wash uphill.

At roughly 1 mile, you will reach Cottonwood Spring—a few scraggly trees at the base of a 10-foot-tall dry waterfall. Climb the waterfall (the hardest part of the hike), and continue following the wash southeast.

Ignore all smaller washes entering from the right, or south.

Roughly 2 miles from the car, look for a distinct butte rising about 200 feet above the wash. Capped with grayish-brown limestone and streaked with red soil, it is both colorful and a major landmark. When you reach the base of this butte (on its west side), turn right (south) and follow the wash that skirts the butte's western edge for a quarter mile until you reach an intersection of drainages, where washes from the left (east) and right (west) converge. The colors and textures of the rocks and soil in this spot are striking in their variety.

From this point, turn right, following the wash that drains from the west. A faint trail parallels the wash high on its northern (south-facing) bank to the crest of a ridge that slopes from the southeast to northwest. At this point Hamblin Mountain rises large in front of you to the south. From this point, drop into the next wash south, then turn left, following the wash up, south, and toward the peak of Hamblin Mountain. After a half mile of hiking up the wash, cairns direct you left (east) as the trail climbs out of the wash to the summit ridge northeast of the peak. Once on the ridge, turn right (southwest) and follow the ridge to the summit. Retrace your steps to return.

Please practice Leave No Trace principles whenever you travel and camp, by sticking to trails, washes, or stone whenever possible (read more about LNT and trail etiquette, page 18).

trip 10 Lake Mead: Northshore Summit Trail

Distance	0.5 mile, out-and-back
Hiking Time	30 minutes to 1 hour
Elevation	+/-400 feet
Difficulty	Moderate
Trail Use	Leashed dogs, good for kids
Best Times	Cool to warm
Agency	Lake Mead National Recreation Area at (702) 293-8907; www.nps.gov/lame
Recommended Maps	*Lake Mead* 1:100,000; *Callville Bay* and *Boulder Canyon* 7.5 minute
GPS Waypoints	Parking area: 36.227° N, 114.621° W
Vehicle	Passenger car OK

HIGHLIGHTS The view from this high point along Northshore Road offers a taste of the many beautiful geologic wonders of this region. From the south, the view sweeps clockwise from Northshore Peak, to the red sandstone of the Bowl of Fire, to the limestone of Muddy Peak and Bitter Ridge, and across Bitter Spring Valley into the Virgin River basin.

DIRECTIONS There are two ways to drive to this hike from Las Vegas: From I-15 at North Las Vegas, take Lake Mead Blvd. east for about 14 miles to the entrance station for Lake Mead National Recreation Area. About 2 miles past (east of) the entrance station, turn left (east) onto Northshore Road. From Henderson and Hwy. 215 south, travel east on Lake Mead Drive for 7 miles. Soon after the entrance station to Lake Mead, turn left (north) onto Hwy. 167 (Northshore Road) and follow this as it leads north then east. The parking area is on the left (north) side of Northshore Road between mile markers 20 and 21.

FACILITIES/TRAILHEAD The closest restrooms are in Calville Bay at mile 11 on Northshore Road. More restrooms and information are available at the Alan Bible Visitor Center and at marinas along Lake Mead between Hemenway and Overton. There are six National Park Service campgrounds in the Nevada portion of Lake Mead National Recreation Area, between Cottonwood Cove (south of Las Vegas and east of Searchlight) and Echo Bay (east of the Valley of Fire State Park), offering more than 600 sites for RVs, cars, and tents. They offer running water, dump stations, picnic tables, barbecue grills, and shade. Backcountry camping is allowed throughout Lake Mead and along the lakeshore, except in developed, restricted, or ecologically sensitive areas. Backpacking and horseback camping

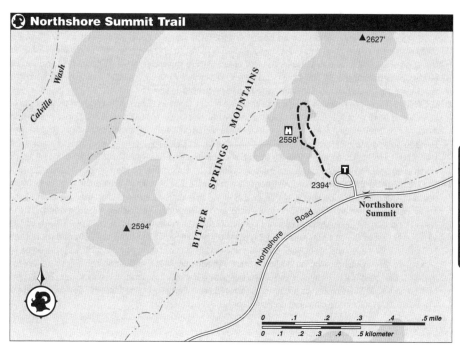

Northshore Summit Trail

is prohibited within 500 feet of any paved road, within 100 feet of any spring or watering device, or in areas signed NO CAMPING. Vehicle camping is allowed only in designated spots.

From the parking area, follow the trail north to the viewpoint. A spur of the trail loops around to a saddle and back to the summit, offering a variety of views along the way. Interesting geology is also apparent at your feet. On the slopes immediately west of the summit, you'll be able to see layers bent by years of pressure and tectonic movement.

Retrace your steps to return.

trip 11   Lake Mead: Pinto Valley

Distance	2 miles or 5 miles, out-and-back
Hiking Time	2 to 5 hours
Elevation	+/-245 feet (short option); +/-800 feet (long option)
Difficulty	Moderate
Trail Use	Leashed dogs, good for kids, backpacking option, map and compass
Best Times	Cool to warm
Agency	Lake Mead National Recreation Area at (702) 293-8907; www.nps.gov/lame
Recommended Maps	*Lake Mead* 1:100,000; *Boulder Canyon* 7.5-minute
GPS Waypoints	Viewpoint: 36.233° N, 114.538° W
Vehicle	Passenger car OK

HIGHLIGHTS Solitude, geological wonder, and fragile desert beauty await in this wide, hidden valley. Although Pinto Valley is less than an hour from the Strip, it can seem 1,000 miles (or 1,000 years) away—as long as you can ignore the many airplanes flying to and from Vegas. Pinto Valley slopes to the southwest and eventually drains to Lake Mead through Boulder Wash. This isolated and fragile landscape is part of the 39,000-acre Pinto Valley Wilderness Area. Please hike in washes or on rocks whenever possible to avoid damaging the fragile cryptobiotic soils.

DIRECTIONS There are two ways to drive to this hike from Las Vegas: From I-15 at North Las Vegas, take Lake Mead Blvd. east for about 14 miles to the entrance station for Lake Mead National Recreation Area. About 2 miles past (east of) the entrance station, turn left (east) onto Northshore Road. From Henderson and Hwy. 215 south, travel east on Lake Mead Drive for 7 miles. Soon after the entrance station to Lake Mead, turn left (north) onto Hwy. 167 (Northshore Road) and follow this as it leads north then east. Park at the unsigned pullout on the left (north) side of road at roughly mile 25.7.

FACILITIES/TRAILHEAD The closest restrooms are in Calville Bay at mile 11 on Northshore Road. More restrooms and information are available at the Alan Bible Visitor Center and at marinas along Lake Mead between Hemenway and Overton. There are six National Park Service campgrounds in the Nevada portion of Lake Mead National Recreation Area, between Cottonwood Cove (south of Las Vegas and east of Searchlight) and Echo Bay (east of the Valley of Fire State Park), offering more than 600 sites for RVs, cars, and tents. They offer running water, dump stations, picnic tables, barbecue grills, and shade. Backcountry camping is allowed throughout Lake Mead and along the lakeshore, except in developed, restricted, or ecologically sensitive areas. Backpacking and horseback camping is prohibited within 500 feet of any paved road, within 100 feet of any spring or watering device, or in areas signed NO CAMPING. Vehicle camping is allowed only in designated spots.

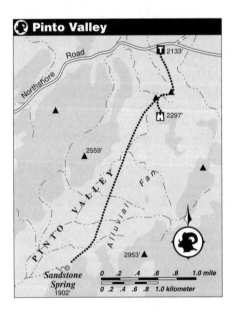

From the car, hike south less than a mile up low hills and washes to the first sandstone formation. There is no trail. Turn right (southwest), then hike past (or through) the next sandstone formation to the top of the low saddle separating the road from Pinto Valley. You'll know by the view of the long valley to the southwest that you've arrived.

This is a perfect place to stop, enjoy the view, have a picnic, and explore the sandstone surrounding you. The bright rocks are petrified sand dunes from the age of the dinosaurs between 65 million and 250 million years ago. Oxidized iron in the rock creates the bright reds and oranges. Called Aztec sandstone locally, these are the same rock formations as at Valley of Fire and at Red Rock Canyon. The lighter buff-colored rock on the higher ridges is limestone dating back as many as 500 million years. In some places, thrust-faulting has pushed this much older rock up and over the younger sandstone.

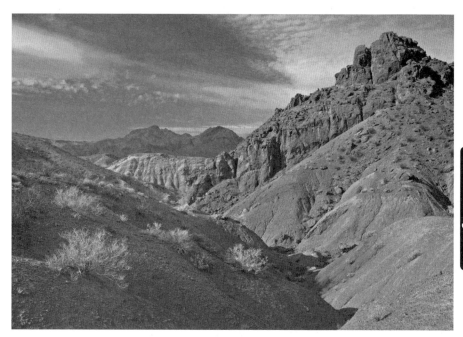

Every turn in the trail offers a unique glimpse into the geologic wonders on Lake Mead's north shore.

trip 12 Lake Mead: Redstone Trail

Distance	0.5 mile, loop
Hiking Time	30 minutes to 1 hour
Elevation	+/-45 feet
Difficulty	Easy
Trail Use	Leashed dogs, good for kids
Best Times	Cool to warm
Agency	Lake Mead National Recreation Area at (702) 293-8907; www.nps.gov/lame
Recommended Maps	Free map at entrance station
GPS Waypoints	Parking area: 36.242° N, 114.516° W
Vehicle	Passenger car OK

HIGHLIGHTS This enjoyable interpretive hike takes you through wonderful red sandstone formed between 65 million and 250 million years ago. Keep an eye out for petroglyphs made by ancient people who lived here long ago.

DIRECTIONS There are two ways to drive to this hike from Las Vegas: From I-15 at North Las Vegas, take Lake Mead Blvd. east for about 14 miles to the entrance station for Lake Mead National Recreation Area. About 2 miles past (east of) the entrance station, turn left (east) onto Northshore Road. From Henderson and Hwy. 215 south, travel east on Lake Mead Drive for 7 miles. Soon after the entrance station to Lake Mead, turn left (north) onto Hwy. 167 (Northshore Road) and follow it north then east to mile marker 27. The signed parking area is on the right (south) side of the road.

FACILITIES/TRAILHEAD Restrooms and picnic tables are available here. More restrooms and information are available at the Alan Bible Visitor Center and at marinas along Lake Mead between Hemenway and Overton. There are six National Park Service campgrounds in the Nevada portion of Lake Mead National Recreation Area, between Cottonwood Cove (south of Las Vegas and east of Searchlight) and Echo Bay (east of the Valley of Fire State Park), offering more than 600 sites for RVs, cars, and tents. They offer running water, dump stations, picnic tables, barbecue grills, and shade. Backcountry camping is allowed throughout Lake Mead and along the lakeshore, except in developed, restricted, or ecologically sensitive areas. Backpacking and horseback camping is prohibited within 500 feet of any paved road, within 100 feet of any spring or watering device, or in areas signed NO CAMPING. Vehicle camping is allowed only in designated spots.

From the parking area, follow the trail south as it winds around the sandstone formations and back to the parking lot.

During the age of the dinosaurs, between 65 million and 250 million years ago, these bright sandstone formations were part of a great sandy desert stretching to what is now southern Colorado. Minerals cemented the shifting sand into stone. Rusted iron molecules give the stone its red color. Geologists call this Aztec sandstone today. It's the same sandstone at Valley of Fire State Park to the north, and at Red Rock Canyon on the west side of Las Vegas Valley.

The Black Mountains to the south are lighter-colored limestone dating back as many as 500 million years. Thrust-faulting has pushed this much older rock up and over the younger sandstone. Erosion has washed away the limestone and sculpted the dunes into these unique shapes.

For thousands of years, ancient peoples lived among rock formations like these, leaving behind mysterious petroglyphs and other artifacts that are fragile, irreplaceable, and protected by state and federal laws. Please *do not touch* petroglyphs or other artifacts. Leave them as you find them so others may enjoy them too.

Most animals living here come out only at night. Look carefully for tracks of lizards, kangaroo mice, beetles, and maybe even kit foxes or coyotes. Bighorn might be watching from the hills to the south.

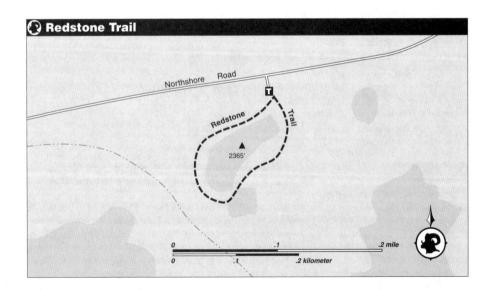

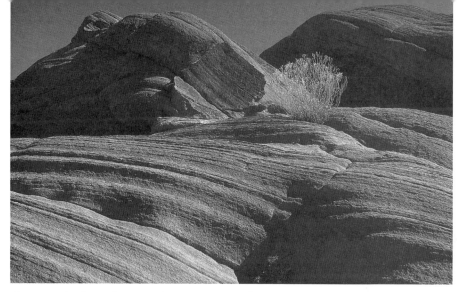

Blowing sand millions of years ago helped create these patterns on the sandstone.

trip 13 Lake Mead: Redstone Peaks

Distance	3 to 4 miles, loop
Hiking Time	3 to 4 hours
Elevation	+/-1200 feet
Difficulty	Difficult
Trail Use	Leashed dogs
Best Times	Cool to warm
Agency	Lake Mead National Recreation Area at (702) 293-8907; www.nps.gov/lame
Recommended Maps	*Lake Mead* 1:100,000; *Boulder Canyon* 7.5-minute
GPS Waypoints	Parking area: 36.242° N, 114.516° W; Summit: 36.230° N, 114.499° W
Vehicle	Passenger car OK

HIGHLIGHTS This hike begins among the picturesque sandstone formations at the Redstone Trail, then scrambles up to sweeping views across the rugged and beautiful Black Mountains on Lake Mead's north shore.

DIRECTIONS There are two ways to drive to this hike from Las Vegas: From I-15 at North Las Vegas, take Lake Mead Blvd. east for about 14 miles to the entrance station for Lake Mead National Recreation Area. About 2 miles past (east of) the entrance station, turn left (east) onto Northshore Road. From Henderson and Hwy. 215 south, travel east on Lake Mead Drive. After about 7 miles, turn left (north) onto Hwy. 167 (Northshore Road) and follow this as it leads north then east. This hike begins at the Redstone Trail parking area, at mile marker 27, on the right (south) side of the road.

FACILITIES/TRAILHEAD Restrooms and picnic tables are available here. More restrooms and information are available at the Alan Bible Visitor Center and at marinas along Lake Mead between Hemenway and Overton. There are six National Park Service campgrounds in the Nevada portion of Lake Mead National Recreation Area, between Cottonwood Cove (south of Las Vegas and east of Searchlight) and Echo Bay (east of the Valley of Fire State Park), offering more than 600 sites for RVs, cars, and tents. They offer running water, dump stations, picnic tables, barbecue grills, and shade. Backcountry camping is allowed throughout Lake Mead and along the lakeshore, except in developed, restricted, or ecologically sensitive areas. Backpack/horseback camping is prohibited within 500 feet of any paved road, within 100 feet of any spring or watering device, or in areas signed NO CAMPING. Vehicle camping is allowed only in designated spots.

From the parking area, follow the Redstone Dunes Interpretive Trail to its highest southeast point, then stop and look up to the southeast. The highest rugged peaks above you are your goal. Now, venture from the trail, heading southeast cross-country. Aim for the eastern (left) side of the smaller ridge in front of you, point 950 on the map. Although there is no official trail, this hike is popular with locals. Your attentive eyes will help you follow a faint climbers' route for the remainder of this hike. Following this route whenever possible will preserve this area's fragile soils and plants, and trekking poles will help you climb and descend this rugged, ankle-breaking landscape.

Once you are at the eastern base of point 950, continue circumnavigating this formation in a clockwise direction, following the drainage between it and the higher peaks to your left. After another quarter mile, look up to your left (south), where you'll see a notch to the right (west) of the prominent peak above you. This is your goal. Start climbing. Once on the ridge, you'll notice several peaks in this neighborhood, all of which are accessible. Each one offers a unique view into the jumbled canyons below. Climb as many as your energy level and desire allow. To return, either retrace your steps, or descend the next drainage to the east of Redstone Peaks.

While drinking in the view to your south, consider the violent geologic events that made this beautiful landscape possible: Between 11 and 15 million years ago, the Cleopatra Mountains to your east and the peaks of Hamblin Mountain to your west were part of a single, large stratovolcano. Enter plate tectonics and the Hamblin Bay Fault, which you crossed hiking from the car, and which ripped the volcano apart, sliding the northern half (Hamblin Mountain) to the west, and the southern half (Cleopatra) to the east. The two halves of this former volcano now sit about 10 miles apart. The basalt peaks on which you stand

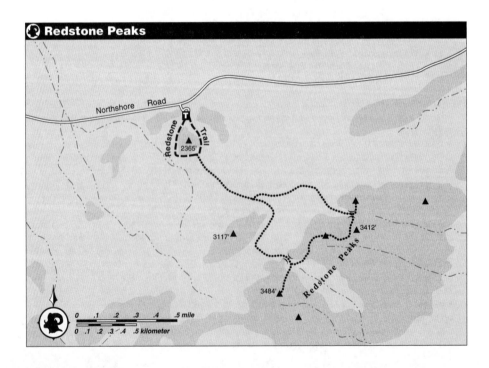

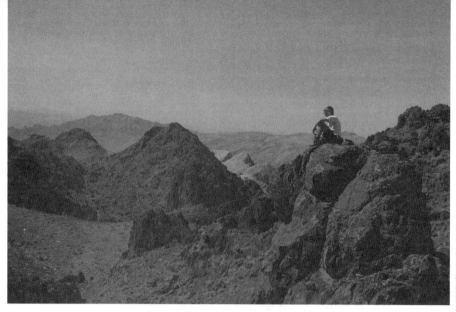

There's a lot of wild, rugged beauty to soak in from the top of Redstone Peaks.

are pieces of the volcano that broke off during all the pushing and shoving.

Millions of years later, and thousands of years ago, ancient peoples lived in this area, leaving behind mysterious petroglyphs and other artifacts that are fragile, irreplaceable, and protected by state and federal laws. Please *do not touch* petroglyphs or other artifacts. Leave them as you find them so others may enjoy them too.

Hike quietly and scan the slopes around you during this hike for a glimpse of the bighorn sheep herds that live in this area.

Please follow Leave No Trace principles whenever you travel and camp, by sticking to trails, washes, or stone whenever possible (read more about LNT and trail etiquette, page 18).

trip 14 Lake Mead: Jimbilnan High Route

Distance	2.5 miles, out-and-back
Hiking Time	2 to 5 hours
Elevation	+/-730 feet
Difficulty	Difficult
Trail Use	Leashed dogs, backpacking option, map and compass
Best Times	Cool to warm
Agency	Lake Mead National Recreation Area at (702) 293-8907; www.nps.gov/lame
Recommended Maps	*Lake Mead* 1:100,000; *Middle Point* 7.5-minute
GPS Waypoints	High point: 36.245° N, 114.454° W
Vehicle	High-clearance or 4WD vehicle recommended

HIGHLIGHTS This cross-country hike leads to soaring views over Lake Mead and the Cathedral Peaks. These mountains are now part of the 19,000-acre Jimbilnan Wilderness Area, designated in 2002. Although the name *Jimbilnan* might sound exotic, it is the brainchild of Jim, Bill, and Nancy, the Park Service employees who developed the inventory and proposal for this wilderness unit as the legislation was being prepared.

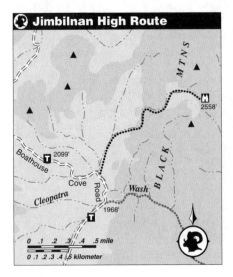

Jimbilnan High Route

DIRECTIONS There are two ways to drive to this hike from Las Vegas: From I-15 at North Las Vegas, take Lake Mead Blvd. east for about 14 miles to the entrance station for Lake Mead National Recreation Area. About 2 miles past (east of) the entrance station, turn left (east) onto Northshore Road. From Henderson and Hwy. 215 south, travel east on Lake Mead Drive for 7 miles. Soon after the entrance station to Lake Mead, turn left (north) onto Hwy. 167 (Northshore Road) and follow this as it leads north then east. Turn right (south) onto the unpaved Boathouse Cove Road about 100 yards before mile marker 30. Follow Boathouse Cove Road south, up and over the summit, then park anywhere between 2 and 3 miles (low-clearance vehicles might have to park at 2 miles) beyond the summit.

FACILITIES/TRAILHEAD The nearest facilities are in Echo Bay, south of mile 35 on Northshore Road. More restrooms and information are available at the Alan Bible Visitor Center and at marinas along Lake Mead between Hemenway and Overton. There are six National Park Service campgrounds in the Nevada portion of Lake Mead National Recreation Area, between Cottonwood Cove (south of Las Vegas and east of Searchlight) and Echo Bay (east of the Valley of Fire State Park), offering more than 600 sites for RVs, cars, and tents. They offer running water, dump stations, picnic tables, barbecue grills, and shade. Backcountry camping is allowed throughout Lake Mead and along the lakeshore, except in developed, restricted, or ecologically sensitive areas. Backpacking or horseback camping is prohibited within 500 feet of any paved road, within 100 feet of any spring or watering device, or in areas signed NO CAMPING. Vehicle camping is allowed only in designated spots, the closest of which are at 1 and 3 miles on Boathouse Cove Road.

From the car, hike north-northeast up the drainage between the peaks to the north and the Black Mountains to the east. Follow the drainages or ridges (whichever you prefer—there is no trail) northeast onto the ridgetops north of Cleopatra Wash and overlooking the Overton Arm of Lake Mead.

This hike into the eastern Black Mountains shows that these mountains are anything but black. Much of this colorful volcanic rock spewed from the Cleopatra-Hamblin Volcano between 13 million and 20 million years ago. Eruptions over time produced lava and ash with differing mineral content and texture, helping to create the variety of shapes and colors you see today.

Eventually, as tectonic forces pulled apart this region to create the Great Basin

Time your hike in spring, and wildflowers will add to the show.

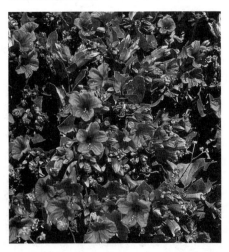

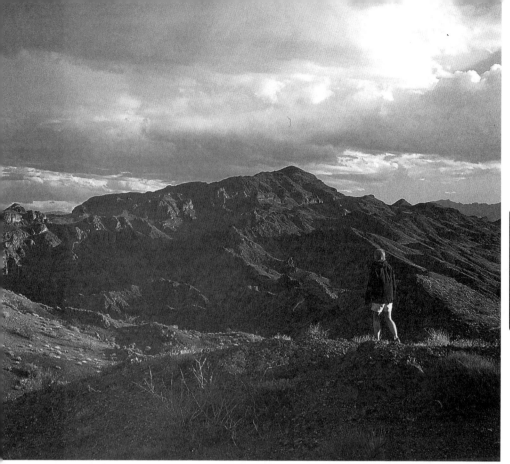

Enjoying the ruggedly beautiful Jimbilnan Wilderness

to the north, a strike-slip fault split the volcano in two and carried the southern half of it 10 miles to the west. This hike explores the remnant northern half of the volcano. The southern remnant is Mt. Hamblin, which is just east of Calville Bay (Trip 9). Even more tilting, faulting, and erosion have given these hills their dramatic appearance.

The views from the ridgetops are splendid and worth the cross-country travel, towering over the Cathedral Cliffs to the northwest, the Overton Arm of Lake Mead to the east, and the jagged peaks of the Black Mountains stretching to the south and west. Reaching the summit of the highest peaks is not recommended, as the crumbly rock makes for dangerous climbing.

When you have finished exploring the ridgetops, retrace your steps to return. Undeveloped car campsites are available at 1 and 3 miles along Boathouse Cove Road.

trip 15 **Lake Mead: Cleopatra Wash**

Distance	5 miles, out-and-back
Hiking Time	2 to 5 hours
Elevation	+/-750 feet
Difficulty	Moderate to difficult
Trail Use	Leashed dogs, backpacking option, map and compass
Best Times	Cool to warm
Agency	Lake Mead National Recreation Area at (702) 293-8907; www.nps.gov/lame
Recommended Maps	*Lake Mead* 1:100,000; *Middle Point* 7.5-minute
GPS Waypoints	Top of Cleopatra Wash: 36.237° N, 114.462° W; Viewpoint over Cleopatra Cove: 36.222° N, 114.430° W
Vehicle	High-clearance or 4WD vehicle recommended

HIGHLIGHTS This hike takes you through a cathedral of volcanic rocks to a dry waterfall over Lake Mead, which is inaccessible without climbing skills and ropes; the hike is worthwhile, even if you can't reach the lake. Cleopatra Wash is aptly named. Its towering hoodoos, spires, and sculpted rock formations of every color suggest exotic lands far away. Since 2002, it has been a part of the 19,000-acre Jimbilnan Wilderness Area, which was named for three Park Service employees—Jim, Bill, and Nancy—National Park Service employees who helped develop the inventory and proposal boundaries for the wilderness designation. Clever.

DIRECTIONS There are two ways to drive to this hike from Las Vegas: From I-15 at North Las Vegas, take Lake Mead Blvd. east for about 14 miles to the entrance station for Lake Mead National Recreation Area. About 2 miles past (east of) the entrance station, turn left (east) onto Northshore Road. From Henderson and Hwy. 215 south, travel east on Lake Mead Drive for 7 miles. Soon after the entrance station to Lake Mead, turn left (north) onto Hwy. 167 (Northshore Road) and follow this as it leads north then east. Turn right (south) onto the unpaved Boathouse Cove Road about 100 yards before mile marker 30. Follow Boathouse Cove Road south, up and over the summit, then park at the designated camping area 3 miles (low-clearance vehicles might have to park at 2 miles) beyond the summit.

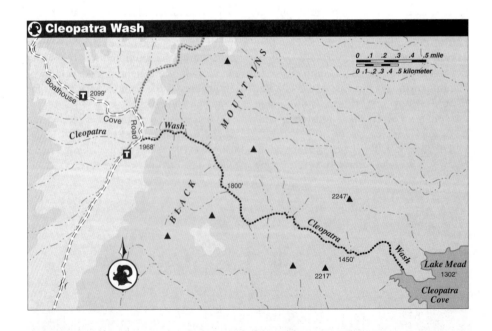

FACILITIES/TRAILHEAD The nearest facilities are in Echo Bay, south of mile 35 on Northshore Road. More restrooms and information are available at the Alan Bible Visitor Center and at marinas along Lake Mead between Hemenway and Overton. There are six National Park Service campgrounds in the Nevada portion of Lake Mead National Recreation Area, between Cottonwood Cove (south of Las Vegas and east of Searchlight) and Echo Bay (east of the Valley of Fire State Park), offering more than 600 sites for RVs, cars, and tents. They offer running water, dump stations, picnic tables, barbecue grills, and shade. Backcountry camping is allowed throughout Lake Mead and along the lakeshore, except in developed, restricted, or ecologically sensitive areas. Backpack/horseback camping is prohibited within 500 feet of any paved road, within 100 feet of any spring or watering device, or in areas signed NO CAMPING. Vehicle camping is allowed only in designated spots, the closest of which are at 1 and 3 miles on Boathouse Cove Road.

From your car, hike east down the wash 2.5 miles to the lake at Cleopatra Cove. The hiking is alternately easy down the sandy wash, and difficult when it comes to negotiating waterfalls, of which there are five or six along the way. Each requires easy scrambling, or offers a way to walk around.

The last waterfall is the most difficult, a 40-foot drop that requires climbing ropes and equipment to climb down.

This drop is a lesson in how quickly landscapes can change in the desert. The first printing of this book described an easy-to-manage 10-foot climb down to the sandbar

Predawn light glows off the water at the mouth of Cleopatra Wash.

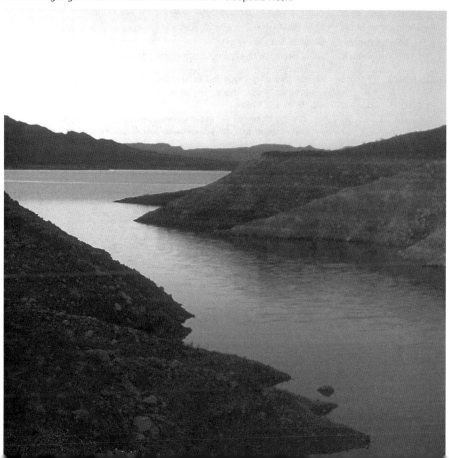

at Cleopatra Cove, which is what I experienced when scouting the trip in 2004. As the water levels dropped in Lake Mead, however, runoff down Cleopatra Wash washed the sandbar away, leaving a much bigger drop and a reminder that desert landscapes can change quickly and dramatically.

Much of this colorful volcanic rock spewed from the Cleopatra-Hamblin volcano between 13 million and 20 million years ago. Soon thereafter (geologically speaking), as tectonic forces pulled apart this region to create the Great Basin to the north, a strike-slip fault split the volcano in two and carried the southern half of it 10 miles to the west, where Mt. Hamblin sits today, just east of Calville Bay (Trip 9). Further tilting, faulting, and other geologic movements helped give the rocks in Cleopatra Wash their topsy-turvy appearance.

Once you have explored the lake and Cleopatra Cove, retrace your steps to return.

trip 16 Buffington Pockets

Distance	Varies
Hiking Time	Varies
Elevation	Varies (2770 feet at dam)
Difficulty	Moderate to very difficult
Trail Use	Leashed dogs, good for kids, map and compass
Best Times	Cold to warm
Agency	BLM Las Vegas (702) 515-5000; www.nv.blm.gov/vegas/
Recommended Maps	*Lake Mead* 1:100,000; *Muddy Peak* and *Piute Point* 7.5-minute
GPS Waypoints	Dam: 36.384° N, 114.690° W
Vehicle	High-clearance or 4WD vehicle recommended

HIGHLIGHTS This hidden wonderland of geology between Valley of Fire State Park and Lake Mead National Recreation Area is great for hiking, climbing, or just enjoying the surroundings.

DIRECTIONS Take I-15 north from Las Vegas. Take exit 75 and drive east toward Valley of Fire on Highway 169. After 3 miles, turn right (southeast) onto the unpaved Bitter Spring Trail Back Country Byway. After 4 miles on the Bitter Spring Trail Back Country Byway, continue straight (east) past the signed intersection for Color Rock Quarry. At roughly 5 miles, veer right (east) at an unsigned fork for another mile to Buffington Pockets. You'll know you're there when you're surrounded by towering, sculpted sandstone formations. Here and there, side roads lead to several informal parking areas and undeveloped campsites.

FACILITIES/TRAILHEAD The nearest facilities are off of I-15 at exit 75. Buffington Pockets is officially Bureau of Land Management backcountry. Camping is allowed anywhere, but please follow state law and Leave No Trace principles by not camping within 200 feet of water. Please also drive only on designated routes and park only in established areas.

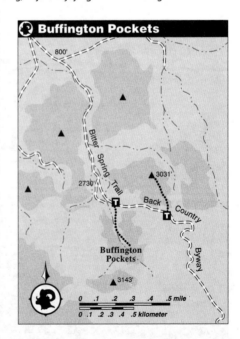

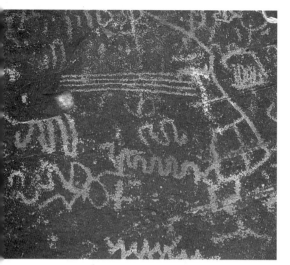

Natives long ago carved these petroglyphs—but what do they mean?

logic wonder—great for picnicking, camping, and exploring. Both easy and difficult routes abound. Like Valley of Fire and Red Rock Canyon National Conservation Area, Buffington Pockets is an area where Jurassic-era (between 65-million- and 250-million-year-old) sandstone meets much older Precambrian limestone (up to 550 million years old), often in amazing and beautiful ways.

For at least 1,000 years and possibly much longer, Native Americans inhabited the region. You might come across signs of these past lives, including agave roasting pits, petroglyphs, campsites, and chipped stone tools. These artifacts are irreplaceable and protected by numerous state and federal laws. *Please do not touch, alter, destroy, or remove any artifacts.* The oil on your skin can damage the natural protective coating on petroglyphs. If you would like to help protect these resources while learning more about them, please volunteer for the BLM's Site Steward program. Call the BLM at the number above for details.

Located in the Muddy Mountains south of Valley of Fire State Park, Buffington Pockets is a vehicle-accessible jumble of geo-

trip 17 Muddy Peak

Distance	8 miles, out-and-back
Hiking Time	6 to 8 hours
Elevation	+/-2850 feet
Difficulty	Most difficult
Trail Use	Leashed dogs, backpacking option, map and compass
Best Times	Cool to warm
Agency	Lake Mead National Recreation Area at (702) 293-8907; www.nps.gov/lame
Recommended Maps	*Lake Mead* 1:100,000; *Muddy Peak* 7.5-minute
GPS Waypoints	Muddy Peak: 36.298° N, 114.692° W
Vehicle	High-clearance or 4WD vehicle recommended

HIGHLIGHTS Muddy Peak is the most difficult trip in this book. Climbers must climb steep, crumbly rocky slopes with sections of high exposure (a high chance of injury or death if you fall) and falling rocks. *Do not attempt this peak unless you are a seasoned, fit, and prepared desert mountaineer.* That said, it's also one of my favorite trips in Southern Nevada. The combination of geology, challenge, and nearly pristine landscape makes it a rewarding journey. Congress designated 48,000 acres of this area as the Muddy Mountains Wilderness Area in 2002.

DIRECTIONS Take I-15 north from Las Vegas. Take exit 75 and drive east toward Valley of Fire on Highway 169. After 3 miles, turn right (southeast) onto the unpaved Bitter Spring Back Country Byway. After 4 miles, follow the byway straight (east) past the signed intersection for Color Rock Quarry. At roughly 5

miles, veer right (east) at an unsigned fork for another mile to Buffington Pockets. Continue east on the byway past Buffington Pockets for another 5 bumpy and twisting miles (always heading southeast at forks) to a right (west) turn off the byway and into a wash that heads 1 mile to the trailhead.
FACILITIES/TRAILHEAD The nearest facilities are at exit 75 on I-15.

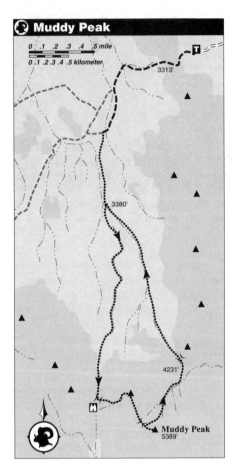

From the trailhead, follow the old jeep trail west up and over the ridge into the next valley. From the ridgetop, follow the trail for 1 mile west past two major washes, then southwest to where it passes between rock formations. After passing the smaller rock outcrop on the left of the road, veer left (southeast) from the road into the wash. Follow the wash south for about 2.1 miles to the far southern end of the valley. Only the first mile or so is on trail. The rest of this hike is cross-country.

As you're hiking south through the main valley toward Muddy Peak, please stick to the washes. Not only are they the easiest and fastest way to navigate this landscape, traveling in them protects the fragile cryptobiotic soils throughout the valley.

As you enter the valley, the sharp profile of Muddy Peak rises southeast of the cliffs at the southern end of the valley. Your goal is the saddle right (west) of the cliffs. As you're hiking, notice the beautiful geology of this valley. The colorful sandstone formations are fossilized sand dunes dating back 65 million to 250 million years to the age of the dinosaurs. The limestone peaks rising above and on top of the sandstone is much older, dating back as many as 600 million years. As a rule, younger rocks lie on top of older rocks. However, Earth's powerful tectonic forces cracked, bent, and thrust the limestone up and over the younger sandstone about 65 million years ago. The thrust fault in this valley is similar to the Keystone Thrust Fault in Red Rock Canyon.

Once you've caught your breath and enjoyed the view on the saddle, turn left (east) and start climbing up the slope. The easiest route (a relative term) is a couple hundred yards to the right (south) of the unnavigable ridgeline. Once you reach the shoulder of the ridge (where you gain a view to the east), follow the ridgeline southeast to the peak, climbing the short rocky points along the way. The final few hundred vertical feet to the peak are the most difficult. The easiest route follows the ridgeline into a manageable climb up the crack to the left of the prominent fin on the peak's northwest corner. You definitely need to use your hands at this point, and you could get hurt if you fall, possibly seriously. Luckily, this pitch is short (only about 10 to 15 vertical feet).

To avoid fateful encounters with falling rocks, send only one climber at a time up or down the most exposed sections, with others waiting below safely out of the way. Once the leader has reached a safe spot, from which no rocks can fall, send other climbers up. Helmets and ropes are good ideas.

Repeat this strategy on the way down and follow your tracks back to the wash and the trail.

For an exciting and beautiful loop back to the main valley and the trailhead, down climb carefully from Muddy Peak, retracing your steps for 0.2 mile, then turn right (east). Traverse the southern (north-facing) slope of the canyon until you find the best route down and north across the canyon. Although this route is difficult, it's no harder than the route up, and you'll be rewarded with juicy views and geology. At 0.6 mile from Muddy Peak, hike up and over the obvious notch (or saddle) on the north ridge of the canyon into the valley through which you hiked on your approach. From the top of the saddle, your route will be obvious: downhill to the north, following the washes back to the jeep track, then right (east) on it to the trailhead and your car.

Looking south from the top of Lovell Wash

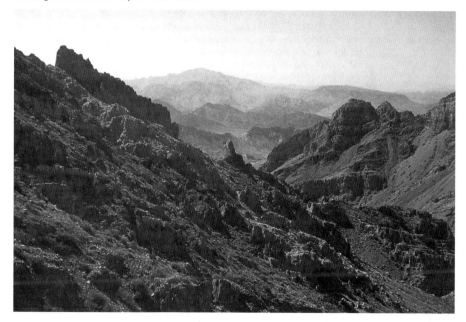

trip 18 Valley of Fire: Atlatl Rock

Distance	0.25 mile or 0.75 mile, out-and-back
Hiking Time	30 minutes to 1 hour
Elevation	+/-40 feet (to Atlatl Rock); +/-130 feet (to overlook)
Difficulty	Easy (with a moderate option)
Trail Use	Leashed dogs, good for kids
Best Times	Cold to warm
Agency	Valley of Fire State Park at (702) 397-2088; www.parks.nv.gov/vf.htm
Recommended Maps	Free *Valley of Fire* map; *Valley of Fire East* and *Valley of Fire West* 7.5-minute
GPS Waypoints	Atlatl Rock: 36.423° N, 114.550° W
Vehicle	Passenger car OK

HIGHLIGHTS Here you'll find beautiful rocks, classic petroglyphs, and a fun scramble up to a view across the Valley of Fire.

DIRECTIONS Take I-15 north from Las Vegas and take exit 75. Drive east on Highway 169 for 14 miles to the park entrance. About 1.5 miles past (east of) the entrance station, turn left (west) on the signed road to Atlatl Rock. The parking area entrance is a half mile farther, on the left (south) side of the road. The visitor center is 2.5 miles east of Atlatl Rock on 169.

For a beautiful loop back to Las Vegas, follow 169 to the east exit of Valley of Fire State Park, then turn right onto Northshore Road, which heads south and west through Lake Mead National Recreation Area back to Las Vegas (allow at least another hour to drive this route).

FACILITIES/TRAILHEAD There are shaded picnic tables and toilets at the trailhead. Water, information, and rangers are available at the visitor center. The park offers two first-come, first-served campgrounds (51 sites) with shaded tables, grills, water, restrooms, and showers. Group campsites are also available, each accommodating up to 45 people. Reservations are required (call 702-397-2088), and the group sites are located near the Beehive rock formations. Backpacking and backcountry camping are not allowed in Valley of Fire State Park.

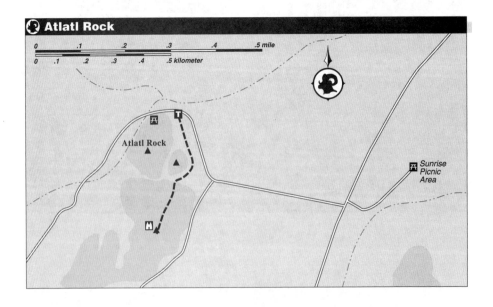

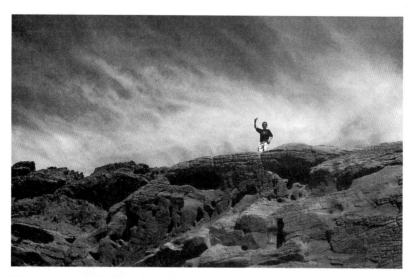

Enjoy the wonderful sandstone at Valley of Fire, but be careful of the fragile petroglyphs.

From the parking lot, head a short distance south and take the 84 steps up to the petroglyph panel on the towering face of Atlatl Rock. Once you come back down the stairs, turn right and walk clockwise around the rock formation, where you'll find more petroglyphs along the way.

Ambitious scramblers who hike south from Atlatl Rock for 100 yards and climb the sandstone southeast to the promontory are rewarded with a nice view of Valley of Fire.

This petroglyph site is named after the atlatl, a handle used to give extra power when throwing a spear. They were nearly ubiquitous hunting tools used by tribes, and artifact atlatls have been found on every continent except Antarctica. The tools date back thousands of years and were the precursors to the bow and arrow, which arrived in the American Southwest sometime between 200 A.D. and 500 A.D.

Look for the atlatl carved on the face of this rock, along with a spear and a bighorn. These designs are pretty easy to understand, as they represent things we can recognize. But what about some of the other designs? Wavy lines, spirals, ladders, headless figures, and other abstract motifs are difficult

for us to understand because we don't recognize them. Perhaps they were calendar markings that lined up with shadows on particular days (such as winter and summer solstice) to help tell time. Perhaps they were clan markings or related to the myths and stories these people told each other.

It's difficult to understand many of these symbols because our minds have been shaped by television, cars, Wal-Mart, restaurants, air-conditioning, and other modern inventions. Some archaeologists believe that Atlatl Rock held special ritual or spiritual significance for the Ancestral Puebloan Indians who carved them. The sheer concentration of petroglyphs on this particular rock supports this theory. The tribes lived in Nevada's only native pueblo (city), which was only 10 miles to the northeast, on the banks of the Virgin River, where Overton is now. Perhaps they came here for special ceremonies or gatherings.

Please take only pictures, and *don't touch the petroglyphs.* The archaeological resources in this area are irreplaceable and very fragile. *Do not touch, alter, destroy, or remove any artifacts,* and please report vandalism to rangers.

trip 19 Valley of Fire: Petroglyph Canyon & Mouse's Tank

Distance	0.5 mile, out-and-back
Hiking Time	30 minutes to 1 hour
Elevation	+/-2080 feet
Difficulty	Easy
Trail Use	Leashed dogs, good for kids
Best Times	Cold to warm
Agency	Valley of Fire State Park at (702) 397-2088; www.parks.nv.gov/vf.htm
Recommended Maps	Free *Valley of Fire* map; *Valley of Fire East* and *Valley of Fire West* 7.5-minute
GPS Waypoints	Trailhead: 36.441° N, 114.516° W Tank: 36.438° N, 114.512° W
Vehicle	Passenger car OK

HIGHLIGHTS Enjoy the geology and petroglyphs at this renegade's hiding spot.

DIRECTIONS Take I-15 north from Las Vegas and take exit 75. Drive east on Highway 169 for 14 miles to the park entrance. Four miles past (east of) the entrance station, turn left (north), pass the visitor center, and continue north on the White Domes Road for 1.25 miles to the signed Mouse's Tank parking area and trailhead on the right (east) side of the road.

For a beautiful loop back to Las Vegas, follow 169 to the east exit of Valley of Fire State Park, then turn right onto Northshore Road, which heads south and west through Lake Mead National Recreation Area back to Las Vegas (allow at least another hour to drive this route).

FACILITIES/TRAILHEAD Toilets and information signs are available at the trailhead. Water, information, and rangers are available at the visitor center. The park offers two first-come, first-served campgrounds (51 sites) with shaded tables, grills, water, restrooms, and showers. Group areas are also available near the Beehive rock formations, each accommodating up to 45 people. Reservations are required (call 702-397-2088). Backpacking and backcountry camping are not allowed in Valley of Fire State Park.

From the car, follow the trail southeast through the wash to the tank. Retrace your steps to return.

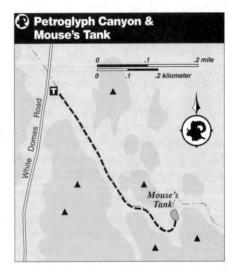

Petroglyph Canyon & Mouse's Tank

According to history (and probably a healthy dose of legend), Mouse was a Southern Paiute living in the region in the 1890s, who allegedly killed two prospectors while drunk in an Indian camp along the Colorado River. He fled into the labyrinth of sandstone west of the river, where he eluded capture for months. A posse finally tracked him down in July 1897 and killed him.

At the end of the trail, you'll see how Mouse survived so long in the desert: He probably got water from the *tinaja* (Spanish for "earthen pot"), or tank, a depression in the sandstone that collects rain.

Mouse wasn't the first to discover these canyons. Along the walls of the trail are petroglyphs, which means tribes had been

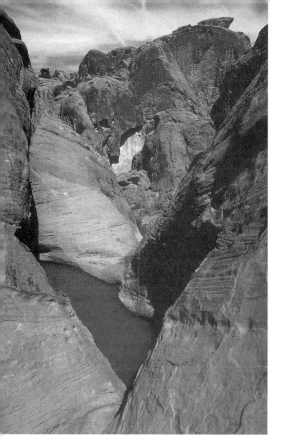

coming to this canyon for hundreds, if not thousands, of years.

Northeast of Valley of Fire is Overton. Between 300 B.C. and 1150 A.D., a large Ancestral Puebloan pueblo sat here on the banks of what is now the Virgin River. Now called Lost City, it was the only major pueblo established in Nevada. Some archaeologists believe that Valley of Fire had ceremonial or religious importance for the people at Lost City.

This area is sacred to the native tribes of this region. Please respect it as you would your own place of worship. The archaeological resources in this area are irreplaceable and very fragile, so admire the petroglyphs from a distance and take only pictures. If you climb on the rocks, be sure to look out for petroglyphs and avoid touching them. Report vandalism to the managing agency listed above.

Eastern Region

Tinajas like Mouse's Tank can be found throughout sandstone country.

trip 20 **Valley of Fire: White Domes**

Distance	2.25 miles, loop
Hiking Time	1 to 2 hours
Elevation	+/-40 feet
Difficulty	Easy to moderate
Trail Use	Leashed dogs, good for kids
Best Times	Cold to warm, early morning or late afternoon
Agency	Valley of Fire State Park at (702) 397-2088; www.parks.nv.gov/vf.htm
Recommended Maps	Free *Valley of Fire* map; *Valley of Fire West* 7.5-minute
GPS Waypoints	Trailhead: 36.485° N, 114.532° W
	Movie set: 36.482° N, 114.533° W
Vehicle	Passenger car OK

HIGHLIGHTS In 1966, Hollywood filmed a classic Western in this park. The natural splendors along this hike might inspire your own lines worthy of a Hollywood script. Here, you'll see a slot canyon (at points only 18 inches wide and 80 feet deep), a natural arch, multicolored sandstone, and interesting patterns of erosion that have created sculptured forms around the trail.

DIRECTIONS Take I-15 north from Las Vegas and take exit 75. Drive east on Highway 169 for 14 miles to the park entrance. Four miles past (east of) the entrance station on 169, turn left (north) onto White Domes Road. Pass the visitor center and continue north on the White Domes Road for 5.5 miles to the signed White Domes parking area on the left (west) side of the road.

For a beautiful loop back to Las Vegas, follow 169 to the east exit of Valley of Fire State Park, then turn right onto Northshore Road, which heads south and west through Lake Mead National Recreation Area back to Las Vegas (give yourself at least another hour to drive this route).

FACILITIES/TRAILHEAD A shaded picnic area and restrooms are available at White Domes. Water, information, and rangers are available at the visitor center. The park offers two first-come, first-served campgrounds (51 sites) with shaded tables, grills, water, restrooms, and showers. Group areas are also available near the Beehive rock formations, each accommodating up to 45 people. Reservations are required (call 702-397-2088). Backpacking and backcountry camping are not allowed in Valley of Fire State Park.

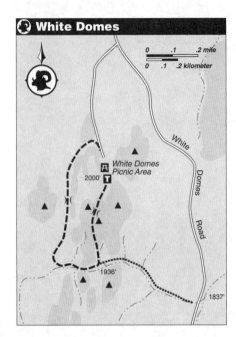

From the parking area, hike a quarter mile downhill to the movie set ruins. Continue downhill into the wash, which runs northwest to southeast. Here, you have two options (both of which I recommend):

A. Turn left (southeast) and follow the wash through the slot canyon for about 0.4 mile. Then retrace your steps.

B. Turn right (northwest) and follow the trail through another slot canyon. After the slot, veer right (north) along the trail, which loops past an interesting arch and between two large sandstone mounds before it returns to the picnic area.

In *The Professionals* (1966), Lee Marvin and Burt Lancaster rescued kidnapped Claudia Cardinale from Jack Palance, with Valley of Fire as a backdrop. The movie set here is left over from that classic Western. It was the last movie set allowed to remain here and adds a bit of Hollywood romance to the hike. (Watch out for cattle rustlers totin' six guns!)

You'll also find plenty of natural beauty on this hike. The surprising reds in the sandstone are the result of iron in the sand

having rusted after being exposed to oxygen. It doesn't take much iron to imbue the rock a fiery red. One part per million can do the trick. The White Domes lack such iron in them.

The rocks' many sculptured forms are a result of erosion and inconsistent cementing in the rock. During the sandstone's formations over millions of years, minerals such as calcium carbonate and lime have cemented the stone together. However, some parts are cemented more firmly than others. When weather comes, it erodes the weakest links, creating the many shapes you see in Valley of Fire.

Although many people credit wind and rain as the primary movers of erosion, much of it is caused by freezing and thawing. In winter, water penetrates the cracks in the rock and then freezes. As the water molecules expand, they pry the rock apart.

These scientific explanations, however, fall short of conveying the true wonders and beauty that result from their actions.

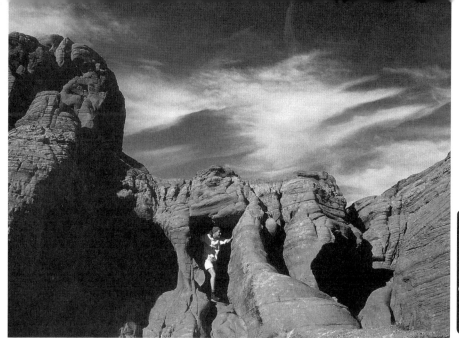

This sandstone wonderland can bring out the kid in anyone.

trip 21 Valley of Fire: Elephant Rock

Distance	0.25 mile, out-and-back
Hiking Time	1 hour
Elevation	+/-50 feet
Difficulty	Moderate
Trail Use	Leashed dogs, good for kids
Best Times	Cold to warm
Agency	Valley of Fire State Park at (702) 397-2088; parks.nv.gov/vf.htm
Recommended Maps	Free *Valley of Fire* map; *Valley of Fire East* 7.5-minute
GPS Waypoints	Elephant Rock: 36.428° N, 114.459° W
Vehicle	Passenger car OK

HIGHLIGHTS During the last ice age, which ended 10,000 years ago, this area was much cooler and wetter, providing habitat for many animals that are now extinct, including saber-toothed cats, giant ground sloths, prehistoric horses and camels, and giant mammoths. The only relic of that time is a giant rock that looks like an ancient mammoth. Elephant Rock is a testament to the many varied stone shapes at Valley of Fire, thanks to the wonders of geology and the erosive power of weather.

DIRECTIONS Take I-15 north from Las Vegas and take exit 75. Drive east on Highway 169 for 14 miles to the park entrance. Continue east on 169 through Valley of Fire for 7 miles to the signed Elephant Rock parking area and trailhead on the left (north) side of the road.

For a beautiful loop back to Las Vegas, follow 169 to the east exit of Valley of Fire State Park, then turn right onto Northshore Road, which heads south and west through Lake Mead National Recreation Area back to Las Vegas (give yourself at least another hour to drive this route).

FACILITIES/TRAILHEAD Information and restrooms are available at Elephant Rock. Water, information, and rangers are available at the visitor center. The park offers two first-come, first-served campgrounds (51 sites) with shaded tables, grills, water, restrooms, and showers. Group areas are also available near the Beehive rock formations on the west end of the park, each accommodating up to 45 people. Reservations are required (call 702-397-2088). Backpacking and backcountry camping are not allowed in Valley of Fire State Park.

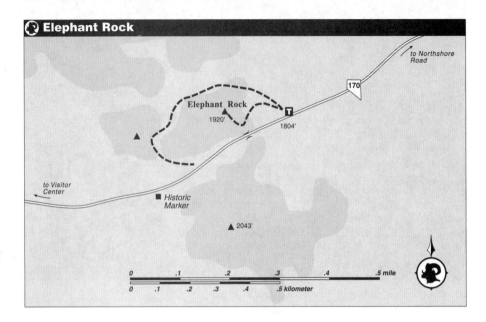

Elephant Rock

to Northshore Road

170

Elephant Rock
1920'

1804'

to Visitor Center

■ Historic Marker

▲ 2043'

| 0 | .1 | .2 | .3 | .4 | .5 mile |
| 0 | .1 | .2 | .3 | .4 | .5 kilometer |

From the parking area, hike west toward the rock formations until the trail soon forks. Follow the left, southerly fork for a couple hundred yards up over the rocks to the road. Elephant Rock stands tall on the right (north) side of the road. (There is a small pullout by the side of the road next to Elephant Rock, if you'd prefer not to walk). Retrace your steps to return.

At the same trail fork west of the trailhead, choose the right, northerly fork to follow the historic Arrowhead Trail around the north side of the rock formations and back to the paved road. This packed-dirt trail, built in 1916, was a favorite adventure for early drivers traveling between Los Angeles and Salt Lake City.

Gold Butte offers an impressive combination of rare plants and wildlife, inspiring geology, archaeology, and pioneer history.

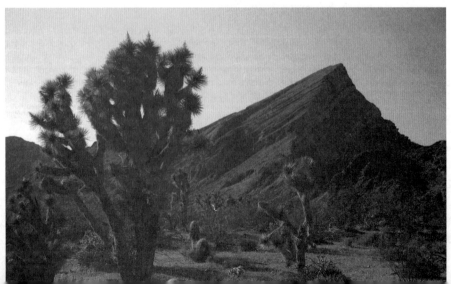

trip 22 Gold Butte: Whitney Pockets

Distance	Varies, out-and-back
Hiking Time	Up to 3 hours
Elevation	Up to +/-150 feet
Difficulty	Easy to moderate
Trail Use	Leashed dogs, good for kids, backpacking option, map and compass
Best Times	Cool to warm
Agency	BLM Las Vegas (702) 515-5000; www.nv.blm.gov/vegas/
Recommended Maps	*Overton* 1:100,000; *Whitney Pocket* 7.5-minute
GPS Waypoints	Whitney Pocket intersection: 36.522° N, 114.138° W
Vehicle	Passenger car OK

HIGHLIGHTS Not necessarily a hiking destination, Whitney Pockets is simply a good place to be—to enjoy the shade, explore the sandstone, and camp surrounded by desert beauty. Nestled among the outcrops are perfect spots to enjoy lunch in the shade or to set up camp at this gateway to Gold Butte.

DIRECTIONS From Las Vegas, take I-15 north to exit 112 to Riverside/Bunkerville. Turn right (east) on Highway 170, cross the Virgin River, then turn right (south) onto the first unsigned, paved road, about 200 yards east of the river. This road, called the Gold Butte Back Country Byway on some maps, winds along the river and then across the slopes southwest of the Virgin Mountains for 19 miles until the colorful and shapely sandstone outcrops announce your arrival at the Whitney Pockets area. The pavement ends at about 20 miles, right before the intersection with the short road that heads north to Whitney Pockets proper.

All of the sandstone outcrops around you have undeveloped campsites and parking places nestled up against them. Campsites and parking areas are also available along the Whitney Pockets side road. Choose your favorite place, and let the exploration begin.

FACILITIES/TRAILHEAD The nearest facilities are in Mesquite, 60 miles northwest on I-15. Undeveloped campsites abound throughout the region. Please camp only on previously established sites, well away from water (wildlife need to access it), and avoid trampling sensitive plants or soils.

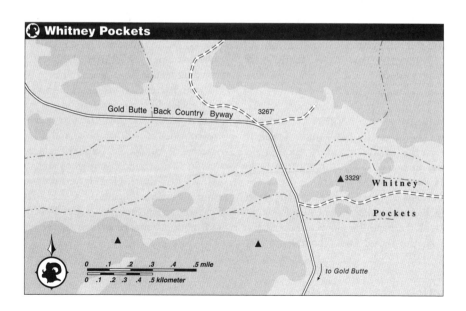

Whitney Pockets

Gold Butte Back Country Byway 3267'

▲3329' Whitney

Pockets

to Gold Butte

0   .1   .2   .3   .4   .5 mile
0   .1   .2   .3   .4   .5 kilometer

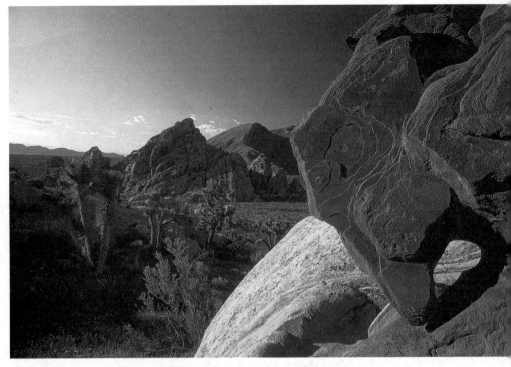

Colorful sandstone monuments make Whitney Pockets a truly special place.

Find a place to park among the sandstone, and explore whichever direction piques your interest.

One of my favorite spots in Nevada is what I call Falling Man Rocks, 2 miles south of Whitney Pockets. To go there, drive 1 mile west of pavement's end, take the unsigned, unmaintained dirt track heading south, aiming for the sandstone outcrop immediately to the north of the volcanic butte and larger (but still minor) peak to the south. Park on the north side of the rocks, then hike south through the rocks to explore.

Perhaps there was more water here long ago, or maybe ancient people simply enjoyed the beautiful alcoves and theaters among the rocks. Look carefully for the many petroglyphs scattered throughout the area. My favorite is Falling Man (you'll recognize him when you see him), who is stylistically unlike any other petroglyph I've seen. It's sad to think that he might tell of someone's long-ago fall from the high cliff above, but he does it so beautifully.

The archaeological resources in this area are irreplaceable and very fragile, so please *do not touch* the petroglyphs. Native Americans consider rock art to be sacred. Please respect it as you would your own place of worship. Report vandalism to the managing agency listed above. Or help protect these resources by donating money or time to the Archaeology Site Stewards: (702) 486-5011 or visit http://nevadasitestewards.org.

Cryptobiotic Soils: Living Dirt

When you're hiking across valley bottoms or open slopes in your explorations, keep your eyes on the dirt under your feet. It just might be alive.

Enormous networks of fungi, bacteria, mosses, and lichens stitch themselves together to create vast communities of life in the top layers of soil. These networks, called cryptobiotic (also cryptogamic or microphytic) soils are desert ecosystems' security forces, helping these ecosystems in many ways.

The crusts act as large sponges, soaking up rainwater before it has a chance to run off. The layers then prevent life-giving water from evaporating away. They also protect fragile plant communities by creating a shield that exotic plant seeds have a hard time penetrating. This crust also prevents soil from blowing away as dust. Scientists estimate that cryptogamic communities dominate up to 70 percent of desert soils on the planet.

All of these benefits disappear, however, when the seal is broken. When large numbers of people, animals, and vehicles travel across these soils, they break down the networks, start erosion, release dust, and allow invasive plants to take root.

When you see a bumpy crust in the soil that looks like it might be fungus or lichen, please avoid walking on it. Please stick to trails and durable surfaces and help the cryptobiotic crusts do their job.

trip 23 Gold Butte: Mud Wash Narrows

Distance	Up to 8 miles, out-and-back
Hiking Time	3 to 5 hours
Elevation	+/-380 feet
Difficulty	Moderate
Trail Use	Leashed dogs, backpacking option, maps and compass
Best Times	Cool to warm
Agency	BLM Las Vegas (702) 515-5000; www.nv.blm.gov/vegas/
Recommended Maps	*Lake Mead* 1:100,000; *Overton Beach* 7.5-minute
GPS Waypoints	Red Bluff Spring: 36.461° N, 114.252° W
Vehicle	High-clearance or 4WD vehicle recommended

HIGHLIGHTS This hike follows a twisting slot canyon leading to a beach on Lake Mead. The wash is susceptible to flash floods, so please do not attempt if thunderstorms threaten.

DIRECTIONS From Las Vegas, take I-15 north to exit 112 to Riverside/Bunkerville. Turn right (east) on Highway 170, cross the Virgin River, then turn right (south) onto the first unsigned, paved road, about 200 yards east of the river. This road, called the Gold Butte Back Country Byway on some maps, winds along the river and across the slopes southwest of the Virgin Mountains for 19 miles until the colorful and shapely sandstone outcrops announce your arrival to the Whitney Pockets area. The pavement ends at about 20 miles, just before the intersection with the short road that heads north to Whitney Pockets proper.

From the end of the pavement at Whitney Pockets, set your odometer to zero and continue east toward Gold Butte. At 6.9 miles, turn right (south) onto a signed, unpaved road toward Devil's Throat and Red Bluff Spring. Zero your odometer again. At about 8 miles, you reach Red Bluff Spring, where you can park. From the car, hike downstream to the narrows.

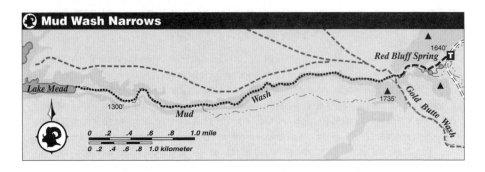

Mud Wash Narrows

Red Bluff Spring
1640'
Lake Mead
1300'
Mud
Wash
1735'
Gold Butte Wash

0 .2 .4 .6 .8 1.0 mile
0 .2 .4 .6 .8 1.0 kilometer

FACILITIES/TRAILHEAD The nearest facilities are in Mesquite, 80 miles northwest on I-15. Undeveloped campsites abound throughout the region. Please camp only on previously established sites, well away from water (wildlife need to access it), and avoid trampling sensitive plants or soils.

From your car, hike down the wash as far as you'd like. Lake Mead is 4 miles away. Retrace your steps to return.

Although the bottom of this 4-mile-long slot canyon is gentle and sandy, hiking in the sometimes-deep sand can be a real workout. Only dedicated, fit hikers should attempt the full 8-mile round-trip. Luckily, you need only walk a short distance to enjoy this canyon.

While you're hiking, notice the conglomerate nature of the canyon walls, made when various types of rocks were caught in previous flows and deposited here. This canyon cuts through sediments placed here by millennia of storm runoff. Each storm carves a new page in the ever-dynamic geologic story of this region.

Notice the large pockets and holes high above you in the canyon walls. Formed by water rushing through during flash floods, they're a convincing argument why you don't want to be here during the next one. *Stay out of all washes and canyons if thunderstorms threaten.*

The conglomerate rock walls of Mud Wash consist of gravel deposited by flash foods eons ago.

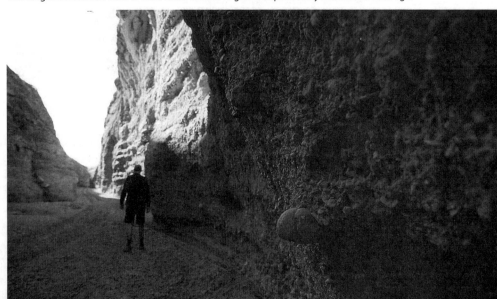

trip 24 Gold Butte: Lime Canyon

Distance	5 miles or more, out-and-back
Hiking Time	1 to 4 hours
Elevation	+/-1700 feet
Difficulty	Moderate
Trail Use	Leashed dogs, backpacking option, map and compass
Best Times	Cold to warm (early morning or late afternoon)
Agency	BLM Las Vegas (702) 515-5000; www.nv.blm.gov/vegas/
Recommended Maps	*Lake Mead* 1:100,00; *Lime Wash* 7.5-minute
GPS Waypoints	Lime Canyon mouth: 36.313° N, 114.250° W
Vehicle	High-clearance or 4WD vehicle recommended

HIGHLIGHTS Lime Ridge is a north-south ridge of sedimentary rock along the western portion of Gold Butte. Lime Canyon cuts east-west through this ridge, then drains to Lake Mead. At its deepest, the canyon walls rise hundreds of feet on both sides of the wash. Congress recognized the unique beauty and solitude of this area by designating the 23,000-acre Lime Canyon Wilderness Area in 2002.

DIRECTIONS From Las Vegas, take I-15 north to exit 112 to Riverside/Bunkerville. Turn right (east) on Highway 170, cross the Virgin River, then turn right (south) onto the first unsigned, paved road, about 200 yards east of the river. This road, called the Gold Butte Back Country Byway on some maps, winds along the river and then across the slopes southwest of the Virgin Mountains for 19 miles until the colorful and shapely sandstone outcrops announce your arrival to the Whitney Pockets area. The pavement ends at about 20 miles, just before the intersection with the short road that heads north to Whitney Pockets proper.

From the end of the pavement at Whitney Pockets, continue east, then south on the Gold Butte Back Country Byway for 20 miles to Gold Butte. At a signed intersection soon after Gold Butte, turn right (northwest) and continue for 3 miles. Turn left (west) onto an unsigned, unpaved jeep track heading down toward the entrance to Lime Canyon, a mile to the west. Park anywhere off the track without damaging vegetation.

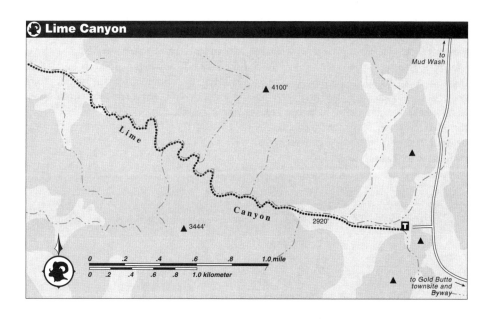

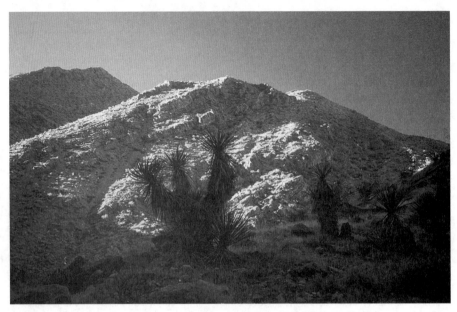

Sunrise hikes allow you to enjoy cool temperatures and magical light.

FACILITIES/TRAILHEAD The nearest facilities are in Mesquite, 80 miles northwest on I-15. Undeveloped campsites abound throughout the region. Please camp only on previously established sites, well away from water (wildlife need to access it) and without trampling sensitive plants or soils.

From the car, follow the jeep track west and downstream for up to 1 mile (depending on where you park) to the canyon entrance, then through the fence. Lime Canyon continues for about 5 miles, until it gives way to an open wash, which slopes gently for another 5 miles to the Overton Arm of Lake Mead. Hike as far as you'd like, then retrace your steps to return. There is no trail, but with the steep canyon walls, you'd have to try hard to get lost.

Lime Canyon makes a wonderful backpacking destination. Just make sure you camp well away from the wash. Not only do you not want to get washed away by a flash flood, but bighorn sheep and other wildlife commute down the wash. Your presence could keep them away from water and survival.

trip 25 Gold Butte: Cottonwood Canyon

Distance	4 miles, out-and-back
Hiking Time	4 to 6 hours or overnight
Elevation	+/-1100
Difficulty	Difficult
Trail Use	Leashed dogs, backpacking option, map and compass
Best Times	Cold to warm
Agency	BLM Las Vegas (702) 515-5000; www.nv.blm.gov/vegas/
Recommended Maps	*Lake Mead* 1:100,00; *Jumbo Peak* 7.5-minute
GPS Waypoints	Parking area: 36.188° N, 114.118° W
Vehicle	High-clearance or 4WD vehicle recommended

Eastern Region

HIGHLIGHTS At 4,631 acres, the Jumbo Springs Wilderness Area is the smallest wilderness in Nevada. But standing in the middle of this rugged, isolated landscape, you'll see why Congress chose to protect this area for posterity. The sculpted granite peaks high in Cottonwood Canyon rival any landscape for sheer beauty. Although it is less than 60 air miles from Las Vegas, this is one of the more rugged and isolated places you can find in Southern Nevada. This trip is designed to put you in the middle of this rugged, beautiful solitude.

DIRECTIONS From Las Vegas, take I-15 north to exit 112 to Riverside/Bunkerville. Turn right (east) on Highway 170, cross the Virgin River, then turn right (south) onto the first unsigned, paved road, about 200 yards east of the river. This road, called the Gold Butte Back Country Byway on some maps, winds along the river and then across the slopes southwest of the Virgin Mountains for 19 miles until the colorful and shapely sandstone outcrops announce your arrival to the Whitney Pockets area. The pavement ends at about 20 miles, just before the intersection with the short road that heads north to Whitney Pockets proper.

At the end of the pavement at Whitney Pockets, set your odometer to zero and continue straight east on the Gold Butte Back Country Byway. After 9 miles, veer right (south) at a junction, following the byway toward the old town site of Gold Butte. At 15.8 miles (about 4 miles north of Gold Butte), veer left (southeast) on a bladed but unsigned dirt road toward Devil's Cove. Follow this rough, dirt

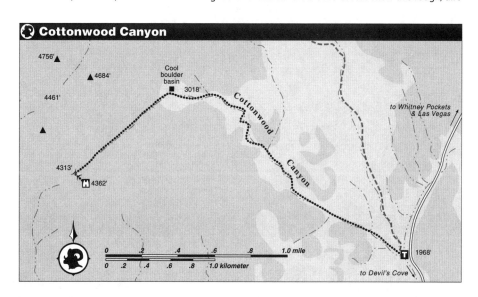

road for 11.5 miles south. (The first 10 miles are passable with two-wheel drive; the final 1.5 miles require high clearance and 4WD.) This road winds over the summit pass, down New Spring Wash to the base of Cottonwood Canyon, at an unsigned intersection with a jeep track heading north. Take a sharp right to head north on that jeep track and park in the first quarter mile.

FACILITIES/TRAILHEAD The nearest facilities are in Mesquite, 90 miles northwest on I-15. Undeveloped campsites abound throughout the region. Please camp only on previously established sites, well away from water (wildlife need to access it) and without trampling sensitive plants or soils.

There is no trail and no sign for this trip. At the car, several canyons and washes come together, threatening to disorient you, but the rugged and beautiful granite peaks of upper Cottonwood Canyon will be clearly visible.

From your car, hike up the canyon toward those peaks, heading west-northwest (do not take the jeep track, which heads north-northwest). Don't let the fact that there are no cottonwood trees anywhere in the vicinity make you think you're in the wrong place; either the canyon was poorly named, or the cottonwoods have long since disappeared.

As you travel up the canyon, you may have to stray onto the slopes above the drainage from time to time to avoid climbing waterfalls. You'll know you have arrived after about 1.5 miles, when you encounter

Exploring Cottonwood Canyon can be very difficult, but the views and surroundings are worth it.

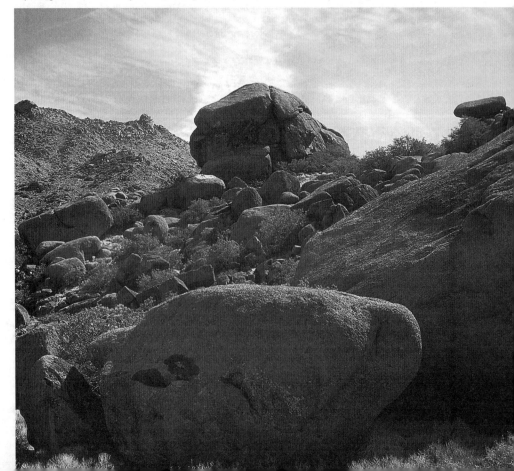

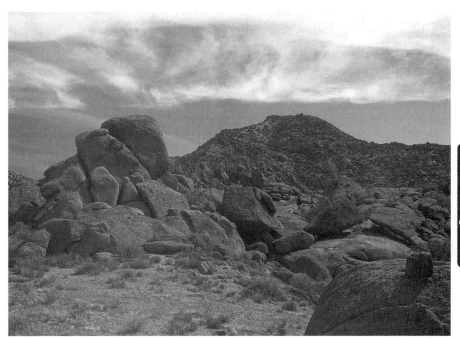

There are no cottonwood trees in Cottonwood Canyon, but its beauty is undeniable.

a theater of jumbled boulders, with the boulder-clad peaks rising above you. Enjoy the scenery, look for hidden springs, and find a place to camp amid the boulders, yucca, and cholla cactus.

Fit, energetic hikers will enjoy the very difficult hike to the top of the canyon, which veers to the left (southwest) for another mile and 1200 vertical feet to the fantastic views waiting at the top of the ridge.

Your pain and suffering on this steep, rugged trip will be rewarded with solitude and the beauty of jaw-dropping geology and varied plant life. Creosote bush, catclaw acacia, ephedra, yucca, and barrel cactus cover the slopes, which are punctuated by giant granitic boulders. From high points, you can see the Grand Canyon beginning to the east.

Retrace your steps to return.

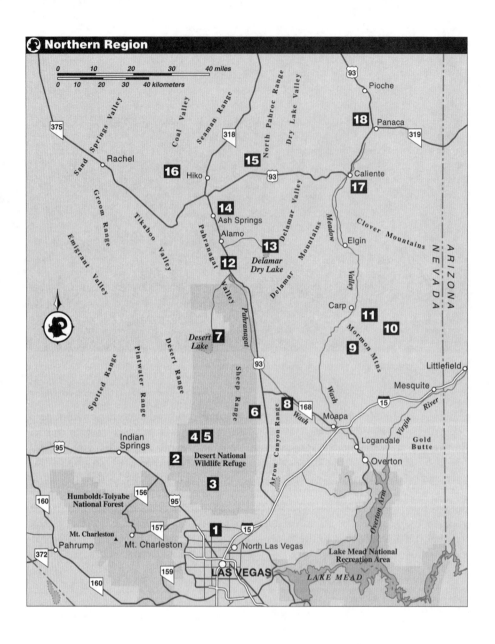

0   10   20   30   40 miles
0   10   20   30   40 kilometers

93   Pioche

375

Sand Springs Valley

Coal Valley

Seaman Range

North Pahroc Range

Dry Lake Valley

18   Panaca

318

15

319

Rachel

16   Hiko

93   Caliente

17

Groom Range

Tikaboo Valley

14   Ash Springs

Alamo

Delamar Valley

Delamar Mountains

Meadow Valley

Clover Mountains

Elgin

NEVADA
ARIZONA

Emigrant Valley

Pahranagat

13

12   Delamar
Dry Lake

Delamar

Carp   11

10

Pahranagat Valley

Desert
Lake   7

9

Mormon Mtns

Littlefield

Spotted Range

Pintwater Range

Desert Range

Sheep Range

93

Mesquite

Wash

15

Indian
Springs

6

8   168
Wash   Moapa

Arrow Canyon Range

95

4   5

2   Desert National
Wildlife Refuge

Logandale   Gold
Butte

Virgin River

Overton

160

Humboldt-Toiyabe
National Forest

156

95

3

Overton Arm

157

1   15

372   Pahrump

Mt. Charleston
Mt. Charleston

North Las Vegas

Lake Mead National
Recreation Area

159

LAS VEGAS

LAKE MEAD

160

chapter 3

Northern Region
INCLUDING DESERT NATIONAL WILDLIFE RANGE

Drive north from I-15 between Las Vegas and the Utah border, and you'll enter some of the least populated, least developed, and strikingly beautiful wild country in Southern Nevada. Here your explorer's curiosity will be rewarded with the Desert National Wildlife Range, Arrow Canyon Wilderness's namesake slot canyon, wonderful wildlife watching at Pahranagat National Wildlife Refuge, and the colorful, eroded cliffs of Cathedral Gorge State Park.

One highlight of this region is the Desert National Wildlife Range (DNWR), the largest national wildlife refuge in the Lower 48, which begins just north of north Las Vegas. The 1.6 million-acre DNWR, known also as Desert Game Range or the Desert Refuge, was designated by President Franklin Roosevelt in 1936 to protect desert bighorn sheep and their habitats. Today, it provides visitors with vast, rugged desert solitude.

In the rain shadow of the Spring Mountains, DNWR gets even less rain than other parts of Southern Nevada, with some low-elevation areas averaging fewer than 4 inches per year. However, some peaks in the DNWR's six mountain ranges rise to nearly 10,000 feet, where precipitation is significantly higher.

Despite the arid climate, DNWR is far from lifeless. Nearly 750 species of plants can be found here, as well as 320 species of birds, 52 species of mammals, 35 species of reptiles, and the endangered Pahrump pupfish. In 2001, there were an estimated 700 bighorn living in DNWR.

Roughly 60 percent of the refuge (the western portion) overlaps with the military's Nellis Air Force Range and is off-limits to the public. The remainder is undeveloped, with primitive roads and no services. For prepared desert travelers, these trips into DNWR lead you to beautiful country, fascinating geology, and secluded pockets of life and discovery you'd never guess were there. If you've never strayed from paved roads, turn to page 20 to learn about special considerations for desert travel.

If you like what you see at the refuge, please consider becoming a volunteer by calling the refuge at (702) 515-5450. The refuge is overwhelmed with visitors and impact from nearby Las Vegas, and they could use the help.

On November 17, 2004, Congress passed the Lincoln County Conservation, Recreation, and Development Act, designating 14 new wilderness areas in the county directly north of Clark County, which is home to Las Vegas. Two of these wildernesses are featured in this book: the Mormon Mountains (Trips 9, 10, and 11), and Big Rocks (Trip 15). Learn more about wilderness in the introduction on page 10. The act also expanded two state parks mentioned in this chapter: Kershaw-Ryan (Trip 17) and Cathedral Gorge (Trip 18).

trip 1 Floyd Lamb State Park: Tule Springs

Distance	Up to 1 mile, loop
Hiking Time	30 minutes
Elevation	2469 feet
Difficulty	Easy
Trail Use	Leashed dogs, good for kids
Best Times	Cold to warm
Agency	Floyd Lamb State Park at (702) 486-5413; www.lasvegasnevada.gov/files/Floyd_Lamb_Park_Brochure.pdf
Recommended Maps	Free map and brochure at entrance station
GPS Waypoints	Main pond: 36.322° N, 115.268° W
Vehicle	Passenger car OK

HIGHLIGHTS This 2,000-acre park offers four small lakes, shaded lawns, picnic facilities, and walking and bike paths that meander through the grounds. Historic stables and other buildings also remain to remind us of its ranching past.

DIRECTIONS From Las Vegas, take Highway 95 north to exit 93 for Durango. Drive northeast on Durango Road for about 1.5 miles, then turn right (east) on Brent Lane, the entrance road for the park.

FACILITIES/TRAILHEAD Restrooms and water are available here.

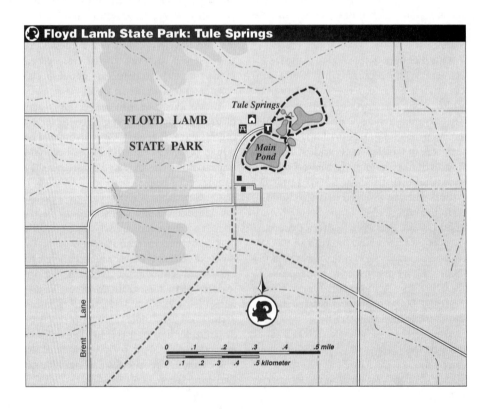

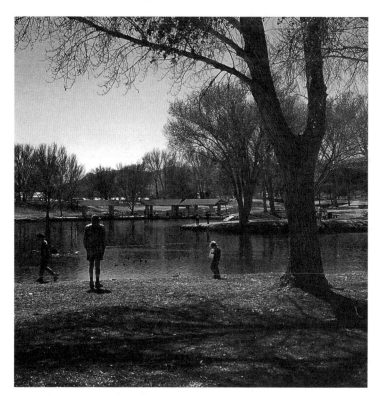

The natural springs feed a splash of green and pleasurable surroundings.

As soon as you get out of your car, meandering paths invite you to stroll around the small, spring-fed lakes in the park. Willows provide comfortable shade, ducks and geese come seeking food, and stress caused by the sprawling frenzy in the Las Vegas Valley melts away.

For thousands of years, the water at Tule (TOO-lee) Springs has attracted animals and humans to this Mojave Desert oasis. Archaeological evidence from the area shows the remains of prehistoric camels and horses, ground sloths, mammoths (all now extinct), and artificial tools dating back about 11,000 years, and possibly much longer.

In the 1940s, Prosper Jacob Goumond acquired the property and established a dude ranch, where people from around the country could come and wait out their six-week residency required by Nevada to get a divorce. The many celebrities coming here to ride horses, swim, and play tennis while taking advantage of Nevada's liberal divorce laws brought notoriety to the state and Tule Springs.

In 1964, the ranch became a city park, named after then-State Senator Floyd Lamb. In 1977, the Division of State Parks acquired the park and has managed it ever since. Despite its official name, many locals still refer to the area as Tule Springs.

trip 2 # DNWR: Corn Creek Nature Trail

Distance	1 mile, loop
Hiking Time	30 minutes to 1 hour
Elevation	2920 feet
Difficulty	Easy
Trail Use	Leashed dogs, good for kids
Best Times	Cold to warm (May and September, sunrise and sunset, for best bird watching)
Agency	Desert National Wildlife Range at (702) 879-6110; www.fws.gov/desertcomplex
Recommended Maps	*Las Vegas* 1:100,000
GPS Waypoints	Parking area: 36°438' N, 115°357' W
Vehicle	High-clearance or 4WD vehicle recommended

HIGHLIGHTS Corn Creek is a refreshing splash of green in the baked brown desert of the Las Vegas Valley. For thousands of years, the natural springs here have attracted animals, birds, and humans. Shady paths around the springs provide opportunities to unwind and enjoy natural beauty and perhaps glimpse wildlife.

DIRECTIONS From Las Vegas, take Highway 95 north about 20 miles, past the exit to Kyle Canyon, to the Desert National Wildlife Range (DNWR) entrance on the right. From there, proceed 4 miles east on the graded dirt entrance road to the Corn Creek Field Station.

FACILITIES/TRAILHEAD Restrooms, information, and water are available at the trailhead, which serves as the visitor center for the Desert National Wildlife Range. For a bird list for Corn Creek, call the refuge (listed above). Red Rock Audubon offers bird hikes to Corn Creek (702-390-9890). Picnicking is prohibited at Corn Creek, but there is a picnic area under cottonwood trees southeast of Corn Creek, about a mile away on Mormon Well Road. Primitive car camping is allowed within 100 feet of designated roads. Please use established sites. All camping is prohibited within a quarter mile of springs, artificial water developments (called guzzlers), and other water sources. Although campfires are allowed, wood collecting is not. Bring your own firewood, and check first with refuge headquarters, as there may be fire restrictions in place.

After signing in (it helps the refuge get funding), walk north past the restrooms and information displays to begin your stroll. A mile of paths meanders by three pools, irrigation ditches, a compound for an endangered pupfish, and historic ranch buildings. (Please do not approach the ranch buildings, as they are now the homes of refuge personnel and their families.)

The paths also take you through land that was once much different. Between 2 million and 10,000 years ago, the climate in

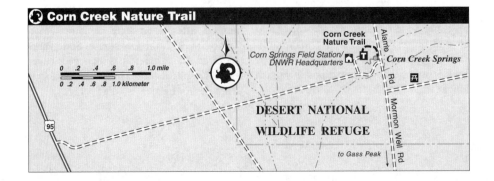

Corn Creek Nature Trail

DESERT NATIONAL WILDLIFE REFUGE

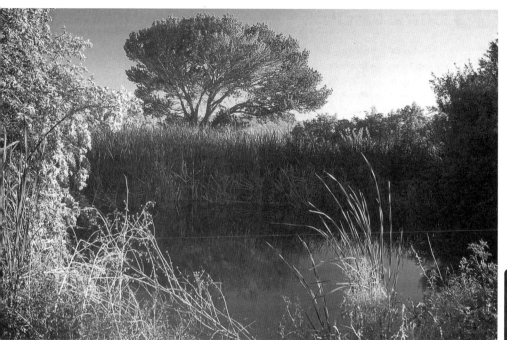

The springs of Corn Creek attract more than 240 bird species.

the Las Vegas Valley was much cooler and wetter, and meadows covered the valley floor. A lake at Corn Creek fed Las Vegas Creek, which meandered past Tule Springs and down to the Colorado River. Fossil records show that mammoths, giant ground sloths, camels, lions, ancient horses, and bison lived in the area.

Ancient peoples lived and hunted at the springs as long as 10,000 years ago. In the 1800s, stagecoaches, pioneers, ranchers, and settlers stopped at the springs on their travels. A ranch was established in the late 1800s. Congress designated the refuge in 1936, then purchased the springs as part of the refuge in 1939.

Today, the springs at Corn Creek are a magnet for many species of birds, which come from the deep desert and high mountains to drink. Migrants stop off to rest here during their travels north in spring and south in autumn. More than 240 species of birds have been recorded on the refuge, and many of these were at Corn Creek, from quail, sparrows, road runners, phainopepla, orioles, and tanagers, to several species of hawks, as well as migrating shore birds. Fruit trees on the property provide food for birds from spring through summer, adding more incentive for them to visit. During bird migration times, which peak in May and September, visit in early morning or late in the afternoon to see them.

After you have explored the spring complex, follow the paths back south to your car.

trip 3 DNWR: Gass Peak

Distance	6 miles, out-and-back
Hiking Time	4 to 6 hours
Elevation	+/-2090 feet
Difficulty	Difficult
Trail Use	Leashed dogs, backpacking option, map and compass
Best Times	Cool to warm
Agency	Desert National Wildlife Range at (702) 879-6110; www.fws.gov/desertcomplex
Recommended Maps	*Las Vegas* 1:100,000; *Gass Peak* 7.5-minute
GPS Waypoints	Gass Spring: 36.425° N, 115.164° W
	Gass Peak: 36.400° N, 115.179° W
Vehicle	High-clearance or 4WD vehicle recommended

HIGHLIGHTS Named after Octavius Decatur Gass, owner of the Las Vegas Ranch and old Mormon Fort in the late 1860s, Gass Peak stands sentinel at the north end of the Las Vegas Valley and marks the boundary between bustling civilization and undeveloped wildlands. Gass, and more than a million acres to the north, are part of the Desert National Wildlife Range, the second-largest wildlife refuge in the U.S. (the largest is the Arctic National Wildlife Refuge in Alaska). An excellent way to enjoy this peak is to climb it on the afternoon of a full moon, watch the sunset over Mt. Charleston and the Spring Mountains, then let the moonlight guide your way back down. Just to be safe, bring a headlamp. Or better yet, camp up top and watch the sunrise, too.

DIRECTIONS From Las Vegas, take Highway 95 north about 20 miles, past the exit to Kyle Canyon, to the Desert National Wildlife Range (DNWR) entrance on the right. From there, proceed 4 miles east on the graded DNWR entrance road to the Corn Creek Field Station. After signing in (it helps the refuge get funding), continue east for a quarter mile, then turn right (south) onto Mormon Well Road. After 4 miles, turn right (south) onto the signed GASS PEAK ROAD. Drive for 12.5 miles, then park at a fork, where a spur road heads southwest toward Gass Spring and a sign warns that the spur is for service vehicles only.

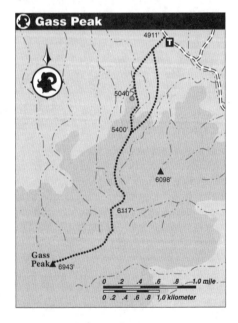

FACILITIES/TRAILHEAD Restrooms, information, and water are available at Corn Creek Field Station. Primitive car camping is allowed within 100 feet of designated roads. Please use established sites. All camping is prohibited within a quarter mile of springs, artificial water developments (called guzzlers), and other water sources. Although campfires are allowed, wood collecting is not. Bring your own firewood, but check first with refuge headquarters about any fire restrictions.

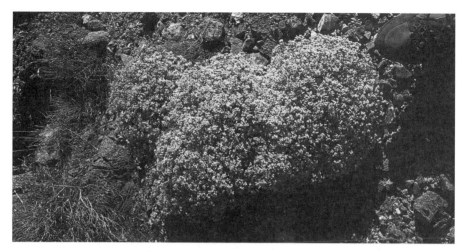

A variety of buckwheat species bring color to the desert.

From your car, hike southwest on the spur road for a few hundred yards to the fork. Take the left (south) fork, which climbs southerly to the base of a minor ridge. Follow the ridge southwest to the main eastern ridge of Gass, about 1 mile away. The right (southwest) fork accesses Gass Spring (which may not have water, depending on the season). While you're hiking, keep your eyes open for fossils of ancient sea life along the way, reminding you that 500 million years ago, this mountain wasn't so dry.

Once on the main eastern ridge of Gass (about the halfway point), take a moment to get your bearings. Look back at your route and your car. On the way back, it won't be so obvious which way you came up, because the small ridges descending to the north are similar.

After admiring the view to the south into the rugged canyons below, follow the main ridge another mile or so west to the summit. The best route doesn't stay on the crest of the ridge but instead weaves north and south across the ridge crest, skirting the minor summits. There are faint use trails along the way, but don't be too concerned if they disappear under your feet, as the general route is obvious.

The easiest final approach to Gass Peak is up the southeast face of the peak. The communications facility at the peak removes any sense of pristine, but the views are worth it, across the wide Vegas sprawl to the Spring Mountains, capped by Mt. Charleston to the west, then north to the Sheep Range and the cliffs of Fossil Ridge.

To return, retrace your steps or make a loop by taking the alternate spur road back to your car.

trip 4 DNWR: Hidden Forest & Deadman Canyon

Distance	10 miles, out-and-back
Hiking Time	6 to 8 hours
Elevation	+/-2170 feet
Difficulty	Moderate
Trail Use	Leashed dogs, backpacking option, map and compass
Best Times	Cold to warm
Agency	Desert National Wildlife Range at (702) 879-6110; www.fws.gov/desertcomplex
Recommended Maps	*Indian Springs* 1:100,000; *Hayford Peak* and *White Sage Flat* 7.5-minute
GPS Waypoints	Wiregrass Spring: 36.633° N, 115.208° W
Vehicle	High-clearance or 4WD vehicle recommended

HIGHLIGHTS Hidden Forest lives up to its name. Driving through the parched landscape of the Las Vegas Valley and the Desert National Wildlife Range, it's hard to imagine that enough water exists here, high in the Sheep Range, to support such a beautiful forest. This area is a perfect example of a "sky island" habitat, in which temperate plant and animal communities, supported by the cool temperatures and higher precipitation at elevation, thrive high above the sere landscape below. Isolated forests such as this are common high in Nevada's many mountain ranges.

DIRECTIONS From Las Vegas, take Highway 95 north about 20 miles, past the exit to Kyle Canyon, to the Desert National Wildlife Range (DNWR) entrance on the right. From there, proceed 4 miles east on the graded dirt entrance road to the Corn Creek Field Station. After signing in (it helps the refuge get funding), continue east for a quarter mile, then turn left (north) onto Alamo Road for 16 miles to the Deadman Canyon and Hidden Forest turnoff on the right. Follow that road east for 3.7 miles to the trailhead.

FACILITIES/TRAILHEAD Restrooms, information, and water are available at Corn Creek Field Station and visitor center. Primitive car camping is allowed within 100 feet of designated roads. Please use established sites. All camping is prohibited within a quarter mile of springs, artificial water developments (called guzzlers), and other water sources. Although campfires are allowed, wood collecting is *not*. Bring your own firewood, but check first with refuge headquarters about any fire restrictions.

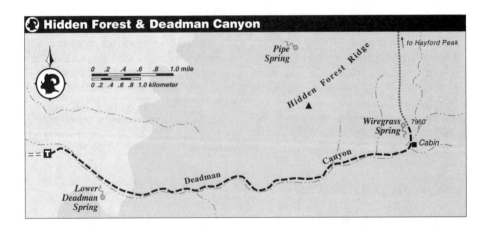

From the car, hike down the trail, through the gate, and into the wash. As soon as you pass through the gate, the plants around you begin to change. After driving through a landscape dominated by yucca and creosote, the desert almond, ephedra, rabbitbrush, pinyon pines, and junipers begin to appear, telling you you've reached 6000 feet in elevation.

Jagged limestone cliffs rise on both sides of the wash. About 500 million years ago, they were sediments at the bottom of a shallow sea. Now they tower above you, steep and rugged, and an indication of the Earth's powerful tectonic forces.

The trail meanders back and forth across the bottom of the wash, at times in parallel trails. There's little worry of getting lost, however, as the steep walls on either side guide you up the valley. The most difficult aspect of this hike is the occasional deep sand and gravel in the wash, which will ensure sore legs the following day.

For prehistoric native peoples, this route was a common commute between the Spring Mountains to the west and the Virgin and Colorado rivers to the east. They likely rested and camped in the shallow caves and shelters along Deadman Canyon. Stone chippings, campsites, and roasting pits hint at these past lives. Please enjoy these cultural remnants respectfully and do not collect or disturb any artifacts.

After about 4 miles, you reach the first of the ponderosa pine trees, followed shortly by white fir. Hiking will seem cooler and more pleasant in this forest above 7000 feet.

After 5.7 miles, you reach a corral, then the old game warden's cabin. Picnic tables invite you to rest, have lunch, and enjoy the sounds of alpine birds and animals, such as towhees, titmice, warblers, thrushes, broadtailed hummingbirds, chipmunks, and rock squirrels.

Hike a quarter mile farther, passing the cabin on the left (north), then head up the side canyon to the north to Wiregrass Spring, where cool water refreshes the landscape. Feel free to sit and enjoy the spring habitat, but do not tarry long. Bighorn sheep and other wildlife depend on this water for survival and will not visit if people are nearby. In 2010 the spring was dry.

To return, retrace your steps.

Desert Bighorn

Before Europeans came to this continent, bighorn sheep ranged from the Rockies to the Sierra Nevada, from Canada into Mexico. Loss of habitat and the bighorn's vulnerability to diseases passed by domestic sheep has reduced their range drastically. Bighorn now live in small numbers in high mountains or refuges.

Over time, bighorns have adapted to desert climates, and they do not need to drink water during the winter, when leafy greens are available. In summer, they must drink at least once every few days. Their nine-stage digestive system allows them to get many nutrients from low-quality food.

During the rut in autumn, the crashing of rams' horns can echo through the canyons, as they collide head-to-head to battle for the right to breed with the females. Here at Wiregrass Spring, you have a good chance of seeing them.

trip 5 DNWR: Hayford Peak

Distance	14 miles, out-and-back
Hiking Time	Long day or overnight
Elevation	+/-4170 feet (from car); +/-2000 feet (from spring)
Difficulty	Difficult
Trail Use	Leashed dogs, backpacking option, map and compass
Best Times	Cool to hot
Agency	Desert National Wildlife Range at (702) 879-6110; www.fws.gov/desertcomplex
Recommended Maps	*Indian Springs* 1:100,000; *Hayford Peak* and *White Sage Flat* 7.5-minute
GPS Waypoints	Wiregrass Spring: 36.633° N, 115.208° W
Vehicle	High-clearance or 4WD vehicle recommended

HIGHLIGHTS On this hike, you travel through beautiful pine forests to great views at the highest point of the Sheep Range.

DIRECTIONS From Las Vegas, take Highway 95 north about 20 miles, past the exit to Kyle Canyon, to the Desert National Wildlife Range (DNWR) entrance on the right. From there, proceed 4 miles east on the graded dirt entrance road to the Corn Creek Field Station. After signing in (it helps the refuge get funding), continue east for a few hundred yards, then turn left (north) onto Alamo Road for 16 miles to the Deadman Canyon and Hidden Forest turnoff on the right. Follow the road east for 3.7 miles to the trailhead.

FACILITIES/TRAILHEAD Restrooms, information, and water are available at Corn Creek Field Station and the visitor center. Primitive car camping is allowed within 100 feet of designated roads. Please use established sites. All camping is prohibited within a quarter mile of springs, artificial water developments (called guzzlers), and other water sources. Although campfires are allowed, wood collecting is not. Bring your own firewood, but check first with refuge headquarters about any fire restrictions.

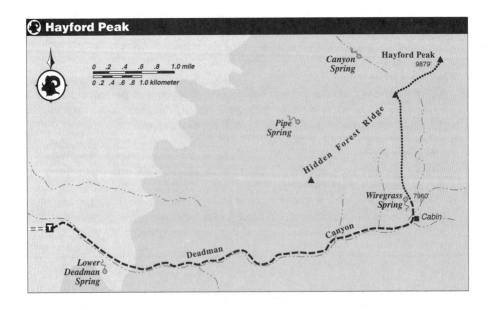

This trip begins at Wiregrass Spring, after you have followed the route to the destination of the previous trip, Hidden Forest.

From the car, hike down the trail, through the gate, and into the wash. Follow the wash 5.7 miles to the corral, then pass the game warden's cabin, and head up the side canyon north to Wiregrass Spring.

From Wiregrass Spring, continue north and uphill, following the ridgelines up. There is no trail above Wiregrass Spring, but with some attention to your map and compass, you shouldn't have any trouble following the ridgeline northeast to the summit.

Hayford Peak makes an obvious landmark to the north. For the first mile beyond the spring, Hidden Forest Ridge to your left (northwest) might lobby for your attention. It, too, would make a fine destination, with great views of the western slope of the Sheep Range, into the Nellis Air Force Range and toward the Nevada Test Site. But if your goal is Hayford Peak, aim for the peak to the north and right (northeast) as you're hiking.

In addition to the views of forested ridges around you, a highlight is the stand of bristlecone pine trees you encounter at about 8800 feet, as you crest the nose of a lesser ridge near the base of Hayford Peak. Most bristlecones are shorter and gnarled because of the harsher conditions at high altitude, but the trees in this stand seem taller and healthier than many at high elevation. Bristlecones can live more than 5,000 years, but the trees in this stand are likely much younger. Interestingly, bristlecones live longest in the highest, harshest conditions, exposed to weather we would find inhospitable.

About 2 miles after you leave Wiregrass Spring, you reach Hayford Peak. The communications tower complex on the summit destroys any sense of pristine solitude, but the views make up for it: The Sheep Range snakes away to the north and south. You can also see Sheep Peak (to the south), the Arrow Canyon Range, the Mormon Mountains, and the Virgin Mountains (to the east). To the west lie the Desert Range, the Nellis Air Force Range, and the Spring Mountains in the distance.

Once you have enjoyed the summit, retrace your steps to return.

trip 6 DNWR: Bookshelf Canyon

Distance	6 miles, out-and-back
Hiking Time	3 to 5 hours
Elevation	+/-720 feet
Difficulty	Moderate
Trail Use	Leashed dogs, backpacking option, map and compass
Best Times	Cold to warm
Agency	Desert National Wildlife Range at (702) 879-6110; www.fws.gov/desertcomplex
Recommended Maps	*Indian Springs* 1:100,000; *Arrow Canyon NW* 7.5-minute
GPS Waypoints	Parking spot: 36.712° N, 114.930° W Canyon mouth: 36.717° N, 114.976° W
Vehicle	High-clearance or 4WD vehicle recommended

HIGHLIGHTS There is no name for this canyon on any map. Nor will it stand out as particularly inviting on any map. However, this canyon offers what no road map can show: stunning geology. I call it Bookshelf Canyon to describe the wonderful limestone layers standing vertically on both walls of the canyon. This hike offers, not only mind-bending geology, but also an encounter with wide-open

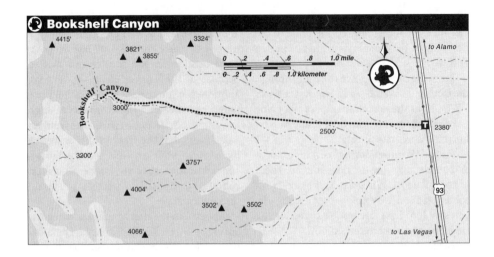

Mojave Desert. Bookshelf is an insignificant part of the 1.6-million-acre wildlife refuge that most people have never visited—just another blank spot on the map. Maybe its anonymity is why I like it. For many years, Bookshelf Canyon was part of the BLM "Fish and Wildlife #2" Wilderness Study Area. In 2002, Congress transferred jurisdiction of this land to the Fish and Wildlife Service, making Bookshelf part of the Desert National Wildlife Range.

DIRECTIONS From Las Vegas, take I-15 north for about 20 miles. Take exit 64, turn left (west), zero your odometer after crossing under the underpass, and follow Highway 93 north toward Pioche and Ely for 26 miles. At 26 miles, park on either side of the road, well off the pavement at the highway's lowest point (elevations are subtle here, but looking north and south along the highway, you'll know you're there—it's OK if you're off by a quarter mile or so).

FACILITIES/TRAILHEAD The nearest facilities are in Las Vegas. Primitive car camping is allowed within 100 feet of designated roads. Please use established sites. All camping is prohibited within a quarter mile of springs, artificial water developments (called guzzlers), and other water sources. Although campfires are allowed, wood collecting is not. Bring your own firewood, but check first with refuge headquarters about any fire restrictions.

Look west-northwest up the bajadas (the gently sloping land between you and the mountains of the Las Vegas Range), and you will see the small entrance to Bookshelf Canyon about 2.5 miles away. Hike under the power lines and directly toward it. There is no trail, but the open vegetation on the bajada makes for easy travel.

After hiking a few hundred yards west of your vehicle, take a moment to orient yourself. In this open country with no prominent landmarks, scale can be deceiving, and cars can disappear in the vast expanse. Here's a tip to keep from losing your car: Draw a mental line directly from the mouth of Bookshelf Canyon, through you and your vehicle to the Arrow Canyon Range rising to the east. Memorize the specific features of the mountains to your east and west where the line meets them. Knowing your car is on this line will help you find it easily on your return.

Walking west across the bajada, you travel over stones covered with a dark brown ceramic sheen, a coating known as desert varnish that bacteria deposit to protect themselves against the harsh sun. Desert varnish was a popular surface on which native peoples carved petroglyphs hundreds, even thousands of years ago (however, no petroglyphs are known to be along this hike—please let me know if you find some!). Scattered creosote and yucca, as well as barrel, beavertail, and cholla cacti, show this bajada is far from lifeless. This gentle, unobtrusive quality of landscape makes up the majority of the Mojave Desert.

After about 2.5 miles, you reach the entrance to Bookshelf Canyon, which is only 20 or 30 feet wide. Inside, vertical fins of limestone jut up to the north and south for the length of the canyon. Five-hundred-million years ago, these layers were simply muck accumulating on the bottom of the sea. Millions of years of tectonic activity later, they're standing on end 5000 feet above sea level in a canyon hundreds of miles from the sea.

Look at the hills north and south of Bookshelf to see the varied configurations of layers. Farther west, the Sheep Range rises behind the Las Vegas Range to 9912 feet at Hayford Peak (Trip 5). To the east, the Arrow Canyon Range rises to 5200 feet and displays one of the more striking faces in Southern Nevada. With this view, it's easy to understand why stratigraphers (geologists who specialize in rock layers) come from around the world to study its lessons about past geological eras.

About a half mile up Bookshelf Canyon, the canyon splits to the north and south. Country beyond here gets less dramatic. This is a good place to have a snack, then hike back to your car.

Tectonic forces have changed ancient seabeds into vertical spines in desert canyons.

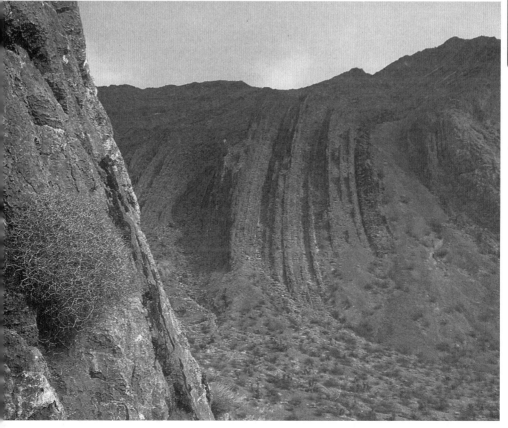

DNWR: Desert Lake Dunes

Distance	Up to 2 miles, out-and-back
Hiking Time	1 to 2 hours
Elevation	+/-150 feet
Difficulty	Easy to moderate
Trail Use	Leashed dogs, backpacking option, map and compass
Best Times	Cold to warm
Agency	Desert National Wildlife Range at (702) 879-6110; www.fws.gov/desertcomplex
Recommended Maps	*Pahranagat Range* 1:100,000
GPS Waypoints	Summit of the dunes: 37.018° N, 115.187° W
Vehicle	High-clearance or 4WD vehicle recommended

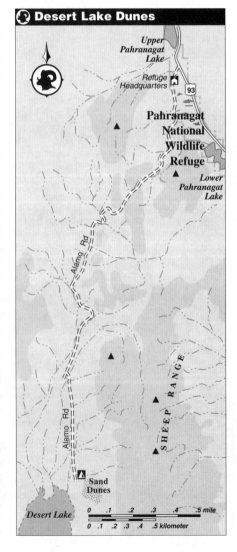

HIGHLIGHTS It may not be vast, but this dune field is fun to explore (although hiking is not required). The soft, shifting sands, vast desert solitude, and rugged beauty are the prime attractions here. It is a good place to camp if you're looking to find yourself in one of the loneliest, most isolated, sun-baked spots in Southern Nevada.

DIRECTIONS From Las Vegas, take I-15 north for about 20 miles. Take exit 64 and follow Highway 93 north toward Pioche and Ely for about 60 miles to the Pahranagat National Wildlife Refuge on your left (west). Less than a mile south of Upper Pahranagat Lake, turn left (west) onto the refuge headquarters access road, which heads southwest. Continue past the headquarters and follow the signs to get you on the Alamo Road (also called the Old Corn Creek Road) toward the Desert National Wildlife Range and Corn Creek Station. Turn right (west) on Alamo Road and continue southwest for 5 or 6 miles to the DNWR boundary.

Zero your odometer at the boundary, then keep driving, ignoring all roads that tempt you away from your southerly bearing. At each road fork, choose the south fork. About 15 miles later, you reach Desert Lake, which is usually dry. The dunes are located at the base of the Sheep Range, at the northeast corner of the dry lake. Turn left (east) on the spur accessing them, drive in (not too far—watch out for deep sand), park, and break out the cooler. Return the way you came.

FACILITIES/TRAILHEAD The nearest facilities are 5 miles north of Pahranagat National Wildlife Refuge on Highway 93. Stock up on everything you need in Las Vegas. Primitive car camping is allowed within 100 feet of designated roads. Please use established sites. All camping is prohibited within a quarter mile of springs,

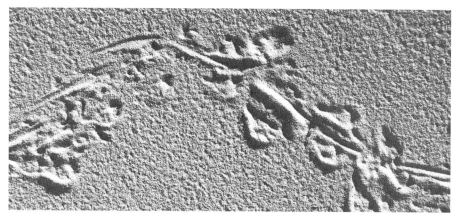

The desert can seem lifeless. These lizard tracks tell otherwise.

artificial water developments (called guzzlers), and other water sources. Although campfires are allowed, wood collecting is not. Bring your own firewood, but check first with refuge headquarters about any fire restrictions.

The dunes sit at the western base of the rugged and beautiful Sheep Range, which stands between the dunes and Highway 93, and at the eastern edge of vast Desert Valley. Five miles to the west, across the lake, is the boundary for the 3.1-million-acre Nellis Air Force Range. The name alone explains why it's off-limits. About 40 miles west-southwest is Frenchman Flat, the site of numerous above- and below-ground nuclear tests between the 1950s and 1990s.

A similar distance to the northwest sits Groom Lake, known to military conspiracy theorists as the site of Dreamland, or Area-51, where the U2, SR-71, and Stealth Bombers were developed. It's also supposedly where the bodies of the aliens who crashed at Roswell, New Mexico, in 1947, are being kept, and where their craft is being reverse-engineered to create technology for our military. If you were ever going to see strange lights in the night sky, this would be the place.

Even if you don't see any, you're sure to have a wonderful sky-watching experience. On full moons, the vast landscape glows a glorious blue (or is that from the nuclear tests?). On new moons, the sky fills with stars as only high-desert skies can—perfect for watching meteor showers and other celestial phenomena.

Northern Region

Another Nevada Dry Lake

Before you pack your water wings, be aware that Desert Lake is not for swimming. Like many "lakes" you'll find in Nevada, it is a playa, a dry lakebed—flat, dusty, expansive. However, when rain comes, Desert Lake collects the runoff from a large watershed, making the lakebed an impassable mucky mess—the reason the U.S. Fish and Wildlife Service has closed Alamo Road south of the dunes, where it crosses the lake toward Corn Creek Station. If you were to get stuck out here, it would be a 20-mile walk back to the highway, in temperatures that can reach 120 degrees. Good thing you're prepared, right? If not, you can read (page 20) while you're stranded.

trip 8 Arrow Canyon

Distance	Up to 8 miles, out-and-back
Hiking Time	Up to 4 hours
Elevation	+/-120 feet
Difficulty	Moderate
Trail Use	Leashed dogs, good for kids, backpacking option
Best Times	Cold to warm
Agency	BLM Las Vegas at (702) 515-5000; www.blm.nv.gov/vegas
Recommended Maps	*Overton, NV* 1:100,000; *Arrow Canyon* 7.5-minute
GPS Waypoints	Canyon entrance: 36.727° N, 114.765° W
Vehicle	Passenger OK; high-clearance or 4WD vehicle recommended

HIGHLIGHTS Tall, narrow slot canyons are common in the canyon country of Utah and Arizona, but there are few in Nevada. Arrow Canyon, 3 miles long and at places only 20 feet wide and 400 feet deep, is one of the Silver State's crown jewels. This hike offers incredible geology, fossils, hints of ancient cultures, and the thrill of hiking through a deep, narrow canyon. As you explore, you'll see why Congress designated the 27,530-acre Arrow Canyon Wilderness Area in 2002. This is not the place to be in a flash flood. If thunderstorms are active anywhere in the sky, hike somewhere else.

DIRECTIONS From Las Vegas, drive north on I-15 to exit 90 (to Moapa/Glendale), and follow Highway 168 west, past Moapa, to mile marker 13. Just west of the mile marker, turn left (south) into what looks like a driveway to a house. As you approach the house, stay to the right. The dirt road takes you past the house to its right (please drive slowly to keep the dust down), then past a small pumping station (low-clearance cars park here; you have to hike an additional mile west in the wash to the canyon). If you have a high-clearance, 4WD vehicle, drive past the pumping station, following the track into the wash, then west for 1 mile to the trailhead/parking area.

Consider this scenic option for the drive home: After your hike, continue west on 168 to Highway 93, then follow it south back to I-15. It adds 15 to 20 minutes to your travel time, but the scenery is worth it. Once you turn south on U.S. 93, you have incredible views east of the colorful layers and rugged face of the Arrow Canyon Range, and west to the Las Vegas and Sheep ranges of the Desert National Wildlife Range.

FACILITIES/TRAILHEAD The nearest facilities are in Moapa or Glendale.

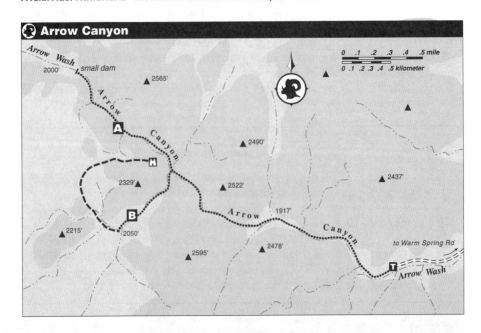

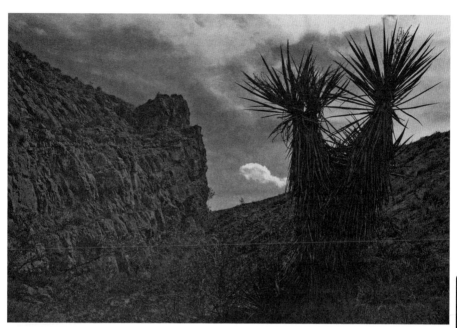

Strata-loving geologists come from around the world to read the stories written in the many layers of the Arrow Canyon range.

From the car, hike west into the canyon. Before you enter the canyon, explore the wonders waiting at its mouth. Look at the rocks around you for fossils of crinoids (sea lilies), brachiopods (lamp shells), corals, and other marine organisms, as well as the roots of the Lepidodendron tree, *Stygmaria*. Many of these date back to the Cambrian period, 500 million years ago, when these jagged rocks were sediments accumulating at the bottom of the ocean.

After 2 miles, the wall opens to a wash on your left (south). Here you have two options:

A. For an easier hike, ignore the wash to the south and continue hiking through the canyon for another mile to a small dam at the head of the canyon, then turn around and retrace your steps.

B. For a moderate hike, follow the wash south out of the canyon for a half mile or so until you see a jeep trail heading west. Follow this route less than a mile until you see another road leading to the right (northwest). This road makes a clockwise U to the west then north back toward the canyon. As you approach Arrow Canyon from the south, veer right (easterly) to climb to a point high on the south rim of the canyon, looking in, where your view of the canyon is worth the heavy breathing.

From here, you can retrace your steps, or continue down the ridge to the west, into the basin above the dam in option A. Then turn right (east), following a trail along the southern edge to the right of the basin. Clamber over the dam into Arrow Canyon, then follow the canyon back to your car.

At the top of Arrow Canyon, in the wide basin upstream from the dam, you will see one of the major problems facing Western landscapes today: invasive, exotic plants.

The Bureau of Land Management has been battling the notoriously invasive tamarisk (also known as salt cedar, or *tamarix ramossisima*). Growing quickly up to 20 feet tall, tamarisk aggressively outcompetes native plants. Because it grows most often along waterways, it seriously impacts critical life zones in the deserts. You may find tamarisk here, or evidence of the BLM's efforts to eradicate it so native plants can gain their foothold again.

Arrow Canyon is at the bottom of Pahranagat Wash, which drains thousands of square miles of watershed. Throughout the area you might find signs of the native people who lived in the area. Some of the petroglyphs may have been carved by Ancestral Puebloans 1,500 to 3,000 years ago, or perhaps even by their predecessors, Desert Archaic peoples between 2,000 and 8,000 years ago.

If you find any archaeological artifacts, please admire them but *do not touch*. State and federal laws protect these artifacts, so they will remain to thrill and educate others. Arrow Canyon is sacred to local tribes. Please respect it as you would your own place of worship.

trip 9 Mormon Mountains: Hackberry Springs

Distance	5 miles, out-and-back
Hiking Time	3 to 5 hours
Elevation	+/-1000 feet
Difficulty	Moderate
Trail Use	Leashed dogs, map and compass, backpacking option
Best Times	Cool to warm
Agency	BLM Las Vegas at (702) 515-5000; www.blm.nv.gov/vegas
Recommended Maps	*Overton, NV* 1:100,000; *Moapa Peak NW* 7.5-minute
GPS Waypoints	Parking area/campsite: 36.897° N, 114.417° W
	Hackberry Springs: 36.917° N, 114.438° W
Vehicle	High-clearance or 4WD vehicle recommended

HIGHLIGHTS Hackberry Springs is in just one of many rugged, winding, and beautiful canyons in the Mormon Mountains. This south-facing valley is dry and best avoided in hot weather, despite the higher elevation. Many species of wildlife are common in this area, including wild horses, burrowing owls, bighorn sheep, and raptors. In November 2004, Congress designated 158,000 acres of the Mormon Mountains as wilderness. In 2005, a wildfire swept through, decimating the native yucca and blackbrush plant community. Native plants can take decades to recover, and these face additional competition from invasive weeds like red brome and cheatgrass.

DIRECTIONS From Las Vegas, take I-15 north to exit 100 to Carp and Elgin. Cross under the freeway, then turn right to follow the paved frontage road for a few miles until it turns to the north and the pavement ends. Zero your odometer at the pavement's end and continue north for 7.3 miles, crossing under the power lines along the way.

Turn left (northwest) onto an unmaintained, unsigned, and easy-to-miss jeep track, which climbs the bajada (gentle slope) to the east of Moapa Peak. Follow the track for about 3.5 miles, ignoring any routes that turn off of it, to an open bench on the left (west) side of a wash. Park here. (And consider camping here, too.)

FACILITIES/TRAILHEAD The nearest facilities are in Glendale off I-15, about 20 miles away.

From the car, drop into the wash and follow it upstream and north. Within a half mile, you pass through an impressive narrow "gate" in the rugged rock formations at the head of the wash.

Upstream from the gate, look for agave roasting pits to the side of the road. These circular mounds of charred white rock are leftovers from native barbecues hundreds, if not thousands, of years ago. Please respect

⊕ Hackberry Springs

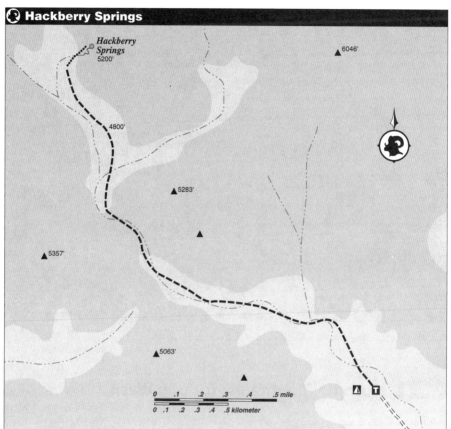

these important artifacts from a distance. Keeping them intact allows others to enjoy them and archaeologists to learn about the people who made them.

Beyond the gate, the wash opens up again and continues northwest. Although the terrain isn't difficult, the deep sand makes for slow and tiring progress. About 2.5 miles from the car, at the head of the valley, you'll see trash and historical artifacts left by generations of ranchers, prospectors, and chucklehead campers who didn't clean up after themselves.

Look for a faint footpath that heads northeast from this area, up a shrub-tangled

side canyon, about a quarter mile to Hackberry Springs, which is tucked deep under overhanging rocks on the south side of the drainage. Last time I was there, it was dripping, but barely.

If you're itching for more, continue up-canyon past the springs for as long as you'd like, where you'll get to know the true, rugged, isolated beauty that permeates the Mormon Mountains. You can also climb the rocky ridge to the east of the stone "gate" back down at the foot of the valley to look for small caves and panoramic views toward Las Vegas Valley.

Retrace your steps to return.

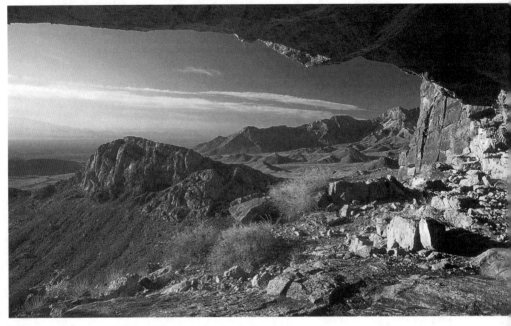

The slopes of the Mormons offer shallow caves and wonderful views.

trip 10 Mormon Mountains: Toquop Wash

Distance	4 to 6 miles, out-and-back
Hiking Time	4 to 6 hours
Elevation	+/-1000 feet
Difficulty	Moderate
Trail Use	Leashed dogs, backpacking option, map and compass
Best Times	Cool to warm
Agency	BLM Ely at (775) 289-1800; www.nv.blm.gov/ely
Recommended Maps	*Overton, NV* 1:100,000; *Davidson Peak* and *Moapa Peak NW* 7.5-minute
GPS Waypoints	Horse Spring: 36.941° N, 114.447° W
Vehicle	High-clearance or 4WD vehicle recommended

HIGHLIGHTS Named after a Southern Paiute word that means "black tobacco" (which refers to a plant that grows in the area), Toquop Wash is one of the more beautiful valleys in the Mormon Mountains. Perhaps it's the shape of the hills, the limestone cliffs high on the peaks, or the open, silent solitude. There is no real destination here. This hike is designed to help you enjoy the beauty of this rugged valley, where the Great Basin meets the Mojave Desert. In November 2004, Congress designated 158,000 acres of the Mormon Mountains as wilderness. In 2005 a wildfire burned the canyon.

DIRECTIONS From Las Vegas, take I-15 north to exit 100 to Carp and Elgin. Cross under the freeway (heading northwest), then turn right to follow the paved frontage road for a few miles until it turns to the north and the pavement ends. Zero your odometer at the pavement's end and continue north (crossing under the power lines). Continue following this graded gravel road it as it veers northeast, over a summit, then north again along the eastern slope of the Mormon Mountains.

At 15.7 miles, turn left (west) onto an unsigned, unpaved road that heads westerly up Toquop Wash. Follow this route for about 6 miles and park by an old corral near the large fork in the canyon.

FACILITIES/TRAILHEAD The nearest facilities are at Glendale off I-15.

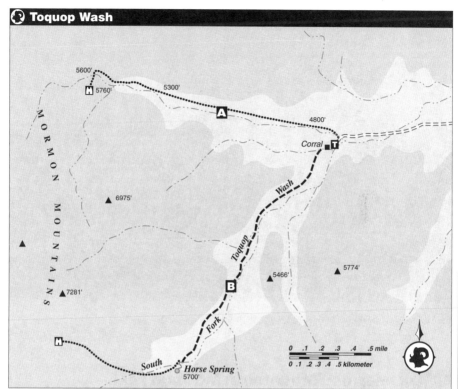

Toquop Wash

The parking area is at the fork of the canyon, so you have two options:

A. Follow the right (northerly) fork to the west as it climbs into the theater of cliffs to the north of Peak 7377. There is no trail, but determined hikers are rewarded with views and rugged solitude wherever they stop.

B. Follow the 4WD route up and into the left (southerly) fork, which climbs another 2 miles until it ends long after it should on very steep slopes. A quarter mile before its end, a spur heads to the left (south) for a couple hundred yards to Horse Spring, which is dry. Ambitious scramblers might want to climb beyond the end of the road for another mile to the top of the ridge to the west. This very difficult, rugged cross-country route rewards the determined with a knockout view of the limestone peaks and winding valleys of the Mormons.

Either route you take, look for the sagebrush, bitterbrush, ephedra, and other high-desert plants growing on the lower slopes, and the pinyon-juniper forests dominating the higher slopes. You may also see agave roasting pits on either side of the road. These circular mounds of charred white rock are left over from native barbecues hundreds or even thousands of years ago. Please respect these important artifacts from a distance.

Many species of wildlife are common in the area, including wild horses, burrowing owls, bighorn sheep, and raptors. While high on the ridge to the west at sunset once, I had a memorable encounter with a barn owl, who circled me closely several times, trying to figure out what I was.

Once you have enjoyed the solitude and beauty of the area, retrace your steps to return.

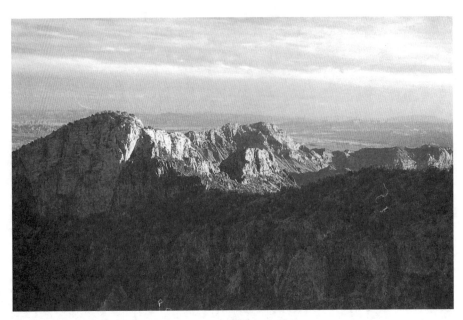

Rocky limestone peaks tower over rugged canyons in the Mormons.

trip 11 Mormon Mountains: Mormon Peak

Distance	8 to 10 miles, out-and-back
Hiking Time	6 to 8 hours
Elevation	+/-3500 feet
Difficulty	Difficult
Trail Use	Leashed dogs, backpacking option, map and compass
Best Times	Cool to warm
Agency	BLM Ely at (775) 289-1800; www.nv.blm.gov/ely
Recommended Maps	*Overton, NV* 1:100,000; *Rox* and *Rox NE* 7.5-minute
GPS Waypoints	Turnoff at Hoya Siding: 36.936° N, 114.654° W
	Ridge at 2 miles: 36.965° N, 114.526° W
	Mormon Peak: 36.973° N, 114.500° W
Vehicle	High-clearance or 4WD vehicle recommended

HIGHLIGHTS This is the crowning point of the Mormon Mountains, which are among the more rugged and remote mountains in Southern Nevada. The drive is remote and rough, with water crossings and deep sand; the hike is cross-country (no trail), with no water or services. Only fit and experienced desert explorers should drive or hike in this area. The only way to approach Mormon Peak is from the west, because steep limestone cliffs circle the peak on all other directions. Read about safe desert driving for tips on how to prepare (page 20). Mormon Peak lies within the 158,000-acre Mormon Mountains Wilderness Area, designated by Congress in 2004.

DIRECTIONS From Las Vegas, take I-15 north and take exit 90 to Moapa and Glendale. Drive west on Highway 168 for 2.8 miles to Meadow Valley Road. Turn right (north), and zero your odometer, and drive past the end of the pavement as it parallels the Union Pacific train tracks. At 10.5 miles, you will find a ROAD CLOSED AHEAD sign posted by Union Pacific. At this point, turn left (west), cross under the tracks, then follow the well-maintained gravel road north as it parallels the tracks on the west side.

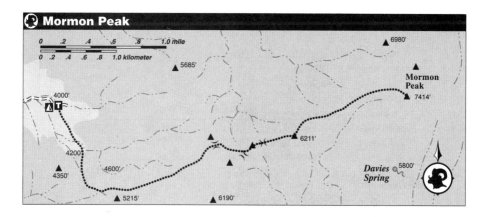

Mormon Peak

0 .2 .4 .6 .8 1.0 mile
0 .2 .4 .6 .8 1.0 kilometer

6980'

▲ 5685'

▲ Mormon Peak

4000'
▲T

▲ 7414'

4200'

6211'

4350'   4600'
▲

Davies Spring ○ 5800'

▲ 5215'   ▲ 6190'

This road first climbs up onto bluffs, then it drops down into Meadow Valley Wash. (Look for migrating songbirds along the water, or raptors riding currents along the cliffs above.)

At 15.5 miles, the road veers east and crosses back under the tracks, before it turns north again to parallel the tracks, this time on the east side. At the crossing, there are several low, muddy spots, smaller routes veering off left and right, and no signs. The road you want winds through the brush and low hills a quarter mile or so east of the tracks. At 19.5 miles, after cresting a berm (and just east of Hoya Siding on the railroad tracks), notice an unsigned jeep track heading east up a wide wash (see UTM coordinates above). Turn here, and follow this unsigned, unpaved road northeast up the bajada (or "alluvial fan") for another 6.5 miles. There are decent parking spots and campsites at 25 and 26 miles.

FACILITIES/TRAILHEAD The nearest facilities are in Glendale or Moapa off I-15.

Follow the road up the valley to the small mine ruins at the east head of the valley. From there, hike due south (now off-trail) and up the smooth bowl onto the southern

You'll begin encountering pinyon pines halfway to the peak.

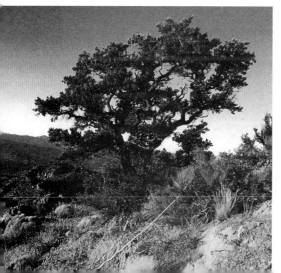

ridge. Once there, follow the ridge east and up (the north-facing slopes just below the ridgeline are easier than the ridgeline itself).

About 2 miles from the valley floor, you top out on a north-south-trending ridge. From this ridge, your route east is visible all the way to the peak. Keep hiking until you're there.

From the peak, you enjoy views across Meadow Valley Wash to the Meadow Valley Mountains to the west, the Sheep and Arrow Canyon ranges to the southwest, the Clover Mountains to the north, the Virgin Mountains to the southeast, and the Las Vegas Valley far to the south. You can also gaze into the rugged interior valleys of the Mormon Mountains.

Retrace your steps to return.

Please follow Leave No Trace principles whenever you travel and camp, by sticking to trails, washes, or stone whenever possible (read more about trail etiquette, page 18).

Northern Region

12 Pahranagat National Wildlife Refuge

Distance	Up to 6 miles, out-and-back
Hiking Time	6 to 8 hours
Elevation	Negligible
Difficulty	Flat and easy
Trail Use	Leashed dogs, good for kids
Best Times	Cool to warm (May and September to see migrating birds)
Agency	Pahranagat National Wildlife Refuge at (775) 725-3417; www.fws.gov/desertcomplex/pahranagat
Recommended Maps	*Pahranagat Range* 1:100,000; free refuge map at information kiosks
GPS Waypoints	Grove Spring: 37.322° N, 115.141° W
Vehicle	Passenger car OK

HIGHLIGHTS In the language of the native Southern Paiute people, *pahranagat* means "valley of shining water," a testament to how precious this stretch of lakes and wetlands is to the people and wildlife of the region. Today, this wetland valley provides essential habitat for wildlife traveling through the parched desert landscape. In 1963, the U.S. Fish and Wildlife Service designated 5,380 acres of Pahranagat Valley's lakes and wetlands as a national wildlife refuge.

DIRECTIONS From Las Vegas, take I-15 north for about 20 miles. Take exit 64 and follow Highway 93 north toward Pioche and Ely for about 70 miles to the wildlife refuge on your left (west). Park here and explore.

FACILITIES/TRAILHEAD The nearest facilities are in Alamo, 5 miles north of Pahranagat National Wildlife Refuge on Highway 93. The refuge contains unimproved camping and picnic areas along Upper Pahranagat Lake, wildlife viewing and hunting platforms, and several miles of access roads and paths for walking and horseback riding.

Upper Pahranagat Lake is a popular spot for picnics, fishing, and watching birds and wildlife.

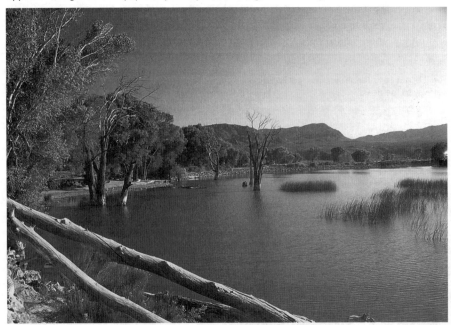

There are no official trails, but you can follow any of the many jeep trails wandering through the refuge. One nice hike is along the west shore of North Pahranagat Lake, south of Grove Spring. From Highway 93 about 1 mile north of North Pahranagat Lake, turn left (west) onto an unsigned unpaved road, then follow it southwest about 0.6 mile to Grove Spring. Here the road takes a sharp turn south and gets much rougher. Please park at least 200 yards from the spring, then hike along the road south. It goes almost 3 miles along the lake to the south end. Walk to the end (or as far as you'd like), then retrace your steps to return.

Located along the eastern edge of the Pacific Flyway (the western migration corridor for birds), the lakes, marshes, and meadows of the Pahranagat Valley provide respite and food for waterfowl, raptors, and songbirds migrating from as far north as the Arctic to as far south as South America. The area is also home to numerous desert wildlife species, including coyote, bobcat, badger, the endangered desert tortoise, jackrabbit, and rattlesnake. Frequent rustling in the bushes as you walk by might make you wonder which of the above species is thrashing about in there.

People have also been drawn to this water for centuries. Look carefully on the rocks around the refuge, and you might find ancient petroglyphs, notably "Pahranagat man" figures, which appear here and nowhere else. Since the mid-1800s, pioneers have also lived, hunted, and ranched in this valley. Several structures on the refuge date to that period.

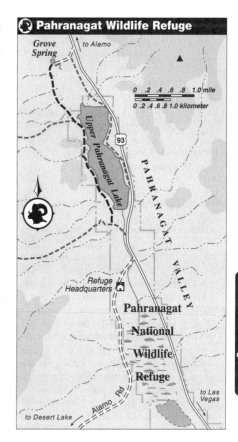

Core samples taken from the lake bottom show these lakes were deeper and surrounded by pine forests as recently as a few thousand years ago. Recent drought has left the lower lakes dry. The core data show this has happened before. Maybe the cycle will come around to wet again, or maybe global warming and Southern Nevada's thirsty and explosive population growth will bring this valley a drier future.

Delamar Dry Lake

Distance	Optional
Hiking Time	Optional
Elevation	Negligible
Difficulty	Flat and easy
Trail Use	Leashed dogs, good for kids, map and compass
Best Times	Cold to warm (at least several days after wet weather)
Agency	BLM Ely at (775) 289-1800; www.nv.blm.gov/ely
Recommended Maps	*Clover Mountains* and *Pahranagat Range* 1:100,000
GPS Waypoints	Lake center: 37.318° N, 114.949° W
Vehicle	High-clearance or 4WD vehicle recommended

HIGHLIGHTS Although there's not much hiking to be done on Delamar Dry Lake, it offers solitude, stark beauty, and a little elbow room on the (usually) dry bed of this ancient lake. When dry, the playa makes a wonderful campsite. If you haven't seen desert stars at their best, plan to camp here on a new moon—you'll be grateful you did. The area's high elevation makes it a cool escape from the Las Vegas heat. However, winter nights can be chilly, with temperatures dropping into the single digits. Avoid driving on the playa after rain. The mud softens, and you could end up stuck up to your axles in goop. It's a long walk out, and an expensive tow to remove your vehicle. After rain, admire it from a distance.

DIRECTIONS From Las Vegas, take I-15 north for about 20 miles. Take exit 64 and follow Highway 93 north toward Pioche and Ely for another 70 miles to the Pahranagat National Wildlife Refuge. A few miles north of Upper Pahranagat Lake, turn right (east) onto the unpaved and very scenic Alamo Canyon Road and follow it east for about 19 miles to the dry lake on your right (south). If the road forks along the way, try to stick to the main, bladed route until you reach the lake bed. Park here and camp. Continue your explorations by driving north along the power line road, which runs north-south to the east of the playa. After about 8 miles, signed roads head east to the ghost town of Delamar, where 3,000 people lived and mined gold in the late 1800s. Return to the power line road, then continue north for another 13 miles until you reach Highway 93 between Caliente and Alamo. Turn left (west) on 93 to return to Vegas (a 2.5-hour drive).

FACILITIES/TRAILHEAD There are no facilities or trailheads at Delamar Dry Lake. The nearest facilities are in Alamo, 20 miles to the west via Alamo Canyon Road.

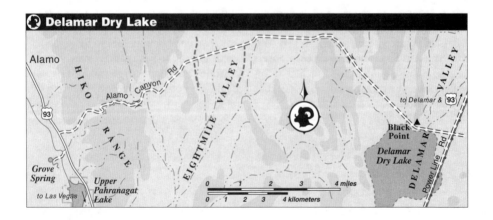

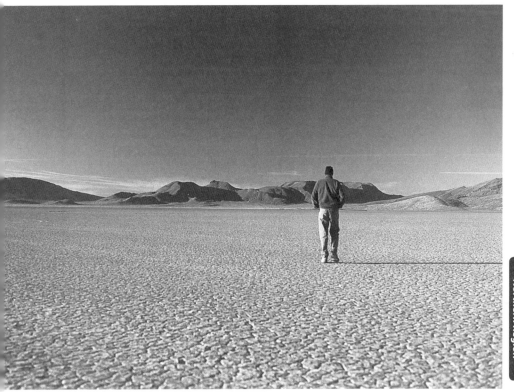

Delamar Dry Lake will cure even the worst case of claustrophobia.

This is not a hike, but a drive to an interesting and beautiful playa (dry lakebed). Such playas scattered throughout Nevada and the Mojave Desert are testaments to the lakes that filled these valleys more than 10,000 years ago, during the last ice age. This and other playas still fill with water after significant rainfall. I visited here once after thunderstorms swept through the area. The entire playa was two inches deep in water. By the next morning, the water had all but disappeared.

Explore the southern tip of the small rocky range to the north of the playa, where ancient petroglyphs indicate that people long ago enjoyed this area, too. Please admire them from a distance. Please *do not touch or damage them* in any way, so people in the future can enjoy them too.

On November 15, 1967, Air Force test pilot Michael Adams launched the experimental X-15 aircraft from Delamar Dry Lake. After topping out at 226,000 feet and making Adams America's 27th astronaut, the plane malfunctioned and crashed on reentry, killing him. Today, amateur rocket clubs use Delamar Dry Lake regularly to launch experimental model rockets of all sizes. The U.S. military also occasionally uses Delamar Dry Lake as an air strip during training exercises.

Delamar Dry Lake is not protected by any laws, so it's important for everyone to clean up after themselves. Please follow Leave No Trace principles when exploring the area and also leave all archaeological artifacts where you found them.

trip 14 Ash Springs

Distance	Up to 1 mile, loop
Hiking Time	1 hour
Elevation	+/-90 feet
Difficulty	Easy
Trail Use	Leashed dogs, good for kids
Best Times	Cold to warm
Agency	BLM Ely at (775) 289-1800; www.nv.blm.gov/ely
Recommended Maps	*Pahranagat Range* 1:100,000
GPS Waypoints	Ash Springs: 37.463° N, 115.192° W
Vehicle	Passenger car OK

HIGHLIGHTS Here you'll find soothing warm springs, endangered fish, and ancient rock art.

DIRECTIONS From Las Vegas, take I-15 north to exit 64, then follow Highway 93 north toward Pioche and Ely to Ash Springs (about 90 miles from Vegas and 7 miles north of Alamo). The warm spring pool is on the right (east) side of 93, across the street from the north end of the gas station, at the end of a short, unsigned, unpaved road.

FACILITIES/TRAILHEAD Restrooms are available here, and other facilities (gas, food, and water) can be found across the street at the gas station.

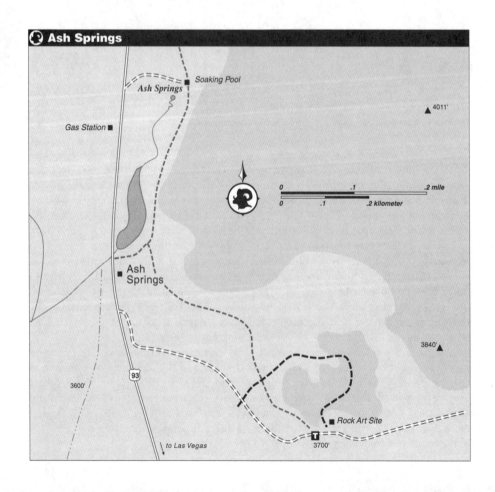

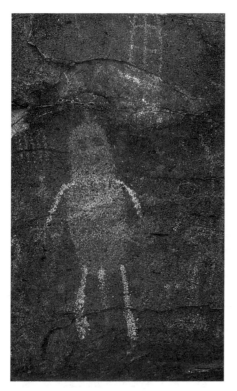

This "Pahranagat man" figure is found only in Pahranagat Valley and nowhere else.

From the car, hike the short 30 feet to the springs. This burbling spring, as well as the entire Pahranagat Valley that runs north-south through this region, have attracted people for thousands of years. If you're looking to relax, grab your bathing suit and ease yourself into the warm water of Ash Springs. Ahhh.

Ash, willow, and mesquite trees grow along the stream by the soaking pool, providing shade for the endangered Pahranagat roundtail chub, which has lived in the Pahranagat Valley and nowhere else on Earth for more than 10,000 years. Please

help it survive by staying out of the creek and enjoying only the soaking pool.

To get to the Ash Springs Rock Art Site, head south on Highway 93 for a quarter mile. On the left (east) side of 93, immediately south of the fence surrounding the springs, follow another unsigned, unpaved access road for a quarter mile, over a cattle guard, to the boulder-strewn slopes above the highway. You could spend hours exploring the rocks here for ancient petroglyphs. There is a self-guided interpretive trail, but no signed trailhead. The BLM publishes an interpretive booklet for this site. Call the number above to order one.

The proximity of water and the abundance of food-grinding surfaces show that this was a popular gathering spot for the Pahranagat people. Some petroglyphs here illustrate bighorn sheep with atlatl spears sticking from their backs. The atlatl was a wooden handle that added speed and distance to spears. Bow and arrows replaced atlatls around 500 A.D., meaning these designs were probably created before then.

Vandalism and litter are common in easily accessible rock art sites. Please be a part of the solution, not a part of the problem, and clean up after yourself. For extra karma points, clean up after others, too. Please *do not touch or damage* any of the rock art. Oil from your skin can make the rock's natural protective covering vulnerable to damage from the sun.

Help preserve rock art so future generations can enjoy it as you did. Please contact the BLM at the number above if you are interested in getting involved with its Archaeological Site Steward program, which organizes volunteers to map, interpret, and monitor this and other archaeological sites throughout the region.

trip 15 Big Rocks Wilderness

Distance	Up to 3 miles, out-and-back or loop
Hiking Time	1 to 4 hours
Elevation	+/-300 feet (option A); +/-600 feet (option B)
Difficulty	Moderate to very difficult
Trail Use	Leashed dogs, good for kids, backpacking option, map and compass
Best Times	Cold to warm
Agency	BLM Ely at (775) 289-1800; www.nv.blm.gov/ely
Recommended Maps	*Caliente* 1:100,000; *Pahroc Spring* and *Hiko NE* 7.5-minute
GPS Waypoints	Corral: 37.648° N, 114.982° W
Vehicle	Passenger car OK (option A); high-clearance or 4WD vehicle recommended (option B)

HIGHLIGHTS Although relatively unknown now, the Big Rocks Wilderness and the larger North Pahroc Range promise to become more popular with hikers. You'll see why, as you explore the many crevices, crags, formations, and canyons in this rugged and picturesque landscape. Innumerable intimate spots of desert solitude await.

DIRECTIONS From Las Vegas, take I-15 north to exit 64, then take Highway 93 north toward Caliente and Ely. About 4 miles north of Ash Springs (about 100 miles from Las Vegas), veer right (easterly) to continue on 93 (the left/west fork leads to Highways 318 and 375). Roughly 13.5 miles east of the intersection of the turnoff to 318, and a half mile east of Pahroc Summit, turn left (north), across a cattle guard and onto an unsigned dirt road. Follow this road for 2 miles to a corral. Zero your odometer, then choose one of the options below:

 A. At a half mile, turn right (east) onto an unsigned jeep track, which leads about 0.2 mile to a large triangular boulder. Park here.

 B. Continue driving north past the corral on the jeep track that winds up the scenic canyon (it quickly becomes high-clearance, or 4WD, only). At 2.5 miles north of the corral, turn right (east) onto an unsigned, unpaved jeep track, which heads a rocky quarter mile to a parking area.

FACILITIES/TRAILHEAD The nearest facilities are in Ash Springs, 20 miles west on Highway 93.

Depending on where you parked, follow the directions below:

 A. From the car, follow the faint hiking trail east and up the hill about a quarter mile to the level bench with scattered boulders, and start exploring. Able and curious hikers might want to explore the very difficult terrain of jumbled boulders of the canyons heading up to the east. Retrace your steps to return.

 B. There are no real trails here, but as you will see, there is a lot of beautiful topography to explore. From the car, follow the gently sloping terrain as it weaves generally northeast between rock formations. After about a mile of walking up pinyon-pine- and juniper-covered slopes, you reach a

Rock climbers affectionately call this area "Mecca."

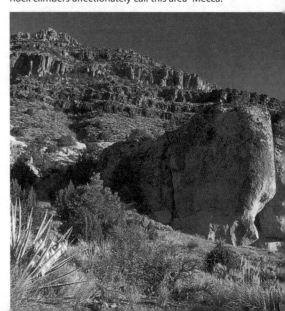

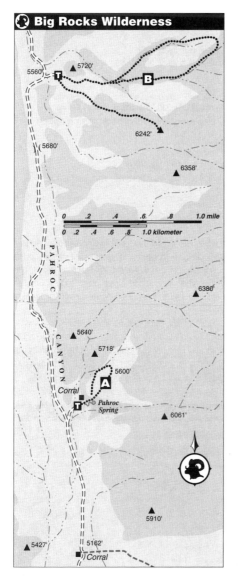

Big Rocks Wilderness

gentle canyon draining to the south. Follow this as it drains southwest, back toward the access road up the canyon, less than a half mile south of your car. There's a lot to explore, so let your curiosity be your guide. Those who don't wish to explore can simply sit and enjoy the ambiance of this majestic landscape.

In Southern Paiute, *pahroc* means "underground water." Rock climbers know this range as Mecca, and they travel from afar to test their bouldering skills on these volcanic boulders and cliffs.

On and under some of the boulders, you'll discover that people have been coming here for centuries. Under some boulders are spacious shelters where people hundreds of years ago escaped the sun. Look carefully, and you'll find both petroglyphs (etched pictures) and pictographs (drawn with pigments). Other petroglyphs are scattered among the jumbled rocks and cliffs higher on the slope and throughout the range. Please enjoy petroglyphs, pictographs, and other artifacts without touching them. They are fragile, sacred to modern Native Americans, and protected by numerous state and federal laws. Please enjoy them from a distance so others may enjoy them in the future.

Northern Region

trip 16 Mt. Irish

Distance	Less than 1 mile (petroglyphs), out-and-back 3 miles (Logan Summit), out-and-back
Hiking Time	1 to 4 hours
Elevation	+/-1100 feet (Mt. Irish)
Difficulty	Moderate (petroglyphs) to most difficult (Mt. Irish)
Trail Use	Leashed dogs, good for kids (petroglyphs only), backpacking option, map and compass
Best Times	Cool to hot
Agency	BLM Ely at (775) 289-1800; www.nv.blm.gov/ely
Recommended Maps	*Pahranagat Range* 1:100,000; *Mt. Irish, Mail Summit,* and *Mt. Irish SE* 7.5-minute
GPS Waypoints	Logan Pass: 37.626° N, 115.409° W
Vehicle	Passenger car OK

HIGHLIGHTS The Mt. Irish Petroglyph Site sits on 640 acres managed by the BLM to promote and protect the area's cultural heritage. There are no trails. Finding petroglyphs here is more like an Easter egg hunt among the rocks. Look carefully, and you will be rewarded. As you look across the slopes, many rock outcroppings promise further adventure to the intrepid. In November 2004, Congress designated much of the area south of the Logan Pass Road as the Mt. Irish Wilderness. Contact the Ely BLM for details.

DIRECTIONS From Las Vegas, take I-15 north for about 20 miles. Take exit 64 and follow Highway 93 north another 75 miles to Alamo, then another 7 miles to Ash Springs (last services). Continue north a few miles to the junction of Highways 93 and 318 and turn left (west) onto 318. At the intersection with Highway 375, keep right (north) to stay on 318, and continue another 2.5 miles (a half mile past

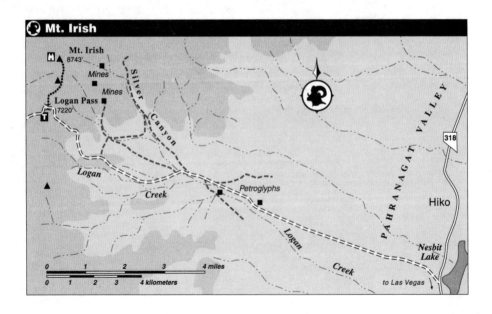

Ponderosa pine forests from high on Mt. Irish

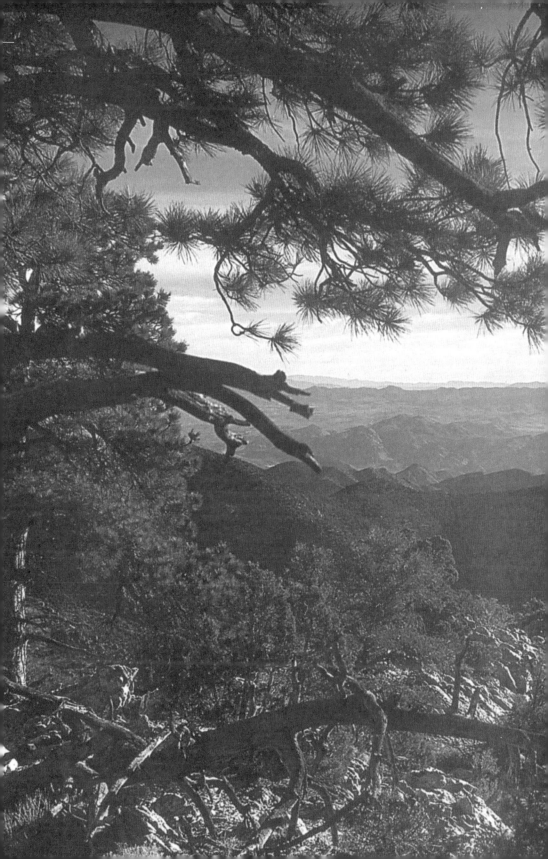

a post office sign on the right) to a gate and the unpaved, unsigned Logan Pass Road on the left (west). After closing the gate behind you, drive west on this bladed dirt road, climbing the slopes of Mt. Irish in front of you.

About 5 miles from 318, look for clusters of rock and signs asking you to protect our precious archaeological heritage (please do!). Park and explore the rocks for petroglyphs. About 7 miles from 318, look for a bladed road veering to the left (southwest). Follow this for a quarter mile to the parking area, and scout the rocks again for petroglyphs.

If you're itching for a difficult but rewarding hike, return to Logan Summit Road and continue following it uphill to the west for 5 miles to Logan Pass. There are no signs, but there are a few undeveloped parking and camping spots on the summit. Choose your favorite and park there.

FACILITIES/TRAILHEAD The nearest facilities are in Ash Springs, about 8 miles south of the bottom of Logan Summit Road, via Highways 318 and 93.

This difficult hike has no trail, signs, or trailhead. From the car, climb the steep slope northeast about 0.8 mile to the top of the white limestone cliff band for soaring views over the valley. Continue northeast along the bench to ponderosa pine trees and more sweeping views. Retrace your steps to return.

The many petroglyphs scattered across the eastern slopes of Mt. Irish, high above the Pahranagat Valley below, help to show how important the "valley of shining water" has been to native peoples for thousands of years. Contact between modern humans and ancient petroglyphs often leads to the destruction of petroglyphs—especially when there is easy vehicle access as there is here on Mt. Irish. I include this site in the book to publicize the importance of these artifacts and encourage people to protect them. Please join me and others who care about this region's cultural heritage to help protect these irreplaceable and fragile treasures. Leave them alone.

trip 17 # Kershaw-Ryan State Park

Distance	Up to 2 miles, loop or out-and-back
Hiking Time	1 to 2 hours
Elevation	+/-220 feet
Difficulty	Moderate
Trail Use	Leashed dogs, good for kids
Best Times	Cold to hot
Agency	Kershaw-Ryan State Park at (775) 726-3564; http://parks.nv.gov/kr.htm
Recommended Maps	*Caliente* 1:100,000
GPS Waypoints	Park entrance: 37.586° N, 114.531° W
Vehicle	Passenger car OK

HIGHLIGHTS This historic pioneer homestead provides shade and beauty, as well as a scenic trail that explores the natural wonders of this rugged canyon.

DIRECTIONS From Las Vegas, take I-15 north to exit 64, then follow Highway 93 north for 150 miles to Caliente. As the road enters town, turn right (south) onto Highway 317 in Rainbow Canyon and follow the signs for 2 miles to the park entrance on the left (east) side of the road.

FACILITIES/TRAILHEAD Restrooms, water, and a picnic area are available here. Other facilities are available in Caliente, 2 miles away.

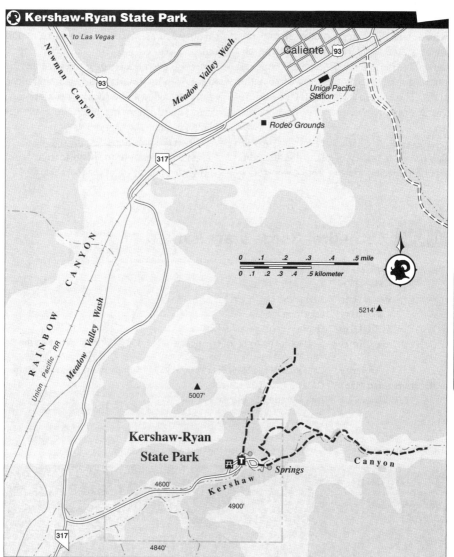

This former homestead in a beautiful canyon is a perfect place to enjoy a picnic or hike on three short trails. In November 2004, Congress passed legislation to expand the park. Check with park officials for details.

From the parking area, follow the Canyon Overlook Trail for 1 mile east up the canyon. The half-mile Horse Spring Trail is a spur off the Canyon Overlook Trail. Heading north from the parking area, the half-mile Rattle-snake Canyon Trail offers another way to explore this beautiful country.

In the 1870s, Sam and Hannah Kershaw homesteaded this picturesque canyon. James Ryan bought the property in 1904, then, in 1926, donated the "Kershaw Gardens" as a public park. The Civilian Conservation Corps developed picnic sites and a wading pond. In 1936, Kershaw-Ryan became a state park.

In 1984, two successive flash floods wiped out the campground, picnic area, water system, and restrooms, forcing closure of the park. In 1997, the park reopened, offering shady picnic areas and three nature trails. The rugged backcountry of the Clover Mountains behind the park is also accessible.

This relatively high, cool canyon provides habitat for a variety of plant life, including riparian species such as cottonwood, dog-wood, willow, and wild grape. Great Basin shrubs such as sagebrush, rabbitbrush, and Indian ricegrass grow on the drier slopes. There are even a few apple trees planted by Kershaw in the 1800s. This welcoming niche of life attracts wildlife such as deer, bobcats, raptors, and migrating birds. It's a perfect place to escape the heat of Las Vegas.

When you're done exploring, head to Caliente to check out the historic train depot and grab a bite to eat at the local cafe.

trip 18 Cathedral Gorge State Park

Distance	Up to 14 miles
Elevation	Up to +/-375 feet
Hiking Time	30 minutes to 5 hours
Difficulty	Easy to moderate
Trail Use	Leashed dogs, good for kids
Best Times	Cold to hot (early morning and late afternoon for dramatic light on the formations)
Agency	Cathedral Gorge State Park at (775) 728-4460; www.parks.nv.gov/cg.htm
Recommended Maps	*Caliente* 1:100,000-scale
GPS Waypoints	Park entrance: 37.803° N, 114.406° W
Vehicle	Passenger car OK

Ancient lake sediments have eroded into a wonderland of shape and shadow.

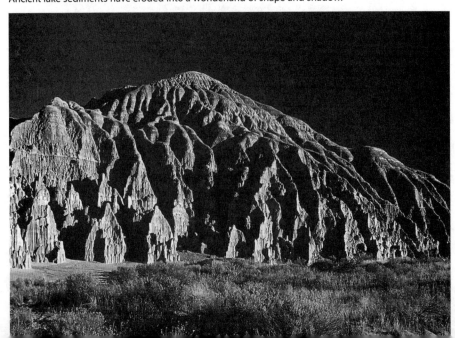

HIGHLIGHTS The strikingly beautiful eroded cliffs of this state park will thrill everyone in your family. Six hiking trails, ranging in distance from 0.15 mile to 7 miles, offer a variety of sights and distances to suit your abilities and desires.

DIRECTIONS From Las Vegas, take I-15 north to exit 64, then Highway 93 for about 170 miles. The park entrance is on the east side of the road, 1 mile north of the intersection of Highways 93 and 319, about 20 miles north of Caliente. A mile inside the park, the entrance road splits. The right (easterly) fork leads to the CCC picnic area. The left (westerly) fork leads to the campground and the group camp and picnic area.

FACILITIES/TRAILHEAD The park has numerous facilities, including a 22-site campground, a shaded picnic area, water, flush toilets, showers, and a dump station. Fees apply to enter the park and to camp.

Several trails offer long, short, easy, and difficult ways to explore this park. From the CCC picnic area, you can access the half-mile Caves Trail, the mile-long trail to Miller Overlook, and the east ends of the half-mile and the 4-mile loop trails. From the campground, you can access the west ends of the half-mile and 4-mile loop trails. All trails are signed and easy to follow. Cathedral Gorge is self-contained, so it is difficult to get lost.

A million years ago, a large, freshwater lake filled the valley, accumulating sediments and gravel on the lake bottom. As the climate warmed, the lake drained, and erosion began to eat through the sediments. Rain, melting snow, and other forms of erosion carved rivulets, cracks, and gullies in the siltstone and clay shale.

Once you have explored the park, head across Highway 93 from the park entrance to the old town site of Bullionville. In the 1870s, it had five stamp mills, an iron foundry, and 500 citizens, but times change.

When you're done, head 8 miles up the road to Pioche, a picturesque historic mining town. Make sure to check out the Million-Dollar Courthouse, shop the antique stores, and have a bite to eat at the Silver Spur. If you have a few more hours to explore, check out the historic train depot in Caliente, or stop

by Kershaw-Ryan State Park, just south of Caliente, on your way back to Vegas.

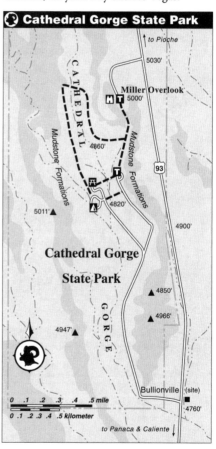

Cathedral Gorge State Park

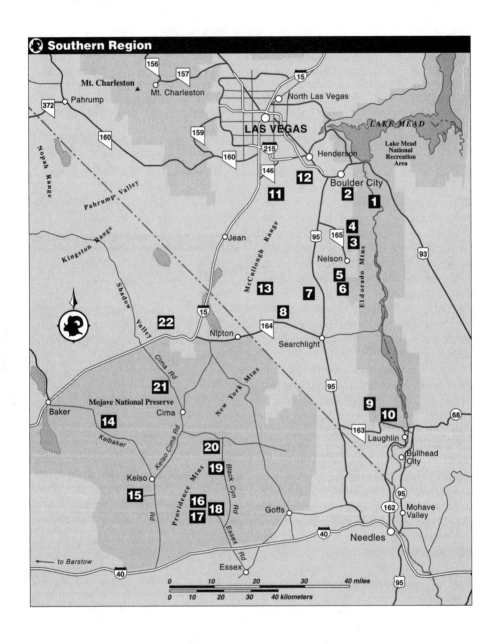

chapter 4

Southern Region

INCLUDING MOJAVE NATIONAL PRESERVE

South of Las Vegas wait myriad natural treasures, from the rugged canyons and colorful mining districts of the Eldorado Mountains along the Colorado River, to peaceful and beautiful Joshua tree forests, to the varied and beautiful landscapes of Mojave National Preserve, just over the border in California. Although millions of people pass these areas every year on Highway 95 and I-15, few leave the pavement to explore the solitude and serene beauty of the area's mountains and canyons.

One of the highlights of this region is the Mojave National Preserve, a great destination for a day or for a weekend.

Mojave National Preserve

Mojave National Preserve, a beautiful and relatively undeveloped park featuring stunning examples of Mojave geology and life, is only a two-hour drive south of Vegas on I-15, just over the border in California. Designated by the 1994 California Desert Protection Act, the 1.5-million-acre preserve sits at the crossroads of three deserts: the Sonoran, Mojave, and Great Basin. Although it may appear desolate, this region is home to more than 300 animal species, 200 species of birds, and more than 400 species of plants.

Elevations range from 1000 to 8000 feet, with geology that varies from lava flows to jumbled granite peaks. These combine with weather to create a wide diversity of habitats for plants and animals, as well as unique and beautiful places to explore, all within a short drive from each other. You're sure to find something to please everyone in your family (unless they crave outlet malls). All of the trips here are accessible with a short hike from your car. Half of the preserve is designated wilderness. Please drive only on designated routes.

Summer temperatures can soar well above 100°F, so the best times to explore are in the cooler months from October to March. Time your visit in spring, and you might catch the Mojave's incredible wildflower displays. Trips 14 through 22 visit some of the most remarkable natural wonders in Mojave Preserve.

Joshua Trees

Among the more beautiful and idiosyncratic residents of the Mojave Desert are Joshua trees, which are common on mid-elevation slopes (3000 to 6000 feet) around Las Vegas. You know you're in the Mojave Desert when you see them. Looking like something out of a Dr. Seuss book, Joshua trees grow in the Mojave and nowhere else on the planet, although relatives may be found as far away as Africa and New Zealand.

Mormon settlers named them after the Biblical prophet Joshua, because they seemed to be waving the settlers on to the promised land in California. Botanists call Joshuas *yucca brevifolia* and place them in the lily family along with grasses and orchids. They're not true trees, because they do not grow rings. But they do grow up to 40 feet tall and live as long as 1,000 years, and have earned at least honorary tree status in many minds.

Joshua trees prefer flat or gently sloping terrain between 2000 and 8000 feet, where it rains between 8 and 10 inches per year. The

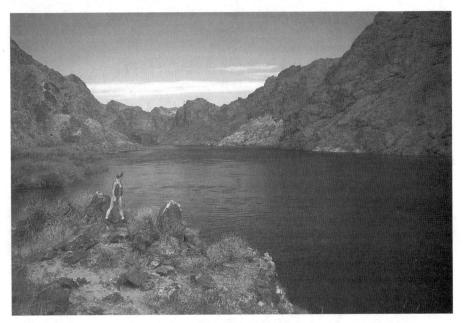

Rugged country, wildlife, and cool water wait along the Colorado River.

largest forest of Joshua trees in the world is in the Cima Dome region of Mojave National Preserve (Trip 21). Like most yuccas, Joshua trees can produce seeds only with the help of the female pronuba moth, which fertilizes the plant while she lays her eggs. Likewise, the moth can reproduce only in yucca, whose seeds become food for her larvae.

Joshua seeds lucky enough to receive just the right amount of rain in winter might sprout to grow a few inches in the first year. At this stage, their shoots are soft and prized by cattle, deer, and rodents; the trees most likely to survive are protected in this young age under cover of a bush. After that, they grow only about a half inch each year.

Pioneer explorer John Frémont called the Joshua "the most repulsive tree in the vegetable kingdom," but modern desert rats are more affectionate toward them. My friend Wally loves them because "they're such wonderful dancers."

trip 1 Kayak or Canoe Float on the Colorado River

Distance	12 miles, point-to-point
Hiking Time	Long day or overnight paddle (optional moderate to most difficult hikes)
Elevation	Negligible
Difficulty	Moderate paddling
Best Times	Cool to warm
Agency	Bureau of Reclamation at (702) 293-8204; www.usbr.gov/lc/hooverdam
Recommended Maps	*Hoover Dam* and *Ringbolt Rapids* 7.5-minute
GPS Waypoints	Hoover Dam Launch: 36.010° N, 114.742° W
	Willow Beach: 35.870° N, 114.660° W
Vehicle	Passenger car OK (and flotation device!)

HIGHLIGHTS Floating the Colorado River below Hoover Dam is a beautiful, unique, and relatively easy way to enjoy the rugged wilderness canyons and wildlife of the Lower Colorado River. Trips between Hoover Dam and Willow Beach, 12 miles downstream on the Arizona side, can be done in one day or overnight. Some people prefer multiple nights because there is so much to explore. The only rapids are Ringbolt Rapids, playful ripples that are dangerous only if you try to capsize in the middle of them.

DIRECTIONS Lower Colorado River floats begin with the outfitters in Boulder City. From Las Vegas, take Highway 93 south to Boulder City. Specific instructions depend upon which outfitter you choose; call them for more information (see numbers on page 219).

FACILITIES/TRAILHEAD The nearest facilities are in Boulder City and at Willow Beach.

The trip begins a stone's throw below Hoover Dam, which towers high above the water. Drifting with the current, you spend most of your time floating between the towering, jagged, and colorful walls of Black Canyon, an experience that is in itself worth the trip. Along the way, the hot springs, side canyons, petroglyphs, remnants of historic developments, and abundant wildlife make the trip truly memorable.

As the major water source of the region, the river attracts many animals and birds. On a recent trip down the river, I watched a rare peregrine falcon sitting a few feet away on the cliffs, a rarer phainopepla songbird feeding the bushes, bighorn sheep eating a

Even beginning boaters will enjoy floating the lower Colorado River.

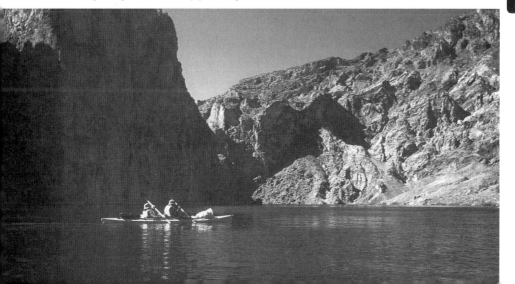

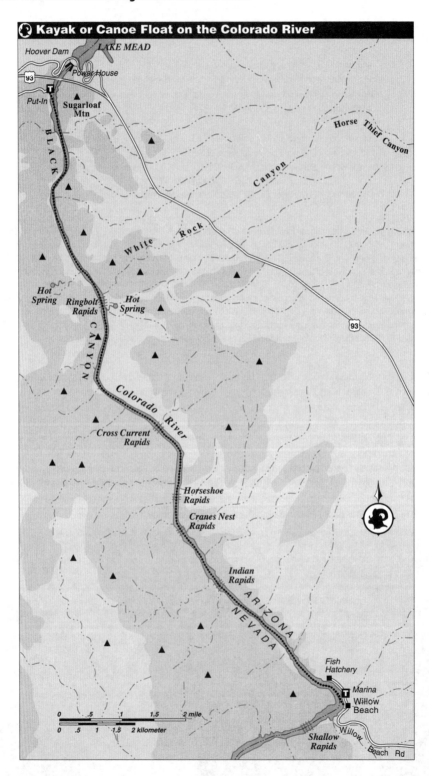

Kayak or Canoe Float on the Colorado River

barrel cactus near the water, and a scorpion under my sleeping pad in the morning—not bad for 24 hours.

Beaches along the way provide opportunities to camp and enjoy beautiful deep canyon nights. Please follow Leave No Trace principles in the canyon, watch for rattlers under rocks and bushes, and shake the scorpions out of your shoes in the morning.

When you reach Willow Beach, your outfitter or scheduled car will pick you up and drive you back to your car in Boulder City.

You must arrange your own launch permit (there is a fee) by calling the Bureau of Reclamation at the number above. Because launch permits are limited, it's important either to arrange them well in advance, or to be flexible about your desired trip dates.

Another option is to reserve a trip with an outfitter (roughly $150 per day per person). The logistical difficulties of arranging your own trip aren't always worth the cheaper price. The price is worth this adventure. For more information from two outfitters in nearby Boulder City, call Boulder City Outfitters (www.bouldercityoutfitters.com) at (800) 748-3702 or Evolution Expeditions (www.evolutionexpeditions.com) at (702) 259-5292.

trip 2 Boy Scout Canyon

Distance	3.4 miles, out-and-back
Hiking Time	3 to 4 hours
Elevation	-/+400 feet
Difficulty	Moderate
Trail Use	Leashed dogs, good for kids, backpacking option
Best Times	Cold to warm
Agency	Lake Mead National Recreation Area at (702) 293-8907; www.nps.gov/lame
Recommended Maps	*Boulder City* 1:100,000; *Boulder City* and *Ringbolt Rapids* 7.5-minute
GPS Waypoints	Trailhead: 35.973° N, 114.769° W
Vehicle	High-clearance or 4WD vehicle recommended

HIGHLIGHTS The Black Canyon along the Colorado River south of Hoover Dam is a jagged, rugged wonderland of volcanic rock. Boy Scout Canyon takes you on a tour of some of the most beautiful geology the region has to offer. As you hike down the wash, rocks of every color rise in hoodoos, spires, fins, and steep canyon walls around you. In places, water has polished the rock into smooth, sensual shapes. Boy Scout Canyon is part of the 17,000-acre Black Canyon Wilderness Area, designated by Congress in 2002. This is *not* the place to be in a flash flood. If thunderstorms are active anywhere in the sky, hike somewhere else.

DIRECTIONS From Las Vegas, take Highway 93 south about 30 minutes to Boulder City. At the intersection with Buchanan, turn right (south) onto Buchanan. After 0.3 mile, turn left (east) onto Adams. Then drive roughly a mile to the cemetery on your right (south). Just past the cemetery, turn right (southeast) onto Utah. Drive past the end of the pavement and under the power lines to the entrance of the transfer station. Just before the transfer station, turn right (southeast) onto an unsigned and maintained dirt road (zero your odometer here), following the signs to the Boulder Rifle and Pistol Club, passing to the right (south) of the pistol range. At 1.3 miles, turn left (northeast) onto an unsigned, unmaintained, and easy-to-miss dirt road, which heads downhill along the eastern fence of the pistol range. Continue on this road as it enters the wash and heads north. At 3.7 miles, you come to a crossroads, where the wash you've been driving crosses the east-west Boy Scout Wash. Park here.

FACILITIES/TRAILHEAD There is no official trailhead. The nearest facilities are in Boulder City.

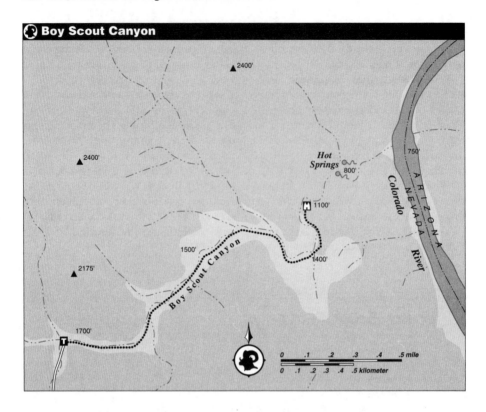

From the car, follow Boy Scout Wash downhill to the east for about 1.7 miles. There is no trail, but there might as well be, as the canyon walls on both sides will keep you from getting lost. A few drops and boulders require scrambling, but most of the walk is along the level bottom of the wash.

You'll know you're near the end when you're standing deep in the narrow canyon, at the top of a 15-foot waterfall (usually dry). Careful scrambling down to the right (south) will get you to the next level, a small, sandy bench above a 10-foot waterfall. (This section is very difficult—*don't attempt unless you're a confident rock scrambler.*) Easier scrambling to the left (north) of the 10-foot waterfall leads to the next small, sandy bench.

Beyond this, you'll need wings, as the final waterfall drops perhaps 200 vertical feet to the bottom of Boy Scout Wash below. If you can't make the final two drops to this point, don't feel disappointed. You can see the view from above the top waterfall.

Standing at the top of the waterfall at the end of the hike, you're level with mountain peaks across the valley, looking over a soaring drop toward the river below. There are hot springs down near the river, but they are best accessed from the river itself.

Retrace your steps to return.

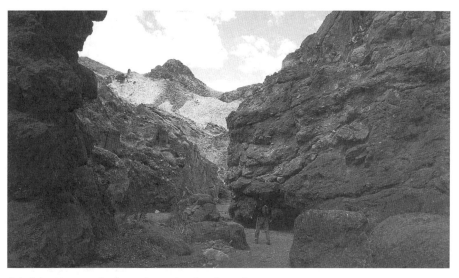

Colorful geology awaits those who explore Boy Scout Canyon.

trip 3 Bridge Spring Arch

Distance	1.5 miles or more, out-and-back
Hiking Time	2 to 4 hours
Elevation	–/+175 feet
Difficulty	Moderate
Trail Use	Leashed dogs, good for kids, backpacking option, map and compass
Best Times	Cold to warm
Agency	BLM Las Vegas at (702) 515-5000; www.nv.blm.gov/vegas
Recommended Maps	*Boulder City* 1:100,000; *Nelson* 7.5-minute
GPS Waypoints	Arch: 35.726° N, 114.818° W
Vehicle	Passenger car OK

HIGHLIGHTS Named after the fabled Incan lost city of gold, the Eldorado Mountains have been some of the richest mining areas in Southern Nevada. Spanish adventurers were said to have discovered gold in these hills in the 1700s. The region's heyday lasted from 1864 to 1930. During this period, the Techatticup Mine, the richest of the region, produced more than $46 million in gold, silver, copper, lead, and zinc. Although you probably won't find gold along the way, the geologic and floral riches of the area will become clear as the colors of the soil change under your feet, reflecting the rich oranges, browns, pinks, and blacks in the jumbled peaks rising overhead. Growing around you are at least six species of cacti, as well as creosote and blackbrush.

Avoid this trip during storms, as flash floods can be a problem. In October 1974, a flash flood up to 30 feet deep roared down the wash, destroying 31 homes and the marina resort at the landing on the Colorado River.

DIRECTIONS From Las Vegas, take U.S. 95 south toward Searchlight. About 19 miles south of the Boulder City interchange (about 40 miles from Vegas), turn left (east) onto Highway 165 toward Nelson. At the top of Rifle Pass, about 9.2 miles from U.S. 95, park at the unsigned, unpaved turnout on the left (east) side of the road.

For an enjoyable side trip (or a road trip worthy in its own right), continue past the trailhead on Highway 165 down Techatticup Wash for 8 miles to Nelson's Landing.

FACILITIES/TRAILHEAD The nearest facilities are in Techatticup or Boulder City.

From the southern end of the parking area, follow a faint hiking trail leading east over a couple of low, sharp ridges. The trail soon enters a gentle wash that drains to the east.

As you enter the canyon, lava and ash tuff rock formations born in volcanic eruptions 10 million to 15 million years ago rise around you. Follow the wash as it heads for the southernmost (right) notch in the ridge to your east. Arrive at the arch in about three-quarters of a mile. In their notebooks on the region, the BLM calls this Gregory Arch, but locals know it as Bridge Spring. And although the oaks and other plants growing in the wash are proof that water does flow, you'll see little more than a trickle at best in the wash upstream.

From the arch, retrace your steps to return. Agile explorers can pursue either of the following two difficult options:

A. Have someone else hike back to the car and meet you at Techatticup (5 miles south then east on 165), where this wash drains. Continue following the wash downstream and east for about 3 miles. You'll enjoy scrambling over the boulders down this narrow canyon to the store at Techatticup. Give yourself an extra hour to complete the hike.

Those of you with the car will enjoy the forest of teddy bear cholla cacti (don't let the name fool you and try to hug one!) west of Techatticup, and the many antiques and other oddities around the store while you wait. Tours of the old mine and kayak rentals are available here. Call (702) 291-0026 or visit www.eldoradocanyonminetours.com.

B. If you're an addict for altitude and views, go to the downhill side of the arch,

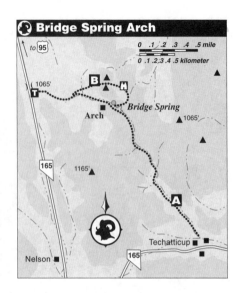

then scramble up the left (north) canyon wall to the top of the unnamed peak directly north of the arch. There's no trail, but the scramble rewards you with a beautiful view into Oak Creek Canyon the Eldorado Wilderness Area to the east. Hike to the small saddle immediately north of the peak, then head west back to the car. The car-to-car distance for this hike is less than 3 miles.

On your drive down Techatticup Wash to Nelson's Landing, about 3 miles east of Nelson, you'll pass greenish, rounded rock outcrops, some of the oldest rocks in Southern Nevada, dating back almost 2 *billion* years.

In the lower reaches of Techatticup Wash, you'll also see several towers of stone called hoodoos, formed when a hard cap protects the softer rock below from being eroded, leaving a tower. Interestingly, geologists can tell from hoodoos that earthquakes have not been active in the area (otherwise the hoodoos would have fallen over).

Creosote

The creosote bush is one of the most successful and abundant residents of the Mojave Desert. Native peoples throughout the Mojave found many uses for it: They kept cool under shade structures built with its branches, and they burned it to keep warm. The branches also became arrows and spears. The lac, a sticky secretion left by insects on its branches, was used to hold spear points in place and plug holes in pottery. They used the bush in tea, ointments, and baths to treat everything from measles, sores, cramps, burns, to stomachaches. Scientists are currently researching creosote for properties that might help treat, and possibly cure, cancer.

Creosote's survival success involves several strategies: Its roots spread both deep and wide to increase its chances of finding water. Its leaves are tiny, which prevents moisture loss from the intense sun and heat. It lacks spines, but it wards off animals with a foul smell and taste. And while it produces seeds, they're not necessary for reproduction. The plant can sprout new growth from a central root cluster that is often centuries old. In fact, botanists have found creosote clones more than 10,000 years old.

Include time to explore the colorful history of Techatticup.

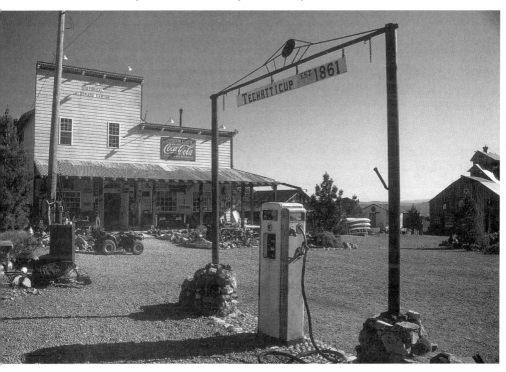

trip 4 Oak Creek Canyon

Distance	4 miles or more, out-and-back
Hiking Time	3 to 5 hours
Elevation	+/-400 feet
Difficulty	Moderate
Trail Use	Leashed dogs, backpacking option, map, and compass
Best Times	Cold to warm
Agency	BLM Las Vegas at (702) 515-5000; www.nv.blm.gov/vegas
Recommended Maps	*Boulder City* 1:100,000; *Nelson* and *Boulder City SE* 7.5-minute
GPS Waypoints	Top of canyon: 35.731° N, 114.819° W
Vehicle	Passenger car OK

HIGHLIGHTS This hike takes you through colorful geology to a rugged, scenic, and isolated canyon in the Eldorado Mountains. Oak Creek Canyon is in the 32,000-acre Eldorado Wilderness Area, designated by Congress in 2002. It is only one of many jagged, winding, and multicolored canyons along the lower Colorado River. The rocks are composed of lavas and tuff born in volcanic eruptions 10 million to 15 million years ago, when a great volcano stood here.

DIRECTIONS From Las Vegas, take U.S. 95 south toward Searchlight. About 9 miles south of the Boulder City interchange (about 40 miles from Vegas), turn left (east) onto Highway 165 toward Nelson. At the top of Rifle Pass, about 9.2 miles from 95, park at the unsigned, unpaved turnout on the left (east) side of the road.

For an enjoyable side trip (or a road trip worthy on its own right), continue past the trailhead on Highway 165 down Techatticup Wash for 8 miles to Nelson's Landing.

FACILITIES/TRAILHEAD The nearest facilities are in Techatticup or Boulder City.

From the southern end of the parking area, follow a faint hiking trail east over a couple of low, sharp ridges. Before dropping into the wash, look at the ridge to the east. To the east-southeast, you can see the notch that leads to Bridge Spring Arch. A half mile north of that notch, to your northeast, lies another lesser notch, the head of Oak Creek Canyon.

You can hike directly to Oak Creek Canyon from the car, but you will find yourself hiking like a roller coaster, up and down east across the drainages that trend north-south.

An easier route is to hike from the trailhead down (east) along Bridge Spring Wash for a half mile or so, then cut left (north) up one of the minor drainages toward Oak Creek Canyon, another half mile north. As you get closer, look for a faint game trail on the slope to the right (south) of the drainage leading to the canyon notch.

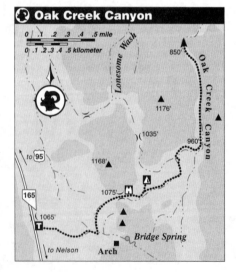

Once you reach the notch, you can see Oak Creek Canyon draining northeast, bordered by a jagged ridge to the east. Oak Creek eventually joins Lonesome Wash and meanders east for 10 miles to the Colorado River.

But you don't have to go that far. There are nice places to stop, eat lunch, and enjoy the view of the canyon within a couple miles of the car. Some minor ridgetops and saddles about a half mile down the canyon would make perfect campsites for backpackers wanting accessible solitude and desert beauty.

If you're out for a dayhike, detour to Bridge Spring Arch on your way to or from Oak Creek Canyon (Trip 3).

Retrace your steps to return.

trip 5 Keyhole Canyon

Distance	0.25 mile, out-and-back
Hiking Time	1 to 2 hours
Elevation	+/-120 feet
Difficulty	Moderate
Trail Use	Leashed dogs, good for kids
Best Times	Cold to warm
Agency	BLM Las Vegas at (702) 515-5000; www.nv.blm.gov/vegas
Recommended Maps	*Boulder City* 1:100,000; *Nelson* 7.5-minute
GPS Waypoints	Canyon: 35.715° N, 114.925° W
Vehicle	High-clearance or 4WD vehicle recommended

HIGHLIGHTS This canyon mouth guards mysterious petroglyphs. If you set a leisurely pace, you can hike to the end of the canyon and back to the car in 15 minutes. But it takes much longer to explore and ponder the hundreds of petroglyphs and occasional pictographs adorning the rocks and walls around the mouth of this canyon. Some are believed to be more than 1,000 years old.

DIRECTIONS From Las Vegas, take U.S. 95 south toward Searchlight. About 16 miles south of the Boulder City interchange (about 45 miles from Las Vegas), turn left (east) onto an unsigned dirt road. After 2.1 miles, turn right (south) onto the road under the second power line. Follow the power line road for 1.8 miles, then turn left (east) for a half mile to the parking area by the canyon mouth.

FACILITIES/TRAILHEAD The nearest facilities are in Boulder City.

From your car, pass through the fence, and you're there. Petroglyphs are everywhere around on the rocks. The canyon continues east for a few hundred yards until it ends at a 30-foot waterfall. Retrace your steps to return.

The sheer number of petroglyphs here show that this was a special place for people long ago. If water was present consistently then, it helps explain why rock art is so prevalent here; petroglyphs are commonly found near springs and water in the Mojave Desert. Like the petroglyphs at Grapevine Canyon to the south, those at Keyhole Canyon may have had ritual significance. Unfortunately, we might never know for sure what these designs mean. It's difficult even to determine who made them, because many peoples passed through this area over the centuries.

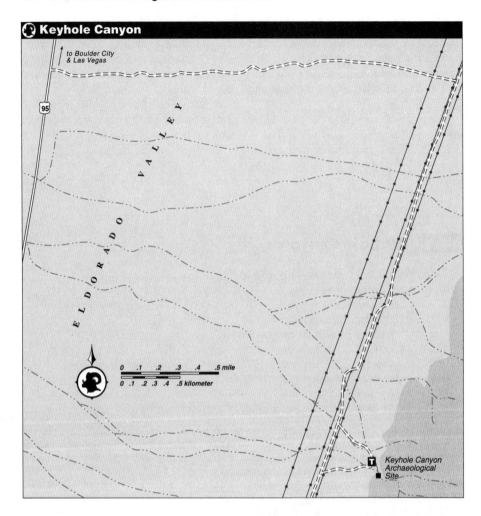

Keyhole Canyon

to Boulder City
& Las Vegas

95

ELDORADO VALLEY

0 .1 .2 .3 .4 .5 mile

0 .1 .2 .3 .4 .5 kilometer

Keyhole Canyon
Archaeological
Site

Keyhole Canyon is a good example of how vulnerable and irreplaceable petroglyphs are. As you gaze around Keyhole Canyon, you can easily see the vandalism that unthinking people have inflicted on these cultural treasures. Graffiti, bullet holes, and burn scars cover many of the petroglyphs.

I included this site to publicize the importance of these artifacts and encourage people to protect them. You can help

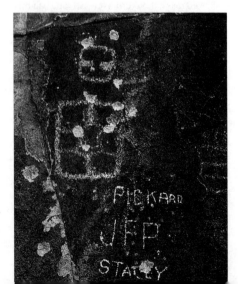

Careless vandals destroyed these
irreplaceable petroglyphs.
Please respect artifacts.

protect these petroglyphs by not touching them, and urging others to respect them. If you want to donate time or money to their protection, call the BLM at the number above for more about local volunteer Archaeological Site Steward programs. If we work together, we can help keep these petroglyphs intact for our children and future generations.

trip 6 Ireteba Peaks

Distance	Up to 3 miles, out-and-back
Hiking Time	1 to 4 hours
Elevation	+/-175 feet (option A); +/-800 feet (option B)
Difficulty	Moderate to most difficult
Trail Use	Leashed dogs, good for kids, backpacking, map and compass
Best Times	Cool to warm
Agency	BLM Las Vegas at (702) 515-5000; www.nv.blm.gov/vegas
Recommended Maps	*Boulder City* 1:100,000; *Nelson* 7.5-minute
GPS Waypoints	Trailhead: 35.649° N, 114.843° W
	North Ireteba Peak: 35.636° N, 114.837° W
Vehicle	High-clearance or 4WD vehicle recommended

HIGHLIGHTS Named for a Mojave Indian guide for the Joseph Ives expedition to this region in 1858, Ireteba Peaks are high, rocky, rugged, and very beautiful. They're also perfect for explorers of every ability and interest level. Even if you don't plan to hike, the granite rock outcrops make for great undeveloped camping. Kids will enjoy scrambling on the rocks, and everyone will savor a picnic in these surroundings. Those who wish can pursue the views to the southeast or the challenge of climbing the peaks to the south. In 2002, Congress designated the 32,745-acre Ireteba Peaks Wilderness to protect the eastern slope of these mountains to the river and provide undisturbed habitat of the lower washes for the endangered desert tortoise and other wildlife.

DIRECTIONS From Las Vegas, take Highway 95 south toward Searchlight. About 21 miles south of the Highway 95 and Boulder Highway interchange on 95 (a little less than 50 miles from Vegas), look for a power line running east-west across 95. Turn left (east) onto the unsigned but maintained power line road and follow it for 7 miles, at which point large granite outcrops begin appearing south of the power line road. Turn right (south) onto an unsigned dirt road that heads south for less than a mile until it ends amid large granite boulders. Park at the southern end of the road. On maps, this trailhead area is 1.5 miles southeast of Knob Hill.

About a quarter mile after turning south from the power line road, another unsigned dirt track veers to the left (southeast) for less than a mile to the old Belmont Phoenix Mine

Southern Region

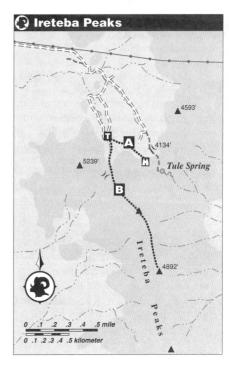

Ireteba Peaks

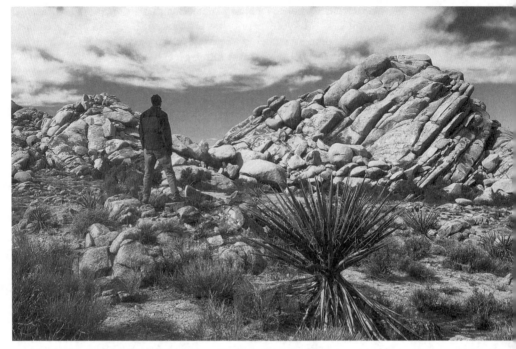

Jumbled granite outcrops are perfect for scrambling and hide-and-seek.

above Tule Spring (which may be dry). This short detour/alternative offers a good view and a decent, undeveloped campsite.

FACILITIES/TRAILHEAD The nearest facilities are in Las Vegas. Sites for car camping here are undeveloped but wonderful.

From your car, hike south to the end of the farthest vehicle route and the Ireteba Peaks Wilderness boundary, which should be marked with a small fiberglass BLM sign, then choose one of two options:

A. For a moderate hike, head southeast cross-country for a quarter mile to the crest of the ridge for a dramatic view of rugged mountains and canyons dropping toward the Colorado River.

B. Fit, ambitious hikers may want to climb 1 mile due south, to the top of the northernmost peak. This very difficult option leads you to scramble over steep boulders up 800 vertical feet to the summit.

As you're hiking, notice how the western slopes of these mountains are relatively gentle, while the eastern slopes drop away precipitously into rugged canyons draining toward the Colorado River. Although beautiful, these rugged canyons and lower washes are best left to the bighorn sheep, eagles, and the fittest, most experienced desert explorers.

Even if you hike very little here, you will love the beauty and ambiance of the jumbled granite boulders. Kids will love to scramble around on the rocks.

To return, retrace your steps to the car.

[trip 7] Highland Range

Distance	Up to 6 miles, out-and-back or loop
Hiking Time	1 to 4 hours
Elevation	+/-600 feet
Difficulty	Moderate to difficult
Trail Use	Leashed dogs, backpacking option, map and compass
Best Times	Cool to warm
Agency	BLM Las Vegas at (702) 515-5000; www.nv.blm.gov/vegas
Recommended Maps	*Boulder City* 1:100,000; *Nelson SW* 7.5-minute
GPS Waypoints	A nice spot for lunch and a view: 35.663° N, 115.030° W
Vehicle	High-clearance or 4WD vehicle recommended

HIGHLIGHTS Only a few miles off Highway 95 and surrounded by power lines, the Highland Range doesn't seem on paper like an obvious destination for a hike. One look at its profile rising jagged against the sky, however, will change your mind. Its multicolored volcanic rocks, scattered yucca, cholla and barrel cacti, and solitude among the rock formations make it one of my favorite spots in Southern Nevada.

DIRECTIONS From Las Vegas, take Highway 95 south toward Searchlight. About 21 miles south of the Highway 95 and Boulder Highway interchange on Highway 95, look for a power line running east-west across 95. Turn right (west) onto the power line road and follow it for 2.9 miles to a junction. Turn right (north) and drive counterclockwise around the ridge for another mile to a gate and a route heading south into the valley. Follow this vehicle route for about a half mile and park.

FACILITIES/TRAILHEAD The nearest facilities are in Las Vegas.

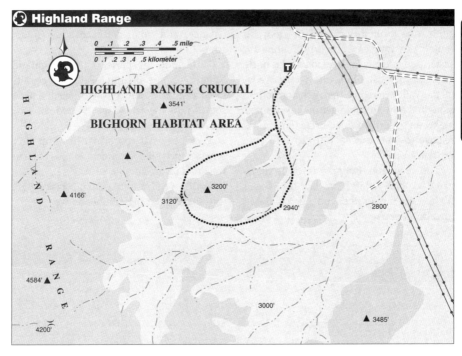

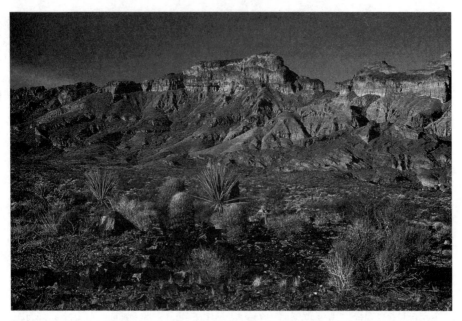

Rocks on the Highland Range erupted from the earth between 5 million and 20 million years ago.

There are no trails in the Highland Range, so your own curiosity and desire will guide your exploration. For an enjoyable route from your car, hike south along the eastern edge of the valley, then hike north back to your car along the western edge of the valley, circling the rock formations along the way. To avoid getting disoriented, make an effort to memorize landmarks relative to your car, so you can find your way back easily.

The Highland Range has been designated crucial habitat for bighorn sheep. It's also home to the endangered desert tortoise. If you're lucky to encounter either of these animals, please respect them from a distance. Their survival rests on a fragile balance, and your presence adds undue stress to their lives.

Unfortunately, parts of the Highland Range are not pristine. People have littered campsites and pushed illegal vehicle routes into the landscape. Please *don't* be like them.

Pack out what you bring, clean up after others, and hike as much as possible in washes and on durable surfaces. If you see litter or a vehicle trespassing, please report it to the BLM at the number above.

trip 8 Wee Thump Joshua Tree Wilderness

Distance	Varies, out-and-back
Hiking Time	1 to 4 hours
Elevation	+/-200 feet
Difficulty	Easy
Trail Use	Leashed dogs, good for kids, backpacking option, map and compass
Best Times	Cold to warm
Agency	BLM Las Vegas at (702) 515-5000; www.nv.blm.gov/vegas
Recommended Maps	*Mesquite Lake* 1:100,000; *Highland Spring* and *McCullough Mountain* 7.5-minute
GPS Waypoints	Corral at turnoff: 35.507° N, 115.056° W
	Dead center: 35.536° N, 115.095° W
Vehicle	Passenger car OK

HIGHLIGHTS If you want a peaceful and beautiful corner of desert solitude, Wee Thump is the place. *Wee thump* is Yuman for "ancient ones," a term that aptly describes the trees in this forest, easily one of the more impressive Joshua tree stands in the state. Congress designated this 6,000-acre wilderness area in 2002. In addition to its status as one of the smallest wilderness areas in Nevada, it is also one of the flattest (most designated wilderness areas in the U.S. are mountainous). The other flat wilderness area is the Black Rock Desert Wilderness Area in northwestern Nevada, but that's a topic for another book.

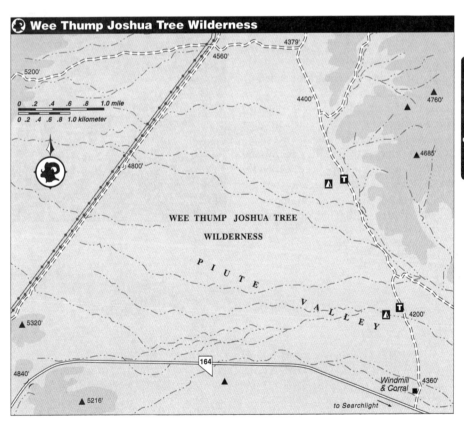

DIRECTIONS From Las Vegas, head south on U.S. 95 about an hour to Searchlight. Turn right (west) onto Highway 164 for 8.4 miles. At the corral and windmill on the right (north) side of the road, turn right (north) onto an unsigned and unmaintained dirt road. Drive through the corral and windmill complex, then continue north on a small, unsigned dirt road. For the next 5 miles or so, everything on your left is the Wee Thump Joshua Tree Wilderness Area. Several places along the way, you'll find unsigned pullouts on the right that you can use to park or as undeveloped campsites.

FACILITIES/TRAILHEAD The nearest facilities are in Searchlight.

There are no trails here, but the open country makes for easy hiking. The beauty is relaxing and sublime. In addition to the Joshuas, you'll find a diverse lowland desert community of plants and animals, including yucca, bunchgrasses, shrubs, and cacti, as well as great horned owls, hawks, coyotes, kit foxes, lizards, bullsnakes, and rattlers. If you're lucky and observant, you might see a gilded flicker, known to occur in Nevada only here. The area is also designated critical habitat for desert tortoise.

Because Wee Thump is surrounded by roads, it would be difficult to get lost here. But don't underestimate it. After a few minutes on this flat landscape with no landmarks, every tree looks like every other, and it's easy to get disoriented. A short morning hike my first time camping here ended up taking much longer as I searched for my car.

To stay found, from your car, choose a compass direction and hike in a straight line for a set time (30 minutes, for example). Stop, have lunch, say hi to the trees around you, then hike in the opposite direction for the same amount of time back to your car. Add security to this system by memorizing the features on the horizon in front of and behind you as you're hiking away from your car.

Motorized vehicles are prohibited in the wilderness, so please restrict your driving to boundary roads and established camp spots. Call the BLM at the number above to report vehicle trespassers.

The pronuba moth helps Joshua trees produce seeds.

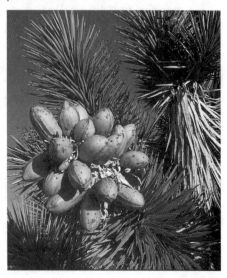

trip 9 Spirit Mountain

Distance	1 mile or 3 miles, out-and-back
Hiking Time	1 to 2 hours or 4 to 6 hours
Elevation	+/-2400 feet
Difficulty	Difficult
Trail Use	Backpacking option, map and compass
Best Times	Cool to warm
Agency	BLM Las Vegas at (702) 515-5000; www.nv.blm.gov/vegas, or Lake Mead National Recreation Area at (702) 293-8990; www.nps.gov/lame
Recommended Maps	*Davis Dam* 1:100,000; *Spirit Mountain* 7.5-minute
GPS Waypoints	Saddle above trailhead: 35.263° N, 114.733° W Beginning of climbers' route: 35.268° N, 114.728° W
Vehicle	Passenger car OK

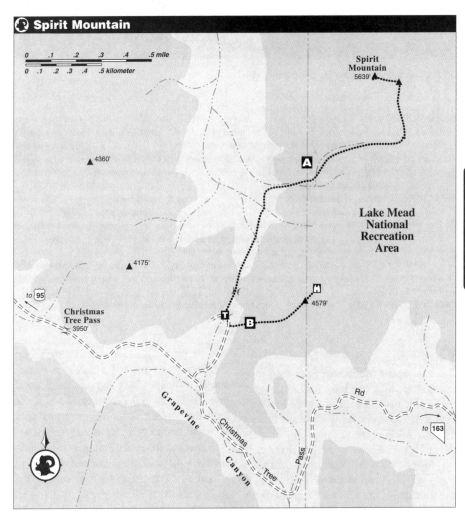

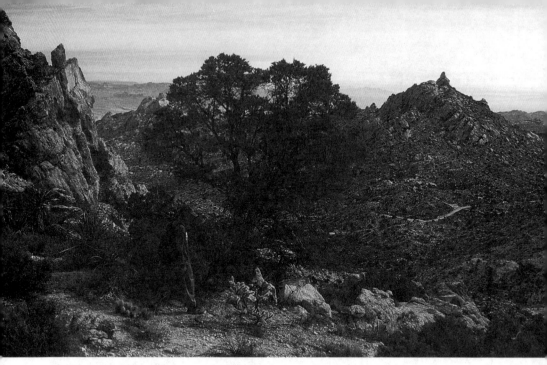

Great views await on Spirit Mountain's south ridge.

HIGHLIGHTS On this trip, you can explore and climb a sacred, geologic wonder. Spirit Mountain is sacred to the Native Americans of this region. It is also on the National Registry of Historic Places. In deference to its many scenic, natural, and cultural values, Congress designated 33,500 acres of this area as the Spirit Mountain Wilderness in 2002. Combined with the Nellis Wash Wilderness to the north and the Bridge Canyon Wilderness to the south, the Spirit Wilderness complex protects more than 58,000 acres of natural landscape.

DIRECTIONS From Las Vegas, head south on U.S. 95 for an hour to Searchlight. Continue south on 95 past Searchlight for another 14 miles. Then turn left (east) onto an unpaved road toward Christmas Tree Pass, 7.3 miles from the highway. A half mile east of the pass, an unsigned dirt road will head north a half mile or so to a series of unofficial campsites and parking areas. Park at one of these or on the main road. There are no signs, nor is there an official trailhead.

When you're done exploring Spirit Mountain, continue east on the Christmas Tree Pass Road for about 5 miles to Grapevine Canyon, then another 2 miles to Highway 163, where a right turn leads back to Las Vegas.

FACILITIES/TRAILHEAD The nearest facilities are in Searchlight, 20 miles north on 95.

From the car, you have two route options:

A. Spirit Mountain: For this 6-mile (round-trip) hike, head north from the spur road (which is a half mile east of Christmas Tree Pass) up and over the low saddle and into the north-south drainage immediately west of Spirit Mountain. Follow that drainage downhill for a half mile, then turn right (east) up the main drainage that leads to the shoulder of the summit ridge, a quarter mile southwest of the peak. This route will challenge your route-finding skills, but keen eyes should be able to find and follow a faint climbers' route marked with cairns (small stacks of rocks). The going gets steep, but if you choose carefully, you should be able to gain the summit ridge without using your hands too much or facing extreme exposure.

Experienced desert mountaineers might look at a map and think the best route from Christmas Tree Pass Road would be the main ridge that climbs north to the summit. That approach, however, is lined with impassable outcrops and ravines.

The summit itself will reward you with inspiring views of the Colorado River snaking north to south and the rugged country of Arizona across the river. Backpackers will find excellent campsites and views on the summit ridge.

Retrace your steps to return.

B. Spirit's south ridge: This 1-mile hike heads toward the main ridge east of the parking area. Too difficult as a route to the summit, this ridge offers great exploring and views. Along the way, you enjoy the many varied plants and rock outcroppings. Once you have enjoyed the views from the ridge, retrace your steps to return.

As you explore either option, watch for rattlesnakes, who are easily startled by poorly placed hands and feet.

Geologically, Spirit Mountain (called Newberry Mountain by some) is a pluton, the fossilized magma chamber left after the rest of an ancient volcano has eroded away. See how its granite rock contrasts with the darker volcanic hills to the north. Scientific explanations aside, the rock formations are awe-inspiring.

Ecologically, Spirit Mountain sits at the crossroads of the Mojave, Sonoran, and Great Basin deserts. Creosote, mesquite, catclaw, yucca, several species of cacti, desert scrub oak, and one of the northernmost populations of smoke tree dominate lower slopes, while pinyon pine and juniper trees find hold in the higher elevations.

Culturally, Spirit Mountain is Avikwame, which figures prominently in the creation of the Colorado- and the Yuman-speaking tribes of the region. The mountain remains sacred to the Native Americans of this region. Please treat it with the same respect you would give your own place of worship.

trip 10 Bridge Canyon Wilderness: Grapevine Canyon

Distance	1 mile, out-and-back
Hiking Time	1 to 3 hours
Elevation	+/-200 feet
Difficulty	Moderate
Trail Use	Good for kids
Best Times	Cool to warm
Agency	Lake Mead National Recreation Area at (702) 293-8990; www.nps.gov/lame
Recommended Maps	*Davis Dam* 1:100,000; *Bridge Canyon* 7.5-minute
GPS Waypoints	Canyon entrance: 35.227° N, 114.685° W
Vehicle	Passenger car OK

HIGHLIGHTS Lying at the foot of Spirit Mountain, which is sacred to native tribes in the region, it's not surprising that Grapevine Canyon offers one of the best petroglyph sites in all of Nevada, with some carvings that may be more than 1,000 years old. In 2002, Congress designated nearly 8,000 acres around Grapevine Canyon as the Bridge Canyon Wilderness Area (named for the next canyon south). Please treat this area with the same respect you would expect in your own place of worship.

DIRECTIONS From Las Vegas, take Highway 95 south for about 90 minutes to State Highway 163, which goes to Laughlin and Davis Dam. Turn left (east) on to 163. After about 12 miles, turn left (north) onto an unpaved road, following the sign to Grapevine Canyon and Christmas Tree Pass. Another 2 miles farther, turn left (west) to the Grapevine Canyon parking area.

Round out your day by driving back to Vegas via Christmas Tree Pass and Spirit Mountain. Instead of turning right (south) from the parking area back to 163, turn left (north) and follow the very scenic road north then west along the south slopes of Spirit Mountain over Christmas Tree Pass and back to 95 south of Searchlight, where a right turn leads back to Las Vegas.

FACILITIES/TRAILHEAD The nearest facilities are in Laughlin or Searchlight.

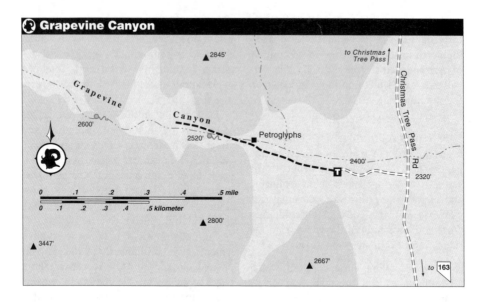

Hike up the wash about a quarter mile to the entrance of the canyon, where the petroglyphs begin. A half mile upstream from the petroglyphs, water springs forth, sustaining wild grapevines and other plants.

Many of the geometric designs at Grapevine Canyon are unlike most petroglyphs elsewhere in Nevada (they look similar to motifs found in Central American artifacts). Because this site is close to the Colorado River, a common cultural travel and trading corridor, it's possible that many peoples and cultures influenced the rock art expressions here. The thickness of many of the lines in the geometric petroglyphs here suggest many people over many years chipped at the same lines to achieve ritual success.

Today, no one knows for sure what these symbols signify, but there are a few leading theories. Petroglyphs often occur near water, illustrating the social and possibly religious significance of life-giving water in the desert. In wet years, a seeping spring up-canyon brings life to this otherwise arid landscape.

Many researchers believe rock art has ritual significance. Sacred Avikwame (Spirit Mountain's Yuman name) towers over this site to the north. Perhaps tribal shamans carved their own dream-state visions into the rock, or used rock art to help initiate others.

Although this is a sacred place rich in Native American history, when Europeans arrived, they disregarded native people's names for this place, renaming it after their own fashion. In 1925, journalist B. M. Bower wrote a letter to then-Nevada Governor James Scrugham, explaining how the area got its name: "I believe the canyon is known locally as Rattlesnake Canyon, but Captain LeBaron asks that the name be made Grapevine Canyon, since there are thousands of grapevines and not so many rattlesnakes, and the local name might have disagreeable effects upon tourists."

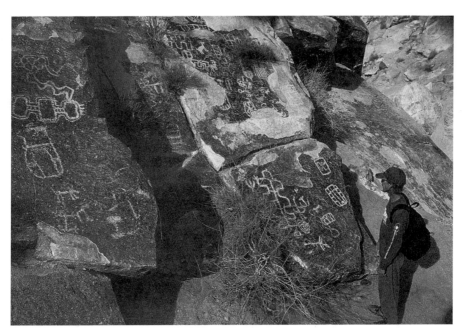

People climbing on the boulders have crushed and destroyed some petroglyphs. Please admire them respectfully.

trip 11 Sloan Canyon National Conservation Area

Distance	4 miles, out-and-back
Hiking Time	1 to 4 hours
Elevation	+/-500 feet
Difficulty	Moderate (difficult in spots)
Trail Use	Leashed dogs, good for kids, backpacking option, map and compass
Best Times	Cold to warm
Agency	Las Vegas BLM at (702) 515-5000; www.blm.gov/nv/st/en/fo/lvfo/ blm_programs/blm_special_areas/sloan_canyon_nca.html
Recommended Maps	*Mesquite Lake* 1:100,000; *Sloan* 7.5-minute
GPS Waypoints	Canyon entrance: 35.227° N, 114.685° W
Vehicle	High-clearance or 4WD vehicle recommended

HIGHLIGHTS One of the best places to see actual written records from people long ago is at the Sloan Canyon National Conservation Area. Scattered along the relatively gentle canyons surrounded by low hills are roughly 1,700 cataloged petroglyphs carved by people from several tribes, including Ancestral Puebloans, Patayan, and Southern Paiute. In 2002, Congress designated the 48,000-acre Sloan Canyon National Conservation Area to protect the petroglyphs in this canyon from sprawl. The BLM plans a trail system and a visitor center in nearby Henderson, with volunteer docents available to offer tours and protect the site from vandals. Contact the BLM at the number above to find out developments.

Southern Region

◯ Sloan Canyon National Conservation Area

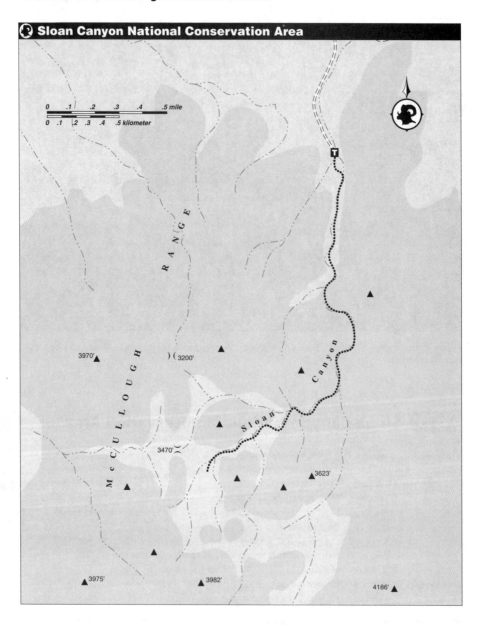

DIRECTIONS Take I-15 south from Las Vegas. Take exit 25 at Sloan and cross under the freeway to its east side, then turn left (north, back toward Vegas) along the frontage road. Less than a half mile north of the exit, turn right (east) onto the unpaved power line road (you'll have to find your way around a gravel pit and electrical substation, but aim for the power line with big brown towers, and you'll get there). Follow the power line several miles. Just past (east of) Tower #84, turn right (south) and follow the track up the gentle slope and into a wash. Follow the wash a few miles to the trailhead in the low hills ahead.

FACILITIES The nearest facilities are in Las Vegas.

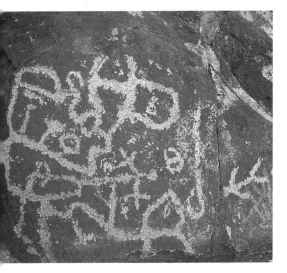

It's fun to ponder the mystery of messages carved thousands of years ago.

From your car, follow the wash south. After the third climb up a dry waterfall (about 1 mile from the first dry waterfall), start looking around you. For the next mile, more than 300 petroglyph panels pepper the rocks on both sides of the wash.

It seems improbable that people could live in the harsh environment of Southern Nevada without air conditioning, but archaeological evidence shows that people have lived in the area for thousands of years. Most of the designs are recognizable etchings of bighorns, lizards, and anthropomorphs (figures resembling man). There are also geometric motifs, such as spirals, meandering lines, grids, and other designs that are harder to interpret. Some are more than 900 years old, but there's also a petroglyph of a cowboy (or a Spaniard?) riding a horse, which clearly dates to post-contact with European cultures.

After you have explored the area and looked at the ancient petroglyphs, retrace your steps back down the wash to return.

Desert Varnish: Is It Really Alive?

While hiking, you might notice rocks covered with a dark reddish or black ceramic-like sheen. This is called desert varnish, and it is created by bacteria living on the rocks. Often only one-hundredth of a millimeter thick, it protects the bacteria from the water loss, intense heat, and solar radiation of the desert.

Ancient people often chose desert varnish as the canvas on which to carve their petroglyphs. Because it can take up to 10,000 years for the varnish to develop a healthy sheen, scientists can estimate the age of petroglyphs and other artifacts by the maturity of the varnish on them.

Despite desert varnish's toughness, oils from our skin can break it down quickly. For this reason, please look but don't touch.

trip 12 Black Mountain

Distance	5 miles, out-and-back
Hiking Time	6 hours
Elevation	+/-2100 feet
Difficulty	Difficult
Trail Use	Backpacking option, map and compass
Best Times	Cool to warm
Agency	Las Vegas BLM at (702) 515-5000; www.nv.blm.gov/vegas
Recommended Maps	*Mesquite Lake* 1:100,000; *Sloan* 7.5-minute
GPS Waypoints	Catchment basin: 35.939° N, 115.077° W
	Peak: 35.931° N, 115.043° W
Vehicle	Passenger car OK

HIGHLIGHTS The view from Black Mountain (5092 feet), the highest point in the North McCullough Range, is sure to clear up anyone's claustrophobia. On clear days, you can see Spirit Mountain to the south; deep into Arizona to the east; Mt. Potosi, Red Rock Canyon, and the Spring Mountains to the west; and the Sheep Range, the Muddy Mountains, and the Mormon Mountains to the north—not to mention all of Las Vegas filling the valley at your feet. In 2002, Congress designated the Sloan Canyon National Conservation Area and North McCullough Wilderness Area, which forever protect the North McCullough Mountains from the encroachment of sprawl.

DIRECTIONS From Interstate 215 south, exit on Eastern Blvd. and drive south (away from the Strip) as it climbs into the Anthem housing development. A half mile south of Green Valley Parkway, veer left onto Anthem Parkway. Another 2 miles farther, turn left (east) onto Somersworth Ave. One mile farther, turn left (east) onto Shadow Canyon Dr. A small trailhead parking area sits on the right about

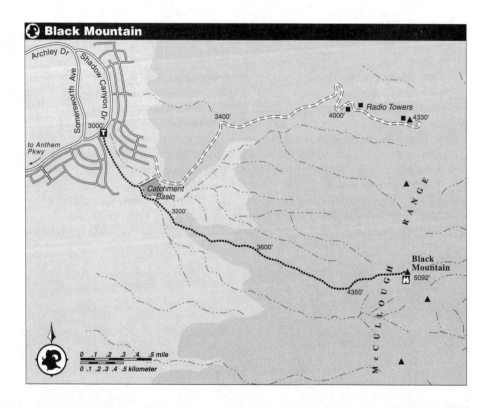

a quarter mile down the hill. From the parking area, follow the paved path up the drainage a half mile to a flood-catchment reservoir.

FACILITIES/TRAILHEAD The nearest facilities are in Henderson.

Once at the catchment reservoir, do not turn left to cross the dam. Instead, continue along the right (west) edge, circling the basin counterclockwise to the back (south) end of the basin. There you'll find the signed

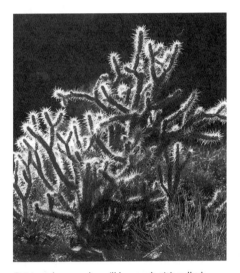

Get too close, and you'll learn why it's called jumping cholla.

BLACK MOUNTAIN TRAIL that climbs a prominent ridge leading east to the summit, which stands tall above you. The trail is mostly easy to follow, but your attention is necessary from time to time to stay on it.

Of all the mountain ranges surrounding the Las Vegas Valley, the North McCullough Range is one of the few with volcanic origins. The scattered black pumice and basalt hint at the eruptions that spewed this rock between 5 million and 20 million years ago. The mature desert varnish on them makes them shine like someone left them in the oven way too long.

The North McCulloughs are typical basin-and-range mountains. Although it may seem steep as you climb the west slope of this mountain, once on top, you'll see you've chosen the easier route to the top. A few steps east of the summit, the mountains fall away into a near-vertical jumble of rock and cliff 2500 vertical feet to the Eldorado Valley below.

Breathe deeply the wide-open vistas, then retrace your steps to return.

Southern Region

Nevada's Mountains: Dip-Slip-Sliding Away

The North McCullough Range is typical Nevada in its shape. Like the great Sierra Nevada, most mountain ranges in the Nevada are long and narrow, running north to south; most also have one side that is gentler and one that is more rugged—the result of plate tectonics: As the Pacific and North American continental plates bump and grind against each other to the west, the Pacific Plate is actually pulling Nevada apart as fast as a couple inches each year. This expansion zone (or rift) is called the Great Basin.

Over the last 20 to 30 million years, the distance between Reno and Salt Lake City has doubled. As the Great Basin expands, smaller plates across Nevada pull apart. Like giant seesaws, these plates teeter up on one side, down on the other, as their edges pull apart from each other. This process has given rise to Nevada's 300-plus mountain ranges, with steep, rugged escarpments meeting low, flatter valley floors at dip-slip faults. The east slope of the North McCulloughs is a perfect example. An estimated 50 million years from now, Nevada's valleys will have dropped enough to turn these mountain slopes into bluffs overlooking an inland sea.

trip 13 McCullough Mountain

Distance	3 miles, out-and-back
Hiking Time	4 hours
Elevation	+/-1720 feet
Difficulty	Difficult
Trail Use	Leashed dogs, backpacking option, map and compass
Best Times	Cool to warm
Agency	Las Vegas BLM at (702) 515-5000; www.nv.blm.gov/vegas
Recommended Maps	*Mesquite Lake* 1:100,000; *McCullough Pass* and *McCullough Mountain* 7.5-minute
GPS Waypoints	Railroad Springs Road: 35.591° N, 115.246° W Cabin: 35.604° N, 115.202° W
Vehicle	High-clearance or 4WD vehicle recommended

HIGHLIGHTS The condition of the access route and the old cattlemen's line shack tell you not many people make it to this corner of Nevada. You'll truly enjoy the solitude as you climb past the spring through pinyon and juniper forest to the summit. McCullough Mountain is part of the 44,245-acre South McCullough Wilderness, designated by Congress in 2002. Note that part of the access road to this hike might be closed (south of the corral and gate) for off-road vehicle races. Call the BLM (number above) to make sure the road is open.

DIRECTIONS From Las Vegas, drive south on I-15 for 30 miles and take exit 1 for Primm. Turn left (east) onto Underpass Road. On the east side of the casinos, before the road heads over an overpass and toward the power plant, veer left through the yellow arrow signs and follow the unsigned and unpaved road east to the railroad. Turn left (north) onto the unmaintained dirt track that parallels the train tracks. After three-quarters of a mile, cross the tracks and follow the power line road northeast about 7.5 miles up the twisty road over Beer Bottle Pass.

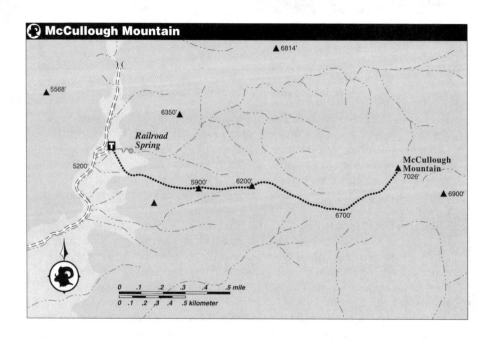

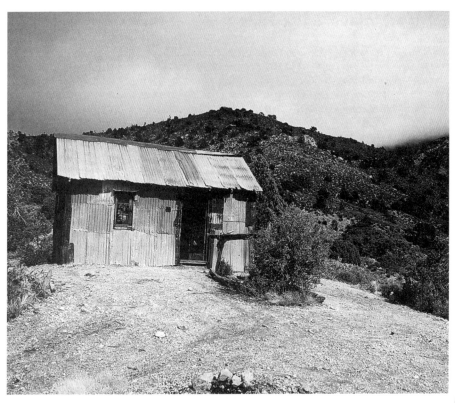

An old rancher's line shack marks the trailhead for McCullough Mountain.

A half mile east of the summit, turn right (south) onto a smaller power line road. At 2 miles, turn left (east) through a corral complex, then right (south) into the wash and to a gate. After closing the gate behind you, follow this deep, sandy route south between the Lucy Grey Mountains on your right (west) and the South McCullough Mountains to your left (east). About 5.5 miles south of the gate, turn left (east) into a small wash a few hundred yards before the well and corral complex (you might have to drive to the well and corral, then turn around and look for the wash). The wash, which doesn't seem like a road at all, takes you to a corrugated tin shack marked Railroad Spring, roughly 11 miles from the main power line road. Park here.

FACILITIES/TRAILHEAD The nearest facilities are in Primm. There is no trail, but the route up the ridge is direct. From the shack, cross the drainage south, then turn left (southeast) to follow the ridgeline east to the peak. Your map and compass should help keep you on route, as many of the ridges look similar.

At the summit, you'll enjoy the contrast between this rugged solitude and the corridors of asphalt and electricity along Highway 95 to the east and I-15 to the west. More beautiful, however, are the views of the McCullough ridgeline stretching to the north and south, the ruggedly beautiful Highland Range to the east, Spirit Mountain to the southeast, and Mt. Charleston far to the northwest.

Retrace your steps to return.

trip 14 Mojave: Lava Beds

Distance	Option A: 1 mile, out-and-back; Option B: 2 miles, out-and-back; Option C: 3 miles, out-and-back or loop
Hiking Time	Options A and B: 1 hour each; Option C: 2 to 3 hours
Elevation	Option A: +/-100 feet; Option B: +/-150 feet; Option C: +/-500 feet
Difficulty	Option A: Difficult; Option B: Moderate; Option C: Difficult
Trail Use	Good for kids, dogs on leash, map and compass
Best Times	Cool to warm
Agency	Mojave National Preserve at (760) 733-4040; www.nps.gov/moja
Recommended Maps	*Trails Illustrated Mojave National Preserve (#256)*
GPS Waypoints	Overlook at option B: 35°180' N, 115°823' W
Vehicle	High-clearance or 4WD vehicle recommended

HIGHLIGHTS These three trips offer three ways to encounter the lava, from intimate (option A) to sweeping (option C). Between 5 million and 20 million years ago, intense tectonic forces were literally ripping the Earth apart in the Mojave region. Here, the crust was thin enough to allow volcanoes to form and molten lava to spew to the surface. Dozens of cinder cones dot the landscape in this area, and each was the site of eruptions and lava flows. Volcanic activity here lasted from 7.6 million years ago to only 10,000 years ago, around the end of the most recent ice age. The black basalt in these flows is so young, geologically speaking, that it seems as though it's still flowing. These flows were designated as wilderness when the 1994 California Desert Protection Act created the preserve.

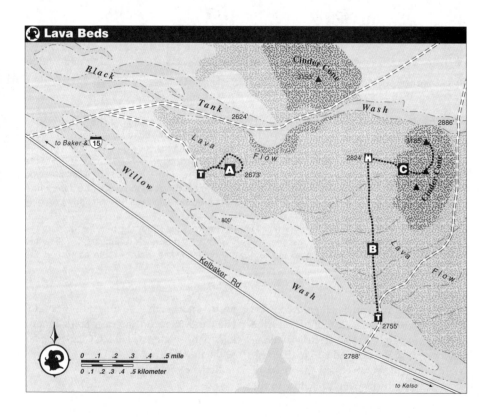

DIRECTIONS From Las Vegas, drive south on I-15 for 90 miles to Baker. After loading up on water, food, fuel, and emergency supplies, turn left (east) on Kelbaker Road into Mojave National Preserve. See below for specific directions to the three options listed here.

FACILITIES/TRAILHEAD Mojave National Preserve is largely undeveloped. Before you enter the preserve, stop by the information center at 72157 Baker Blvd. in Baker for a free map, advice, and travel tips from the rangers there. Food and gas are available only on the edges of the preserve, along I-15 to the north and I-40 to the south. Water is available only at the Cima post office, in the north-central portion of the preserve, via Kelbaker and Kelso-Cima roads from Lava Beds; at the Mitchell Caverns in Providence Mountains State Recreation Area, in the southern portion of the preserve, via Kelbaker Road, I-40, and Essex Road; and at the Hole-in-the-Wall Campground, in the center of the preserve, via Kelbaker, Kelso-Cima, and Black Canyon roads. Make sure you stock up on all necessities before you enter the preserve.

Year-round campgrounds are located at Hole-in-the-Wall, Mid Hills, and at Providence Mountains State Recreation Area. Sites are first-come, first-served. Primitive camping is also allowed at established sites off paved roads. Collecting firewood of any kind is forbidden in the preserve. Bring your own wood, and build fires only in established fire rings.

Choose from the following three routes for this trip:

A. At 15 miles southeast of Baker on Kelbaker Road, turn left (northeast) onto an unsigned, unpaved road. After a half mile, turn right (east-southeast) onto an unsigned, unpaved jeep track. After 200 yards, choose the left (northernmost) fork

The lava beds still seem to be oozing across the landscape.

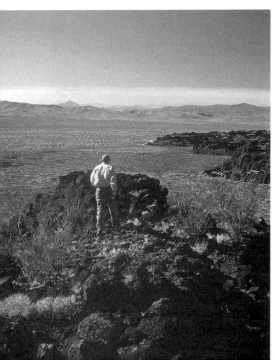

and follow it for less than a half mile to an appealing parking place at the edge of the lava flow. There is no trailhead, and there are no signs. From your car, hike north onto the lava flow as far as you'd like, then back out again. This trip is an intimate exploration of the rugged nature of this lava, which may be only 10,000 years old (infantile in geologic terms). Take care walking on its rough, sharp surface.

B. At 17 miles east of Baker on Kelbaker Road, turn left (north) on an unsigned, unpaved dirt track, which heads north. After 0.2 mile, stop in an unsigned parking spot. From the car, hike north cross-country (not along the road) for about a mile to a small outcrop on the shoulder of the cinder cone to the east of the flow. This moderate hike is the easiest of the three options, and leads through creosote and cactus to an inspiring view over the lava field. Retrace your steps to return.

C. From the overlook in option B, scramble to the top of the nearest cinder cone to the east, then walk to its northern point for a panoramic view of the cinder cones of the region. This side trip adds a difficult mile to your trip. Retrace your steps to return.

Southern Region

trip 15 Mojave: Kelso Dunes

Distance	3 miles, out-and-back
Hiking Time	1 to 2 hours
Elevation	+/-430 feet
Difficulty	Moderate
Trail Use	Leashed dogs, good for kids
Best Times	Cold to warm
Agency	Mojave National Preserve at (760) 733-4040; www.nps.gov/moja
Recommended Maps	*Trails Illustrated Mojave National Preserve* (#256)
GPS Waypoints	South dune summit: 34.898° N, 115.732° W
Vehicle	Passenger car OK

HIGHLIGHTS Kelso Dunes are a testament to how wet this area was 10,000 years ago, at the end of the last ice age. Silver and Soda lakes filled the valley bottoms to the west, and the climate was cooler and wetter. Now those lakes have dried (except for right after big storms), and their sediments have blown and settled here over thousands of years to create these dunes. Tiny rose quartz grains contribute to the dunes, giving them a soft, rosy glow. When the sand is dry and the humidity low, climb to the top and take a nice leap onto a steep face, then listen. The millions of grains of sand rubbing together produce a low hum, making Kelso Dunes one of the many singing sand dunes in the world.

DIRECTIONS From Las Vegas, drive south on I-15 for 90 miles to Baker, then turn left (east) on Kelbaker Road into Mojave National Preserve. Drive 41 miles, past Kelso Depot to the signed turnoff to Kelso Dunes. Turn right (west) and drive 4 miles to the trailhead.

FACILITIES/TRAILHEAD Mojave National Preserve is largely undeveloped. Before you enter the preserve, stop by the information center at 72157 Baker Blvd. in Baker for a free map, advice, and travel tips from the rangers there. Food and gas are available only on the edges of the preserve, along I-15 to the north and I-40 to the south.

Water is available only at the Cima post office, in the north-central portion of the preserve, via Kelbaker and Kelso-Cima roads from Lava Beds; from the Mitchell Caverns in Providence Mountains State Recreation Area, in the southern portion of the preserve, via Kelbaker Road, I-40, and Essex Road; and from the Hole-in-the-Wall Campground, in the center of the preserve, via Kelbaker, Kelso-Cima, and Black Canyon roads. Make sure you stock up on all necessities before you enter the preserve.

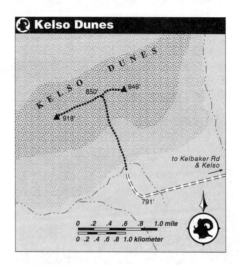

Year-round campgrounds are located at Hole-in-the-Wall, Mid Hills, and at Providence Mountains State Recreation Area. Sites are first-come, first-served. Primitive camping is also allowed at established sites off paved roads. Collecting firewood of any kind is forbidden in the preserve. Bring your own wood, and build fires only in established fire rings.

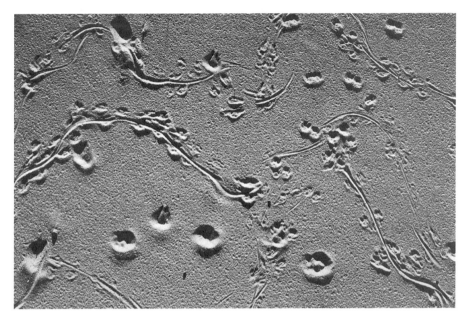

The sand tells stories of wildlife activity at night.

From the trailhead, hike north across the sand, following the trail to the low saddle between the two sandy summits. Once at the saddle, turn left (west) and climb a half mile to the summit.

As you hike, look for animal tracks or animals themselves. At sunrise or sunset, the dunes are a good place to see wildlife—perhaps a kit fox heading back to her den after a night of hunting, or a kangaroo rat grabbing a few last leafy bites before returning underground for the day.

If you're not lucky enough to see wildlife firsthand, you can see how active these creatures are by reading the stories they leave written on the sand. Step off the trail to find a section humans haven't walked on, and if it isn't too windy, you'll see numerous tracks crisscrossing each other, telling tales of the many different journeys taken over these sands.

Kelso Dunes are home to more than 100 species of plants and animals, including the Kelso Dune Jerusalem cricket, which is found here and nowhere else on Earth. Although sand recovers easily after being walked on, the plants that live there don't. Please *don't* walk on the plants.

Either retrace your steps to return, or slide and tumble right down the face.

trip 16 Providence Mountains State Recreation Area: Mitchell Caverns

Distance	1.5 miles, out-and-back
Hiking Time	1½ hours
Elevation	+/-200 feet
Difficulty	Moderate
Trail Use	Good for kids
Best Times	October to May
Agency	Providence Mountains State Recreation Area at (760) 928-2586; www.parks.ca.gov/default.asp?page_id=615
Recommended Maps	None needed
GPS Waypoint	Mitchell Caverns' visitor center: 34.943° N, 115.513° W
Vehicle	Passenger car OK

HIGHLIGHTS Nature's creative forces are sure to please any visitor to Mitchell Caverns. Stalactites, stalagmites, columns, shields, helictites, coral pipes, and cave popcorn might make you think you're in some strange science fiction movie, or on a distant world altogether. Visitors on hot days will wish the tour were longer, as the caverns' constant 65°F is a refreshing respite from the scorching heat outside.

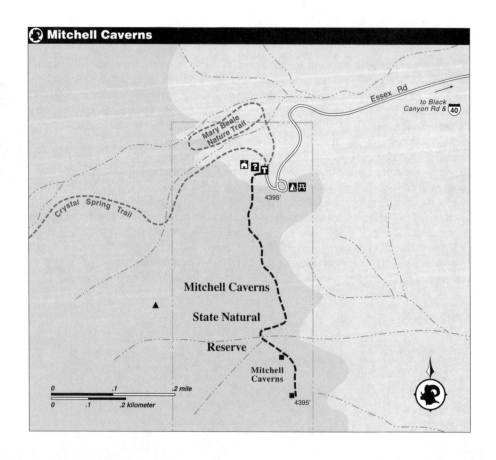

DIRECTIONS From Las Vegas, drive south on Highway 95 for 90 minutes to I-40 at the far southern tip of the state. Turn right (west) onto I-40 and drive for 25 miles. Turn right (north) onto Essex Road, following the signs to Providence Mountains State Recreation Area and Mitchell Caverns. Ten miles north of I-40 on Essex, veer left (westerly) at the fork (the right fork is Black Canyon Road to Hole-in-the-Wall) and continue another 6 miles up to the caverns, trailhead, and campground.

FACILITIES/TRAILHEAD Rangers, phones, restrooms, a campground (with six sites), water, and a gift shop are available here.

To see the caverns, you have to take a tour. Call the number above for details. The tour explores El Pakiva and Tocopa caves. A third cavern, Winding Stair Cave, is dangerous, closed to the public, and often used by search and rescue crews to practice cave rescue techniques.

Named after Ida and Jack Mitchell, who began offering cave tours in 1934, the caverns became a state park in 1956 and remain the only limestone caves in the California park system. When Mojave National Preserve arrived in 1994, this state recreation area became totally surrounded by the preserve.

Limestone caves like Mitchell Caverns are formed when rain picks up carbon dioxide as it falls through the air and soaks into the soil. This process creates a weak carbonic acid that dissolves limestone, slowly eating away tunnels and chambers. Once caverns have formed, calcium carbonate precipitates out of slow-moving water in the cave, creating the wonderland of cave formations (speleotherms) you see in Mitchell Caverns.

trip 17 Mary Beale Nature Trail

Distance	0.5 mile, loop
Hiking Time	30 minutes
Elevation	+/-100 feet
Difficulty	Easy to moderate
Trail Use	Good for kids
Best Times	October to May
Agency	Providence Mountains State Recreation Area at (760) 928-2586; www.parks.ca.gov/default.asp?page_id=615
Recommended Maps	None needed
GPS Waypoint	Trailhead: 34.943° N, 115.513° W
Vehicle	Passenger car OK
Note	Cougars have been seen in this area, and while attacks are rare, please follow the precautions on page 6.

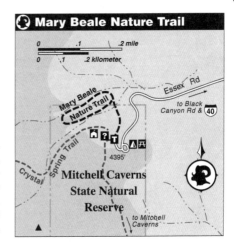

Mary Beale Nature Trail

HIGHLIGHTS Named after a naturalist who dedicated her life to studying the plants of the Mojave, this trail is an informative and only mildly challenging route through the rocky slopes and washes next to the campground. A self-guided brochure will tell you about various plants and animals along the way. A

Southern Region

bench set perfectly about halfway along the trail is a perfect place to enjoy the beauty and solitude of the Mojave Desert.

DIRECTIONS From Las Vegas, drive south on Highway 95 for 90 minutes to I-40 at the far southern tip of the state. Turn right (west) onto I-40 and drive for 25 miles. Turn right (north) onto Essex Road, following the signs to Providence Mountains State Recreation Area and Mitchell Caverns. Ten miles north of I-40 on Essex, veer left (westerly) at the fork (the right fork is Black Canyon Road to Hole-in-the-Wall) and continue another 6 miles up to the caverns, trailhead, and campground.

FACILITIES/TRAILHEAD Rangers, phones, restrooms, a campground (with six sites), water, and a gift shop are available here.

From the top of the parking area, turn right (north) and walk past the visitor center and residences to the trailhead. The Mary Beale Nature Trail is down the hill from the Crystal Spring Trail, and takes a meandering loop across the slopes before it heads back to the trailhead.

Subtle beauty appears whenever you look closely in the desert.

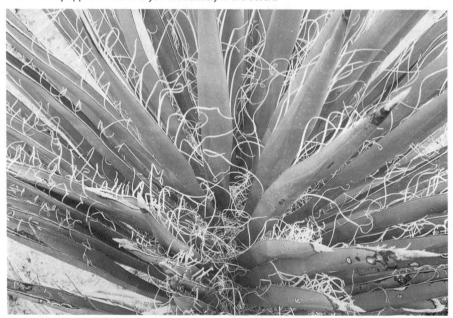

trip 18 Crystal Spring Trail

Distance	2 miles, out-and-back
Hiking Time	1 to 3 hours
Elevation	+/-520 feet
Difficulty	Moderate
Trail Use	Good for kids
Best Times	October to May
Agency	Providence Mountains State Recreation Area at (760) 928-2586; www.parks.ca.gov/default.asp?page_id=615
Recommended Maps	None needed
GPS Waypoint	Crystal Spring: 34.942° N, 115.522° W
Vehicle	Passenger car OK
Note	Cougars have been seen in this area, and while attacks are rare, please follow the precautions on page 6.

HIGHLIGHTS Here you can explore the rugged geology and diverse plants on high Mojave Desert mountain slopes.

DIRECTIONS From Las Vegas, drive south on Highway 95 for 90 minutes to I-40 at the far southern tip of the state. Turn right (west) onto I-40 and drive for 25 miles. Turn right (north) onto Essex Road, following the signs to Providence Mountains State Recreation Area and Mitchell Caverns. Ten miles north of I-40 on Essex, veer left (westerly) at the fork (the right fork is Black Canyon Road to Hole-in-the-Wall) and continue another 6 miles up to the caverns, trailhead, and campground.

FACILITIES/TRAILHEAD Rangers, phones, restrooms, a campground (with six sites), water, and a gift shop are available here.

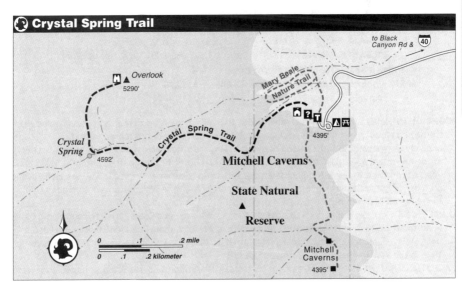

From the top of the parking area, turn right (north) and walk past the visitor center and residences to the trailhead. The trail climbs northwest to the spring, then farther to a lookout.

Crystal Spring provides the water for Providence Mountains State Recreation Area. The trail to the spring offers a scenic tour of the slopes of the mountains in the Mojave Desert. As you hike, notice how the plants around you change as you move into the transition zone between cactus-yucca scrub and pinyon pine-juniper woodland.

The rocks around you are limestone and dolomite, the product of ancient seabed sediments and millions of years of pressure and tectonic movement. They stand in contrast to the Granite Mountains to the southwest and the volcanic mounds of Mid Hills and Hole-in-the-Wall, adding to the geologic diversity of Mojave National Preserve.

The overlook beyond the spring offers a wonderful view east over the desert—perfect to watch the rising sun's rays paint the rugged slopes of the Providence Mountains, or to escape the heat in the shade of late afternoon.

Retrace your steps to return.

trip 19 Mojave: Hole-in-the-Wall & Rings Trail

Distance	Up to 3 miles, loop
Hiking Time	1 to 2 hours
Elevation	+/-150 feet
Difficulty	Moderate (difficult on Rings Trail)
Trail Use	Good for kids
Best Times	Cold to warm
Agency	Mojave National Preserve at (760) 255-8801; www.nps.gov/moja
Recommended Maps	Free *Mojave Preserve* map
GPS Waypoints	Rings Trail Trailhead: 35.043° N, 115.398° W
Vehicle	Passenger car OK

HIGHLIGHTS Hole-in-the-Wall was created about 18.5 million years ago, when a volcano exploded in the nearby Woods Mountains. The resulting cloud of gas, ash, and debris roared across the landscape at nearly the speed of sound, carrying boulders as large as 60 feet across and smothering everything in the 66-square-mile blast zone with rock and ash so hot it fused together instantly. Millions of years of wind and weather have eroded these rocks into the shapes we see today. Bob Holliman, a member of Butch Cassidy's gang, reportedly named Hole-in-the-Wall, because it reminded him of their hideout in Wyoming.

DIRECTIONS From Las Vegas, drive south on I-15 for 65 miles to Cima Road. Turn left (south) onto Cima Road and drive 18 miles to Cima. Turn right (south) onto Kelso-Cima Road for 5 miles. Turn left (east) onto Mojave Road for 6 miles. Turn right (south) onto Black Canyon Road and drive 10 miles to the Hole-in-the-Wall Trailhead and information center.

FACILITIES/TRAILHEAD Rangers, a visitor center, 35-site campground, restrooms, phones, and water are available here.

A cathedral of eroded volcanic tuff awaits at Hole-in-the-Wall.

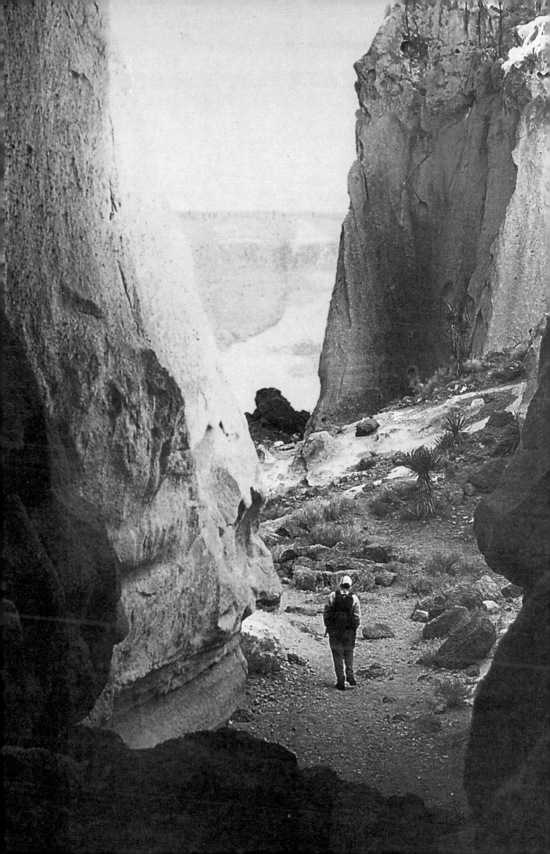

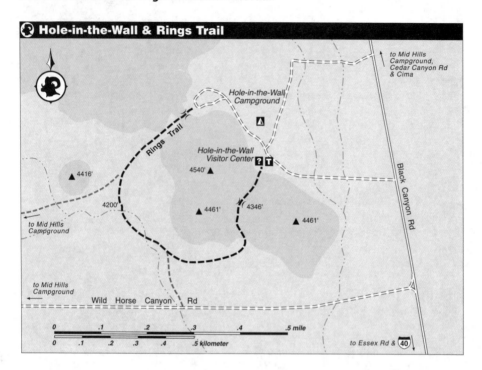

The Hole-in-the-Wall Nature Trail heads south from the information center, then loops clockwise around the Hole-in-the-Wall hills for 1.5 miles to the bottom of the Rings Trail, a quarter mile from the information center by the campground. You can also hike west from the information center to the campground and signed RINGS TRAIL TRAILHEAD, where the most dramatic fun waits.

Hole-in-the-Wall offers a colorful labyrinth of slot canyons, spires, ledges, windows, and passageways. It makes wonderful exploring for kids and kids-at-heart, although everyone should avoid getting too close to dangerous cliffs.

On the Rings Trail, there are two sections of ring ladders, each dropping 10 to 15 feet of the total 150-foot drop to the bottom of Banshee Canyon. Although the rings have my highest difficulty rating, anyone who can negotiate schoolyard monkey bars or a rope ladder should do just fine on these with care and concentration. You'll be happy you did, as the Rings Trail drops you into the heart of the labyrinth you see from above, where the sights and exploring are at their best.

Climbing up or down the Rings Trail is not necessary to enjoy the area. The overlook just a few yards to the left (south) of the top of the Rings Trail offers a view into the geological playground in the canyon below.

trip 20 Mojave: Mid Hills to Hole-in-the-Wall Trail

Distance	8.4 miles, point-to-point
Hiking Time	4 to 6 hours
Elevation	+2000 feet from Hole-in-the-Wall; -2000 feet from Mid Hills
Difficulty	Moderate
Trail Use	Leashed dogs, backpacking option, map and compass
Best Times	Warm to hot
Agency	Mojave National Preserve at (760) 255-8801; www.nps.gov/moja
Recommended Maps	Free *Mojave Preserve* map; *Trails Illustrated Mojave National Preserve* (#256)
GPS Waypoints	Upper trailhead: 35.123° N, 115.432° W
	Lower trailhead: 35°037′ N, 115°406′ W
Vehicle	Passenger car OK

HIGHLIGHTS This beautiful point-to-point hike climbs (or descends) through views and colorful geology in Gold Valley.

DIRECTIONS This trail is point-to-point with two trailheads. From Las Vegas, drive south on I-15 for 65 miles to Cima Road. Turn left (south) onto Cima Road and drive 18 miles to Cima. Turn right (south) onto Kelso-Cima Road for 5 miles. Turn left (east) onto Mojave Road for 6 miles. Turn right (south) onto Black Canyon Road.

For the north trailhead, drive south on Black Canyon Road for 3 miles to Wild Horse Canyon Road. Turn right (west), following the sign to Mid Hills Campground. After 2 miles, turn left (south) to the signed and unpaved parking area by the windmill, opposite the entrance to the Mid Hills Trailhead.

For the south trailhead, drive 11 miles south on Black Canyon Road to the south entrance to Wild Horse Canyon Road (1 mile south of the entrance to the Hole-in-the-Wall information center and campground). Drive west on Wild Horse Canyon Road for a half mile to the signed, unpaved trailhead on the right (north) side of the road

To hike this trail point-to-point, leave cars at either end, or arrange for someone to pick you up at the far end.

FACILITIES/TRAILHEAD Rangers, a visitor center, a 35-site campground, restrooms, phones, and water are available at Hole-in-the-Wall (4400 feet). At Mid Hills (a cooler 5600 feet), there are 26 campsites, pit toilets, picnic tables, fire rings, and limited water. The road to Mid Hills Campground is not paved and is not recommended for large RVs or trailers.

This hike is best done from Hole-in-the-Wall (south) to Mid Hills (north). Climbing is easier on the knees and ankles, but it's admittedly a harder workout for the heart and lungs. Hiking north also keeps the sun out of your eyes and gives you a more intimate view of the plants and geology along the way.

From the south trailhead, hike north on the signed trail through the open shrubs and yucca. About a quarter mile southwest of the dramatic cliffs of Banshee Canyon, you will come to a fork. Take the right (easterly) fork for a dramatic side trip into the slots and shadows of Banshee Canyon and the bottom of the Rings Trail. Or choose the left (westerly) fork and follow the trail north across open slopes and past towering formations for 8.4 miles through Gold Valley to the north trailhead.

Along the way, the trail intersects numerous jeep roads and fence lines that crisscross Gold Valley. Well-placed signs, however, guide you. When in doubt, head north. Even if you take a wrong turn, you can't get too lost, as this trail follows a narrow corridor between Black Canyon and Wild Horse Canyon roads.

As you hike, notice how the plant community changes, from cholla, yucca, and barrel cactus in the lowlands to sagebrush, pinyon pine, and juniper in the hills.

If you'd like a sense of the trail without hiking the entire distance, each trailhead offers shorter, rewarding out-and-back options. From the south (lower) trailhead, the fantastically sculpted Banshee Canyon is less than 1 mile away. From the north (upper) trailhead, a 1-mile hike up the trail takes you to wonderful views of the Providence Mountains and good lookouts over the valley, where you can have a snack before turning back.

Each end of the trail offers shorter out-and-back options.

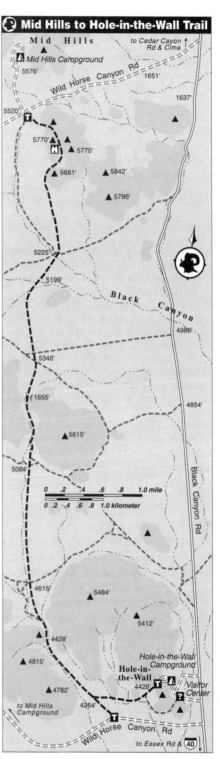

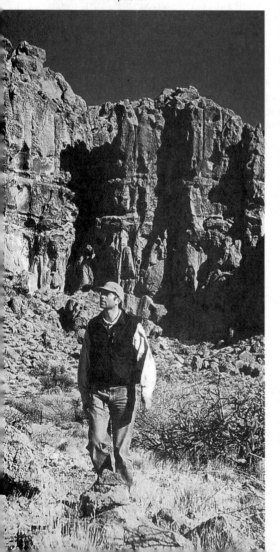

trip 21 Mojave: Teutonia Peak & Cima Dome

Distance	Up to 4 miles, out-and-back
Hiking Time	1 to 3 hours
Elevation	+/-700 feet
Difficulty	Moderate (most difficult to summit)
Trail Use	Leashed dogs, good for kids, backpacking option
Best Times	Cool to warm
Agency	Mojave National Preserve at (760) 255-8801; www.nps.gov/moja
Recommended Maps	Free *Mojave Preserve* map; *Trails Illustrated Mojave National Preserve* (#256)
GPS Waypoints	Teutonia Peak: 35.300° N, 114.562° W
Vehicle	Passenger car OK

HIGHLIGHTS If I were itchin' to get out of town and had two hours until sunset, one of my top destinations would be Teutonia Peak. From the Joshua trees, cholla cactus, and yuccas to the outrageous granite formations along Teutonia's main ridge, the scenery will calm and bring beauty to the most unsettled souls. For those unable or unwilling to make the difficult climb up the final feet to Teutonia Peak, the lower rock formations are still worthwhile—and a great place to camp if you're backpacking. Plus, the Joshua tree forest at Cima Dome in Mojave National Preserve is the largest and densest in the world. That alone is reason enough to visit.

DIRECTIONS Take I-15 south from Las Vegas for 65 miles to Cima Road in California. Exit and head south on Cima Road for 12 miles to the signed trailhead on the right (west) side of the road. Fill your tank before leaving the freeway.

FACILITIES/TRAILHEAD Restrooms are available here. Mojave National Preserve is largely undeveloped. Before you enter the preserve, stop by the information center on Baker Road in Baker for a free map, advice, and travel tips from the rangers there. Food and gas are available only on the edges of the preserve, along I-15 to the north and I-40 to the south. Water is available only at the Cima post office, 6 miles south of the trailhead on Cima Road. Water and information are available at the Hole-in-the-Wall Campground, south of the trailhead via Cima, Kelso-Cima, Mojave, and Black Canyon

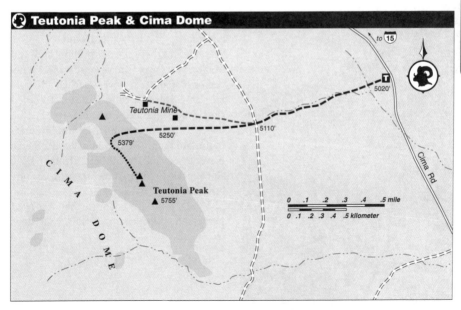

Teutonia Peak & Cima Dome

to (15)

Teutonia Mine

5020'

5110'

5250'

5379'

Teutonia Peak
▲ 5755'

C I M A   D O M E

Cima Rd

0 .1 .2 .3 .4 .5 mile
0 .1 .2 .3 .4 .5 kilometer

Southern Region

roads. Sites are first-come, first-served. Primitive camping is also allowed at established sites off paved roads. Collecting firewood of any kind is forbidden in the preserve. Bring your own wood, and build fires only in established fire rings.

Follow the trail west up the gentle slope through Joshua trees. Trail signs point the way through fences and crossroads, to the rocky main ridge, about a mile away. Then climb the ridge south toward the peak. Cairns mark the route, but you'll be able to find your way even if you don't see the cairns.

After another mile, you reach the top of Teutonia Peak. The view includes the ruggedly beautiful Ivanpah Mountains to your east, Clark Mountain and a distant Telescope Peak in Death Valley to the north,

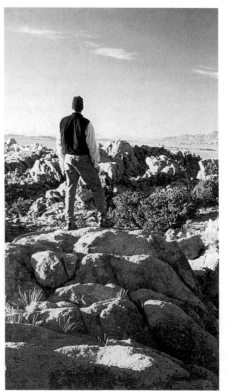

Enjoying the geology of Teutonia Peak

Joshua trees grow about a half inch each year.

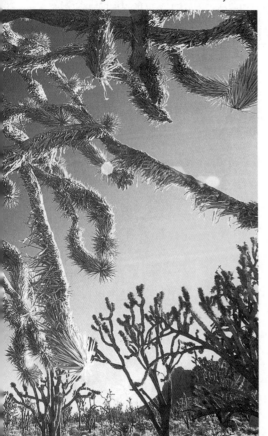

and Mid Hills and the Providence Mountains to the south. To the west rises the enormous, rounded Cima Dome.

Sometime between 80 million and 180 million years ago, Cima Dome was a chamber of magma that never reached the surface as a volcanic flow. Instead, it cooled slowly into granite. Colliding continental plates forced this chamber up until it was a mountain range (in the same way the Sierra Nevada formed). Wind and weather have since eroded Cima Dome down to its current symmetrical profile.

When you have taken in the view (and perhaps the setting sun), retrace your steps to return.

trip 22 Mojave: Clark Mountain

Distance	3 miles, out-and-back or loop
Hiking Time	3 to 5 hours
Elevation	+/-1750 feet
Difficulty	Most difficult
Trail Use	Dogs and children not recommended
Best Times	Cool to warm
Agency	Mojave National Preserve at (760) 255-8801; www.nps.gov/moja
Recommended Maps	Clark Mountain 7.5-minute; Trails Illustrated Mojave National Preserve (#256)
GPS Waypoints	Picnic area and trailhead: 35.300° N, 114.562° W
	Summit: 35.525° N, 115.588° W
Vehicle	High-clearance vehicle recommended

HIGHLIGHTS This desert peak just across the state line in California offers a challenging climb and soaring views from the top. Although officially part of Mojave National Preserve, Clark Mountain sits across I-15 to the north of the main preserve complex, without signs, services, or other reminders of its status as part of the National Park system.

DIRECTIONS Take I-15 south from Las Vegas for about 1 hour. About 15 miles after crossing into California, exit at Mountain Pass. At the top of the off-ramp, turn right (north), then immediately left (west) onto Clark Mountain Road (zero your odometer here). Your goal is the prominent canyon on the southeast side of Clark Mountain, beyond the communications towers to your northwest.

To get there, follow Clark Mountain Rd. as it heads west along I-15. After one mile, at a cattle guard, pavement turns to gravel and the road veers to the northwest toward a communications

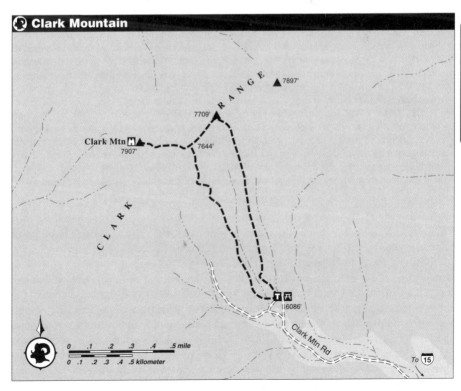

Clark Mountain

7897'

7709'

Clark Mtn 7907'

7644'

C L A R K   R A N G E

T | 6086'

Clark Mtn Rd

0 .1 .2 .3 .4 .5 mile
0 .1 .2 .3 .4 .5 kilometer

To 15

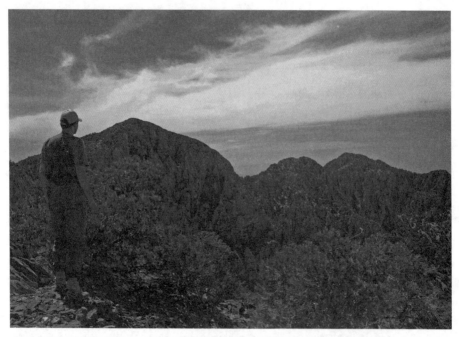

From the summit ridge, dazzling views appear through the cliffs to the next valley north.

tower. A half mile farther, the road veers sharply right to head northeast along the northern edge of a large mine tailing pile. At 2.2 miles, the road veers left to follow a wash north and away from the tailing pile. At 3.8 miles, the road crosses under a power line, then veers left (west), climbing out of the wash. At 4.3 miles, follow the right (north) fork, then quickly after, the left (west) fork. The road drops into a drainage, veers south, then switchbacks, climbs back up, and heads northwest again.

A mile later, you enter the canyon. At 5.7 miles, ignore the right (east) fork; at 6.1, ignore the left (west) fork. Then you arrive at the picnic area, which is your trailhead.

FACILITIES/TRAILHEAD The picnic area offers picnic tables, garbage cans, and BBQ pits, but no water or restrooms. The nearest services are available back at the state line on I-15, or farther west toward Baker, California. For more information on Mojave National Preserve, stop by the information center on Baker Road in Baker (30 miles west on I-15) for a free map, advice, and travel tips from the rangers there. Primitive camping is allowed at established sites off paved roads. Collecting firewood of any kind is forbidden in the preserve. Bring your own wood, and build fires only in established fire rings.

This hike is not a trail, but rather a general route. Directly above and behind the BBQ pits, look for a small social trail that heads up the drainage north toward the ridge east of the summit. The north-south-trending ridges on either side (east and west) of this wash are the best ways up to the summit ridge. I recommend climbing the ridge to the east (climber's right), then returning down the ridge to the west (climber's left). The west ridge has a lot of soft dirt and scree, making it hard to climb but easier to descend.

After gaining the main east-west ridge, turn left (west) and follow it toward the summit. (The peak to the east isn't as high as Clark Mountain, but it offers fine views and reward in its own right, without the climb up cliffs between you and the summit.) The crest of the ridge is jagged and rocky, so going is easier by hiking below along the south side of the rocks.

Where this east-west ridge meets the north-south cliff band that climbs from the south is the most difficult part of the hike: a 50-foot climb up through the cliff band. Be careful. Once above this climb, the journey becomes a hike again and not a rock climb, continuing west, then north to the summit. (Those who do not wish to climb through this cliff band can abandon this summit bid, but enjoy fine views from the peak to the east, mentioned above). Along the way to the summit, enjoy views through notches in the cliffs down into the canyon to the north, where remnant white fir trees still cling to the high, cooler north-facing slopes.

The easiest route down is to climb back down through the cliff, then follow the bottom of the cliff band as it leads you south. You then veer left and drop east into the drainage, which leads directly back to the picnic area. There may be a few dry waterfalls to descend, but you'll be well-prepared after scrambling through the cliffs above.

Like Clark County, Nevada (home to Las Vegas), Clark Mountain is named in honor of William Andrews Clark, a Montana senator who helped bring the Los Angeles and Salt Lake Railroad—and subsequent economic development—through this region in the late 1800s and early 1900s.

And like many limestone mountains in southern Nevada, 600 to 700 million years ago, the jagged cliffs of Clark Mountain were once ooze settling on the bottom of a shallow sea. The limestone comes from the accumulation of shells and coral from that era. Colliding continental plates has pushed this mountain far above sea level. Despite the elevation and miles from the sea, keep your eyes open for fossil seashells as you hike.

It's hard to believe these soaring cliffs were once muck at the bottom of the sea.

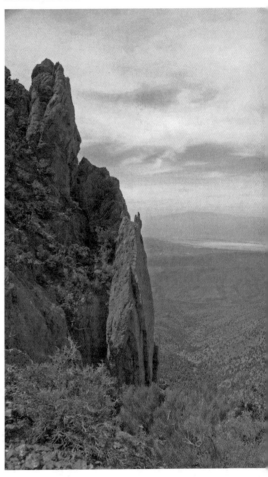

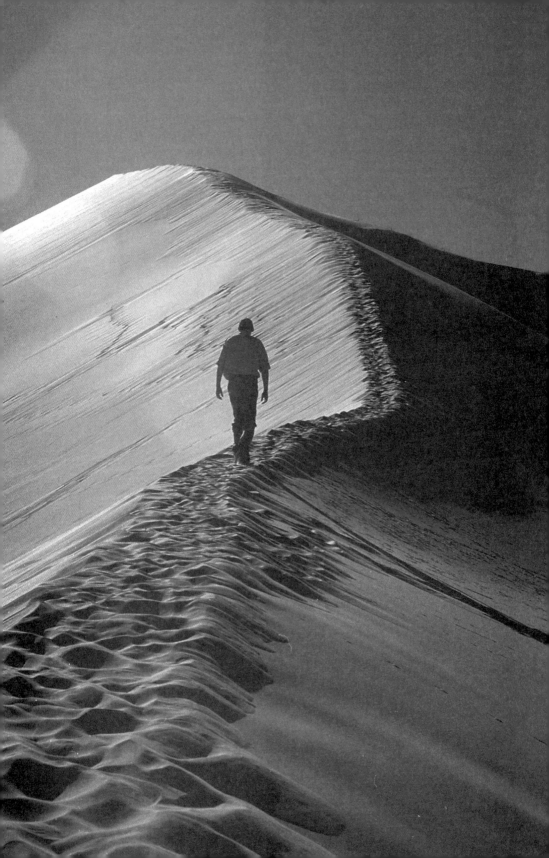

Best Trips by Theme

Best Places to Go First

WESTERN
Trip 1: Sandstone Quarry to Calico Tanks
Trip 9: Ice Box Canyon
Trip 10: Pine Creek Canyon
Trip 23: Mary Jane Falls
Trip 25: Cathedral Rock

EASTERN
Trip 18: Atlatl Rock
Trip 19: Petroglyph Canyon & Mouse's Tank
Trip 20: White Domes

Best Paved Drives

WESTERN
Trips 1–11: Red Rock Canyon National
Conservation Area: 13-Mile Scenic Loop
Trips 31–42: Death Valley National Park

EASTERN
Trips 18–21: Valley of Fire State Park
Trips 6–15: Lake Mead National Recreation Area:
Northshore Road

Best Unpaved, 4WD Drives

WESTERN
Trip 32: Titus Canyon

EASTERN
Trips 16–17: Bitter Spring Trail Back Country
Byway

Best Easier Peaks

WESTERN
Trip 2: Turtlehead Peak
Trip 15: Blue Diamond Hill

EASTERN
Trip 4: River Mountains

Best Undeveloped Camping

EASTERN
Trip 22: Whitney Pockets

NORTHERN
Trip 15: Big Rocks Wilderness

SOUTHERN
Trip 6: Ireteba Peaks
Trip 8: Wee Thump Joshua Tree Wilderness

Best Challenging Peaks

WESTERN
Trip 8: Bridge Mountain
Trip 26: Mt. Charleston

SOUTHERN
Trip 9: Spirit Mountain

Best Developed Camping

WESTERN
Trips 17 & 26: Spring Mountains National
Recreation Area: Dolomite or Kyle canyons

EASTERN
Trips 18–21: Valley of Fire State Park:
Campground B

SOUTHERN
Trip 20: Mojave National Preserve:
Mid Hills

Best Places to Find Water

WESTERN
Trip 9: Red Rock Canyon, Ice Box Canyon

SOUTHERN
Trip 1: Kayak or Canoe Float on the Colorado
River

Mojave National Preserve: Kelso Dunes (Southern Region: Trip 15)

Best Places to Watch the Sunset

WESTERN
Trip 15: Blue Diamond Hill
Trip 42: Dante's View

EASTERN
Trip 4: River Mountains

SOUTHERN
Trip 21: Teutonia Peak & Cima Dome

Best Forests

WESTERN
Trip 17: Upper Bristlecone Trail
Trip 26: Mt. Charleston, South Loop Trail

SOUTHERN
Trip 8: Wee Thump Joshua Tree Wilderness

Best Canyons

WESTERN
Trip 10: Pine Creek Canyon
Trip 20: Fletcher Canyon
Trip 32: Titus Canyon
Trip 40: Sidewinder Canyon

EASTERN
Trip 7: Anniversary Narrows

NORTHERN
Trip 8: Arrow Canyon

Best Places to Take Kids

WESTERN
Trip 5: Children's Discovery Trail

EASTERN
Trip 19: Petroglyph Canyon & Mouse's Tank

SOUTHERN
Trip 16: Mitchell Caverns
Trip 19: Rings Trail

Best Places to See Petroglyphs

EASTERN
Trip 18: Atlatl Rock

SOUTHERN
Trip 10: Grapevine Canyon
Trip 11: Sloan Canyon

Best Places to See Wildlife

EASTERN
Trip 1: Wetlands Park Nature Preserve

NORTHERN
Trip 2: Corn Creek Nature Trail
Trip 12: Pahranagat National Wildlife Refuge

SOUTHERN
Trip 1: Kayak or Canoe Float on the Colorado River

Recommended Books & Websites

Archaeology

Welsh, Liz, and Peter Welsh. *Rock-Art of the Southwest: A Visitor's Companion.* Berkeley: Wilderness Press, 2000. An informative introduction to the peoples, styles, science, and uncertainty behind rock art.

Desert Travel

Alden, Peter, and Peter Friederici. *National Audubon Society Field Guide to the Southwestern States.* New York: Alfred A. Knopf, 1999. This book covers Arizona, Nevada, New Mexico, and Utah, but it's a great introduction to the most common things you'll encounter in the Mojave Desert, from stars to geology, plants, animals, birds, reptiles, and their habitats.

Desert USA, www.desertusa.com. On this informative, well-organized website, you can learn almost anything having to do with the deserts of the Southwest. This site has helped me greatly in my research on the Mojave Desert.

Grubbs, Bruce. *Desert Hiking Tips: Expert Advice on Desert Hiking and Driving.* Helena: Falcon Press, 1998. A compact and informative guide to desert travel.

Geology

Lake Mead Geology, U.S. Geological Survey and National Park Service, www2.nature.nps.gov/geology//usgsnps/lmnra/lmnra1.html. An interesting and informative introduction to Lake Mead geology.

Death Valley Geology, U.S. Geological Survey and National Park Service, www2.nature.nps.gov/geology//usgsnps/deva/deva1.html. An interesting and informative introduction to Death Valley geology.

Tingley, Joseph, et al. *Geologic Tours in the Las Vegas Area* (Nevada Bureau of Mines and Geology, Special Publication 16). Reno: Nevada Bureau of Mines and Geology, 2001. This publication offers excellent explanations of the geology of Southern Nevada and is a wonderful companion to many of the hikes offered in this book.

Plants

Clinesmith, Larry, and Elsie Sellars. *Plants of Red Rock Canyon.* Las Vegas: Red Rock Canyon Interpretive Association, 2003. This short but colorful guide will help you identify some of the most prominent plants at Red Rock Canyon and throughout the Mojave Desert.

Rhode, David. *Native Plants of Southern Nevada: An Ethnobotany.* Salt Lake City: University of Utah Press, 2002. This is the most comprehensive book on the trees, shrubs, grass, and flowers of Southern Nevada. Despite its academic-sounding title and high price, it's organized well, with photos and concise explanations in plain English about the natural history of these plants and how Native Americans used them.

Stewart, Jon Mark. *Mojave Desert Wildflowers.* Albuquerque: Jon Stewart Photography, 1998. A beautiful guide to many of the blooms you'll find in Southern Nevada.

Agencies &
Information Sources

BUREAU OF LAND MANAGEMENT

Ely Field Office
1700 North Industrial Way
Ely, NV 89301
(775) 289-1800
www.blm.gov/nv/st/en/fo/ely_field_office.html

Las Vegas Field Office
4701 North Torrey Pines Drive
Las Vegas, NV 89130
(702) 515-5000
www.nv.blm.gov/vegas

Red Rock Canyon National Conservation Area
HCR 33, Box 5500
Las Vegas, NV 89124
(702) 515-5350
ww.blm.gov/nv/st/en/fo/lvfo/blm_programs/
blm_special_areas/red_rock_nca.html

FISH AND WILDLIFE SERVICE

Ash Meadows National Wildlife Refuge
P.O. Box 2660
Pahrump, NV 89041
(702) 372-5435
www.fws.gov/desertcomplex/ashmeadows

Desert National Wildlife Refuge
1500 North Decatur Blvd.
Las Vegas, NV 89108
(702) 646-3401
www.fws.gov/desertcomplex/desertrange

Pahranagat National Wildlife Refuge
Box 510
Alamo, NV 89001
(775) 725-3417
www.fws.gov/desertcomplex/pahranagat

FOREST SERVICE

Mt. Charleston Ranger District
4701 North Torrey Pine Drive
Las Vegas, NV 89130
(702) 515-5400
www.fs.fed.us/r4/htnf/districts/smnra/index.shtml

NATIONAL PARK SERVICE

Death Valley National Park
P.O. Box 579
Death Valley, CA 92328
(760) 786-3200
www.nps.gov/deva

Lake Mead National Recreation Area
601 Nevada Highway
Boulder City, NV 89005
(702) 293-8907
www.nps.gov/lame

 Alan Bible Visitor Center
 151 Lakeshore Scenic Drive
 Las Vegas, NV 89101
 (702) 293-8990

Mojave National Preserve
222 E. Main St., Suite 202
Barstow, CA 92311
(760) 733-4040
www.nps.gov/moja

STATE PARKS

Cathedral Gorge State Park
P.O. Box 176
Panaca, NV 89042
(775) 728-4460
www.parks.nv.gov/cg.htm

Floyd Lamb State Park: Tule Springs
9200 Tule Springs Road
Las Vegas, NV 89131
(702) 486-5413
www.lasvegasnevada.gov/files/Floyd_Lamb_Park_
Brochure.pdf

Kershaw-Ryan State Park
HC 64 Box 3
Caliente, NV 89008
(775) 726-3564
www.parks.nv.gov/kr.htm

Nevada State Parks Headquarters
1300 South Curry St.
Carson City, NV 89703
(775) 687-4384
www.parks.nv.gov

Spring Mountain Ranch State Park
P.O. Box 124
Blue Diamond, NV 89004
(702) 875-4141
www.parks.nv.gov/smr.htm

Valley of Fire State Park
P.O. Box 515
Overton, NV 89040
(702) 397-2088
www.parks.nv.gov/vf.htm

Glossary

agave roasting pit A ring of ashes and charred rock used as an underground barbecue pit by ancient peoples. Agave plants were often cooked in them, but remains of squash, roots, bighorn sheep, rabbit, and other foods have also been found. Single pits were often used for multiple roasts over many years, evidenced by their great size. Learn more about the prehistoric peoples who made agave roasting pits in the introduction (see page 8).

alluvial fan/alluvium (a-LOO-vee-um) The fan-shaped collection of rocks and soil deposited by rains at the mouth of desert canyons.

bajada (ba-HA-da) The deposits of rock and soil sloping from the steep face of mountains to the valley bottom. Although alluvial fans form only at canyon mouths, bajadas may be anywhere along a mountain range.

cairn (CARE-n) A small stack of rocks used to mark a cross-country route that doesn't have a trail. Beware, the cairns you follow might have been placed by someone who was lost, so use them in conjunction with your own route-finding skills.

caliche (ka-LEE-chee) A hard, white layer in the soil made of calcium carbonate, typical in arid places like the Mojave Desert. Brief, heavy rains dissolve calcium carbonate in the soil. The water then evaporates, and the calcium carbonate precipitates as caliche.

cross-country Traveling across terrain without a trail.

guzzler An artificial water development built for wildlife.

Leave No Trace (LNT) A school of wilderness ethics that teaches specific actions we can take to lessen the impact we have on the landscapes we visit. Read more about LNT in the introduction on page 18, or go to www.lnt.org.

metamorphose/metamorphic rock Formed when extreme pressure, heat, or chemical action change the molecular structure of rock over time.

riparian areas Areas along springs, streams, washes, rivers, and lakes, where water nourishes abundant and often sensitive plant and animal life.

road A vehicle route that is either paved or machine-maintained. Understand that a sudden storm can make any road impassable.

route When there are no trails, your desired route (to a peak or a spring, for example) may lead you up a ridge or canyon, cross-country. Some routes may be marked by cairns. Others may be visible, but they're not established enough to be called a trail.

scree Loose, small rocks covering a slope.

sky islands Plant and wildlife habitats that are high in the mountains, separated by other mountain habitats by wide, inhospitable valleys. This separation leads to species isolation and, after many thousands of years, the evolution of distinct species characteristics and endemic species.

talus Rock debris covering a slope. Talus is bigger than scree.

tectonic Powerful, earth-moving forces associated with colliding continental plates.

track An unmaintained vehicle route, such as a jeep track. Soils in the desert can be fragile, and it may take little more than the passing of a single vehicle to create a track. Be wary of driving on tracks that aren't described in the book. You may end up with a damaged vehicle, and you could also impact the soils, wildlife habitat, and the ecosystem.

trail A definite path along the ground. May be maintained either by humans or animals. Many of the best routes in the Mojave are game trails made by bighorn sheep, deer, or wild horses. Be careful, however, as many game trails have a way of disappearing under your feet.

wash A shallow, wide drainage, usually dry until a flash flood roars through.

wilderness More than just wild country. Congressionally designated wilderness areas are established to preserve the natural character of the land and keep human influence to a minimum. Wilderness keeps air and water clean, protects wildlife and their habitat, and provides recreational opportunities for people. When exploring, please follow Leave No Trace principles (see above and page 18) to help keep our wilderness areas wild and beautiful for generations to come. Read more about wilderness in the introduction on page 10.

About the Author

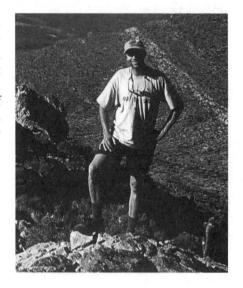

In his work as the outdoors editor for the *Reno Gazette-Journal* and now as the associate director for Friends of Nevada Wilderness, native-Nevadan Brian Beffort has explored the wide valleys, soaring peaks, and twisting canyons of Nevada. Some of his favorite landscapes are in Southern Nevada, near Las Vegas. He lives in Reno with his wife and son.